CARBON NANOTUBES FOR BIOMEDICAL APPLICATIONS AND HEALTHCARE

CARBON NANOTUBES FOR BIOMEDICAL APPLICATIONS AND HEALTHCARE

Edited by

Chin Hua Chia, PhD

Swati Gokul Talele, PhD

Ann Rose Abraham, PhD

A. K. Haghi, PhD

AAP | APPLE ACADEMIC PRESS

First edition published 2024

Apple Academic Press Inc.
1265 Goldenrod Circle, NE,
Palm Bay, FL 32905 USA

760 Laurentian Drive, Unit 19,
Burlington, ON L7N 0A4, CANADA

CRC Press
2385 NW Executive Center Drive,
Suite 320, Boca Raton FL 33431

4 Park Square, Milton Park,
Abingdon, Oxon, OX14 4RN UK

Library and Archives Canada Cataloguing in Publication

Title: Carbon nanotubes for biomedical applications and healthcare / edited by Chin Hua Chia, PhD, Swati Gokul Talele, PhD, Ann Rose Abraham, PhD, A.K. Haghi, PhD.
Names: Chia, Chin Hua (PhD), editor. | Talele, Swati Gokul, editor. | Abraham, Ann Rose, editor. | Haghi, A. K., editor.
Description: First edition. | Includes bibliographical references and index.
Identifiers: Canadiana (print) 20230497934 | Canadiana (ebook) 20230497969 | ISBN 9781774913352 (hardcover) | ISBN 9781774913642 (softcover) | ISBN 9781003396390 (ebook)
Subjects: LCSH: Carbon nanotubes. | LCSH: Nanomedicine.
Classification: LCC TA455.C3 C37 2024 | DDC 620.1/93—dc23

Library of Congress Cataloging-in-Publication Data

CIP data on file with US Library of Congress

ISBN: 978-1-77491-335-2 (hbk)
ISBN: 978-1-77491-364-2 (pbk)
ISBN: 978-1-00339-639-0 (ebk)

About the Editors

Chin Hua Chia, PhD
Professor, Materials Science Program, Department Applied Physics, Universiti Kebangsaan Malaysia, Selangor, Malaysia

Chin Hua Chia, PhD, is a full Professor at the Department of Applied Physics, Faculty of Science and Technology at Universiti Kebangsaan Malaysia (National University of Malaysia), Malaysia. He is a recipient of the Young Scientist Award from the National University of Malaysia and the Malaysian Solid-State Science and Technology (MASS) in 2012 and 2014, respectively. He also received the Distinguished Lectureship Award from the Chemical Society of Japan (CSJ) in 2017. He is a member of several professional organizations and has published several book chapters and more than 200 articles in professional journals. He has also presented at many professional meetings. His core research focuses on metallic nanomaterials syntheses, with a particular emphasis on structure control to tailor the properties of the materials in determining their performances for environmental remediation applications, such as wastewater treatment, supercapacitor, and hydrogen production.

Swati Gokul Talele, PhD
Assistant Professor, Department of Pharmaceutics, Sandip Institute of Pharmaceutical Sciences, Savitribai Phule Pune University, Pune, Maharashtra, India

Swati Gokul Talele, PhD, is currently serving as an Assistant Professor in the Department of Pharmaceutics at Sandip Institute of Pharmaceutical Sciences. She has 18 years of experience in research along with teaching. She has published more than 20 research papers in various reputed international and national journals as well as more than 30 review papers. She has also presented research work at several conferences and has received several awards. She has authored the book titled Natural Excipients and has many chapters and books in progress. She has supervised many MPharm students and is currently associated with many research projects. She also worked as a college examination officer (CEO) for more than three years and is a member of the university examination committee. Dr. Talele has delivered interactive talks at continuous education programs for registered pharmacists and is a life member of the Association of Pharmacy Teachers of India (APTI) and a member of the Indian Pharmaceutical Congress Association (IPCA). Her interests are in the field of nanotechnology, natural polymers, herbal formulations, and radiolabeling-based bio-distribution studies.

Ann Rose Abraham, PhD
Assistant Professor, Sacred Heart College (Autonomous), Thevara, Kochi, Kerala, India

Ann Rose Abraham, PhD, is currently an Assistant Professor at the Department of Physics, Sacred Heart College (Autonomous), Thevara, Kochi, Kerala, India. She has expertise in the field of condensed matter physics, nanomagnetism, multiferroics, and polymeric nanocomposites, etc. She has research experience at various reputed national institutes, including Bose Institute, Kolkata, India; SAHA Institute of Nuclear Physics, Kolkata, India; UGC-DAE CSR Center, Kolkata, India. She has collaborated with various international laboratories. She is a recipient of a Young Researcher Award in physics and Best Paper Awards–2020 (2021). She served as Assistant Professor and Examiner at the Department of Basic Sciences, Amal Jyothi College of Engineering, under APJ Abdul Kalam Technological University, Kerala, India. Dr. Abraham is a frequent speaker at national and international conferences. She has a good number of publications to her credit in many peer-reviewed high-impact journals of international repute. She has authored many book chapters and edited more than 10 books with Taylor and Francis, Elsevier, etc. Dr. Abraham received her MSc, MPhil, and PhD degrees in Physics from the School of Pure and Applied Physics, Mahatma Gandhi University, Kerala, India.

A. K. Haghi, PhD

Professor Emeritus of Engineering Sciences, Former Editor-in-Chief, International Journal of Chemoinformatics and Chemical Engineering; Member of the Canadian Research and Development Center of Sciences and Culture

A. K. Haghi, PhD, has published over 250 academic research-oriented books as well as over 1000 research papers published in various journals and conference proceedings. He has received several grants, consulted for several major corporations, and is a frequent speaker to national and international audiences. He is the Founder and former Editor-in-Chief of *the International Journal of Chemoinformatics and Chemical Engineering,* published by IGI Global (USA), as well as *Polymers Research Journal,* published by Nova Science Publishers (USA). Professor Haghi has acted as an editorial board member of many international journals. He has served as a member of the Canadian Research and Development Center of Sciences and Cultures (CRDCSC) and the Research Chemistry Center, Coimbra, Portugal. Dr. Haghi holds a BSc in urban and environmental engineering from the University of North Carolina (USA), an MSc in mechanical engineering from North Carolina A&T State University (USA), and an MSc in applied mechanics, acoustics and materials from the Université de Technologie de Compiègne (France), and a PhD in engineering sciences from Université de Franche-Comté (France).

Contents

Contributors

Surendra Agrawal
Associate Professor in Quality Assurance, Shobhaben Pratapbhai Patel School of Pharmacy and Technology Management, SVKM'S NMIMS (Deemed to be University), Vile Parle (W), Mumbai, Maharashtra, India

Pankaj Aher
Department of Pharmaceutical Chemistry, Loknete Dr. J. D. Pawar College of Pharmacy, Manur, Kalwan, India

Eknath Ahire
Department of Pharmaceutics, MET's Institute of Pharmacy, Affiliated to Savitribai Phule Pune University, BKC, Adgaon, Nashik, Maharashtra, India

Mir Intaj Ali
Central Institute of Petrochemicals Engineering and Technology (CIPET), Institute of Petrochemicals Technology (IPT), Bhubaneswar, Patia, Odisha, India

Mir Sahanur Ali
Department of Polymer Science and Technology, University of Calcutta, Kolkata, West Bengal, India; Center for Research in Nanoscience and Nanotechnology, Acharya Prafulla Chandra Roy Sikhsha Prangan, University of Calcutta, Saltlake City, Kolkata, West Bengal, India

Mir Sahidul Ali
Department of Polymer Science and Technology, University of Calcutta, Kolkata, West Bengal, India

T. R. Anilkumar
Inter-University Center for Evolutionary and Integrative Biology, University of Kerala, Kariavattom, Trivandrum, Kerala, India

Harshada U. Bagul
Department of Pharmaceutics, Sandip Institute of Pharmaceutical Sciences, Nashik, Maharashtra, India

Akash M. Bhoite
Department of Pharmaceutics, Sandip Institute of Pharmaceutical Sciences, Nashik, Maharashtra, India

Avinash V. Borgaonkar
Assistant Professor, Department of Mechanical Engineering, Pimpri Chinchwad College of Engineering (PCCOE), Pune, Maharashtra, India

Dipankar Chattopadhyay
Department of Polymer Science and Technology, University of Calcutta, Kolkata, West Bengal, India; Center for Research in Nanoscience and Nanotechnology, Acharya Prafulla Chandra Roy Sikhsha Prangan, University of Calcutta, Saltlake City, Kolkata, West Bengal, India

Chin Hua Chia
Materials Science Program, Department of Applied Physics, Faculty of Science and Technology, Bangi, Selangor, Malaysia

Siew Xian Chin
Materials Science Program, Department of Applied Physics, Faculty of Science and Technology, Bangi, Selangor, Malaysia; ASASIpintar Program, Pusat GENIUS@Pintar Negara, Universiti Kebangsaan Malaysia, Bangi, Selangor, Malaysia

Md. Shahariar Chowdhury
Faculty of Environmental Management, Prince of Songkla University, Hat Yai, Songkhla, Thailand

Shanaika Devadiga
Shobhaben Pratapbhai Patel School of Pharmacy and Technology Management, SVKM'S NMIMS (Deemed to be University), Mumbai, Maharashtra, India

Shilpa Gajbhiye
Department of Pharmaceutics, MET's Institute of Pharmacy, Affiliated to Savitribai Phule Pune University, BKC, Adgaon, Nashik, Maharashtra, India

Shweta S. Gedam
Sandip Institute of Pharmaceutical Sciences, Mahiravani, Nashik, Maharashtra, India

Pravina N. Gurjar
Sharadchandra Pawar College of Pharmacy, Otur, Pune, Maharashtra, India

Anil G. Jadhav
Department of Pharmaceutics, Sandip Institute of Pharmaceutical Sciences, Mahiravani, Nashik, Maharashtra, India

Bony K. John
School of Chemical Sciences, Mahatma Gandhi University, Kottayam, Kerala, India

Greeshma Sara John
Department of Physics, CMS College (Autonomous), Kottayam, Kerala, India; Nanotechnology and Advanced Materials Research Center, CMS College (Autonomous), Kottayam , Kerala, India

Neenamol John
School of Chemical Sciences, Mahatma Gandhi University, Kottayam, Kerala, India

Athira Maria Johnson
Department of Physics, CMS College (Autonomous), Kottayam, Kerala, India; Nanotechnology and Advanced Materials Research Center, CMS College (Autonomous), Kottayam, Kerala, India

Sara Jones
Rajiv Gandhi Center for Biotechnology, Thiruvananthapuram, Kerala, India

Sanjay Kshirsagar
Department of Pharmaceutics, MET's Institute of Pharmacy, Affiliated to Savitribai Phule Pune University, BKC, Adgaon, Nashik, Maharashtra, India

K. V. Arun Kumar
Department of Physics, CMS College (Autonomous), Kottayam, Kerala, India; Nanotechnology and Advanced Materials Research Center, CMS College (Autonomous), Kottayam, Kerala, India

Umesh Laddha
Department of Pharmaceutics, MET's Institute of Pharmacy, Affiliated to Savitribai Phule Pune University, BKC, Adgaon, Nashik, Maharashtra, India

Kam Sheng Lau
Materials Science Program, Department of Applied Physics, Faculty of Science and Technology, Bangi, Selangor, Malaysia

Sunil Mahajan
Department of Pharmaceutical Chemistry, MGV's Pharmacy College, Panchavati, Nashik, Maharashtra, India

Abhisek Majhi
Department of Polymer Science and Technology, University of Calcutta, Kolkata, West Bengal, India

Beena Mathew
School of Chemical Sciences, Mahatma Gandhi University, Kottayam, Kerala, India

Jincy Mathew
School of Chemical Sciences, Mahatma Gandhi University, Kottayam, Kerala, India

Maria Mathew
Department of Chemistry, CMS College, Kottayam, Kerala, India

Souvik Mukherjee
Department of Pharmacy, Guru Ghasidas Central University, Bilaspur, Chhattisgarh, India

Jonathan Tersur Orasugh
Department of Chemical Sciences, University of Johannesburg, Doorfontein, Johannesburg, South Africa; DST-CSIR National Center for Nanostructured Materials, Council for Scientific and Industrial Research, Pretoria, South Africa; Department of Textile Technology, Kaduna Polytechnic, Tudun-Wada, Kaduna, Nigeria

Utkarsha P. Patil
Department of Pharmaceutics, Sandip Institute of Pharmaceutical Sciences, Nashik, Maharashtra, India

Rony Rajan Paul
Department of Chemistry, CMS College, Kottayam, Kerala, India

Shital B. Potdar
Department of Chemical Engineering, National Institute of Technology, Warangal, Telangana, India

Nurul Hazwani Aminuddin Rosli
Materials Science Program, Department of Applied Physics, Faculty of Science and Technology, Bangi, Selangor, Malaysia; Physics Department, Center for Defense Foundation Studies, Universiti Pertahanan Nasional Malaysia, Kuala Lumpur, Malaysia

Ashwini Sermasekaran
Shobhaben Pratapbhai Patel School of Pharmacy and Technology Management, SVKM'S NMIMS (Deemed to be University), Mumbai, Maharashtra, India

Sanjana Subramanian
Rajiv Gandhi Center for Biotechnology, Thiruvananthapuram, Kerala, India; Vellore Institute of Technology (VIT), Vellore, Tamil Nadu, India

Khemchand Surana
Department of Pharmaceutical Chemistry, Shreeshakti Shaikshanik Sanstha, Divine College of Pharmacy, Satana, Nashik, Maharashtra, India

P. Arjun Suresh
Department of Physics, CMS College (Autonomous), Kottayam, Kerala, India; Nanotechnology and Advanced Materials Research Center, CMS College (Autonomous), Kottayam, Kerala, India

Gokul Talele
Department of Pharmaceutical Chemistry, MGV's, Pharmacy College, Panchavati, Nashik, Maharashtra, India

Swati G. Talele
Department of Pharmaceutical Chemistry, Sandip Institute of Pharmacy, Nashik, Maharashtra, India

Nilima Thombre
Department of Pharmaceutics, MET's Institute of Pharmacy, Affiliated to Savitribai Phule Pune University, BKC, Adgaon, Nashik, Maharashtra, India

N. V. Unnikrishnan
School of Pure and Applied Physics, Mahatma Gandhi University, Kottayam, Kerala, India

Swati K. Vetal
Sandip Institute of Pharmaceutical Sciences, Mahiravani, Nashik, Maharashtra, India

Jei Vincent
Materials Science Program, Department of Applied Physics, Faculty of Science and Technology, Bangi, Selangor, Malaysia

Abbreviations

2D	two-dimensional
3D	three-dimensional
AC	alternate current
ACE2	angiotensin-converting enzyme 2
Ach	acetylcholine
AD	Alzheimer's disease
AFP	alpha-fetoprotein / auto fluorescent protein
ALP	alkaline phosphatase
ASOs	Antisense oligonucleotides
BBB	blood-brain barrier
BPE	bipolar electrode
BSA	bovine serum albumin
CA	contrast agents
CBNs	carbon-based nanomaterials
CCD	charge-coupled device
CEA	carcinoembryonic antigen
CEA	carcinoembyronic antigen
CEC	N-carboxyethyl chitosan
CK-MB	creatine kinase MB
CNFs	carbon nanofibers
CNS	central nervous system
CNTs	carbon nanotubes
CNT-SPEs	CNT-screen printed electrodes
Cs	chitosan
CT	computed tomography
CTCs	circulating tumor cells
cTnI	cardiac troponin I
CV	cyclic voltammetry
CVD	cardiovascular diseases / chemical vapor deposition
DCMD	direct contact membrane distillation
DDS	drug delivery systems
DHP	dihexadecyl phosphate
DNDs	detonation nano-diamonds
DOS	density of states

DOTA	1,4,7,10-tetraazacyclododecane-1,4,7,10-tetraacetic acid
DOX	doxorubicin
DPV	differential pulse voltammetry
DRG	dorsal root ganglia
DT	digital tomosynthesis
DTPA	diethylenetriaminepentaacetic dianhydride
DWNTs	double-walled nanotubes
EB	Evans blue
ECM	extracellular matrix
EDA	ethylenediamine
EDC/NHS	1-ethyl-3-(3-dimethylaminopropyl) carbodiimide/ N-hydroxy succinimide
EGF	epidermal growth factor
EIS	electrochemical impedance spectroscopy
EpCAM	epithelial cell adhesion molecule
EPO	erythropoietin
EPPGE	edge plane pyrolytic graphite electrode
EPR	enhanced permeability and retention
FA	folic acid
FAK	focal adhesion kinase
f-CNTs	functionalized carbon nanotubes
FDG	fluorodeoxyglucose
FE	field emission
FET	field-effect transistors
FITC	fluorescein isothiocyanate
f-MWNT	functionalized multi-walled carbon nanotubes
FNDs	fluorescent nano-diamonds
FRET	fluorescence resonance energy transfer
GCE	glassy carbon electrode
Gd	gadolinium
GFP	green fluorescent protein
GM-CSF	granulocyte macrophage colony-stimulating factor
GNPs	gold nanoparticles
GNRs	graphene nanoribbons
GNT	gold nanotubes
GNW-MWCNTs	gold nanowires-incorporated MWCNTs
GO	graphene oxide
Gox	glucose oxidase
GQDs	graphene quantum dots

GSH	glutathione
HCC	hepatocellular carcinoma
HER2	human epidermal growth detail receptor 2
HIV	human immunodeficiency virus
HMME	hematoporphyrin monomethyl ether
hMSCs	human MSCs
HUVEC	human umbilical vein endothelial cells
ICG	indocyanine green
ICP-CVD	inductively coupled chemical vapor deposition
IgE	immunoglobulin E
IgG	immunoglobulin G
ISFETs	ion-sensitive field-effect transistors
KARs	kinase interest newshounds
LBL	layer-by-layer
LBP	lobaplatin
LcL	luciola cruciate luciferase
LECs	lymphatic endothelial cells
LOC	lab-on-a-chip
LOD	limit of detection
LRP1	lipoprotein receptor-related protein-1
LSPR	localized surface plasmon resonance
LSV	linear sweep voltammetry
LYVE-1	lymphatic endothelial hyaluronan receptor-1
MA	methacrylic acid
MAbs	monoclonal antibodies
MB	methylene blue
MDR	multi-drug resistant
MF	micro-filtration
MIPs	molecularly imprinted polymers
miRNAs	microRNAs
MOSFETs	metal-oxide-semiconductor field-effect transistors
MR	magnetic resonance / methylene red
MRI	magnetic resonance imaging
MSC	mesenchymal stem cells
MSP	mesoporous silica
MTAC	[2-(methacryloyloxy) ethyl] trimethylammonium chloride
MWCNT	multi wall carbon nanotubes
NDs	nano-diamonds

NF	nano-filtration
NIPAM	N-isopropyl acrylamide
NIR	near infrared
NIR	near-infrared radiation
NIR-II	near infrared II
NO	nitric oxide
NPs	nanoparticles
NRVMs	neonatal rat ventricular myocytes
NSCs	neural stem cells
NTs	nanotubes
OPN	osteopontin
PA	photoacoustic
PAI	photoacoustic imaging
PAT	photoacoustic tomography
PB	Prussian blue
PCA	principal component analysis
PCL	poly(ε-caprolactone)
PCLF	poly(caprolactone fumarate)
PDA	polydopamine
PDMS	polydimethylsiloxane
PDT	photodynamic therapy
PECVD	plasma enhanced chemical vapor deposition
PEG	poly(ethylene glycol)
PEG-gSWCNT	PEG- graft single-walled
PEI	poly ethyleneimine
PEI-SWCNTs	polyetherimide-modified SWCNTs
PET	position emission tomography
PLCL	poly (l-lactic acid-co-caprolactone)
PLGA	poly(lactide-co-glycolide)
PLK1	polo-like kinase
PL-PEG	phospholipid-polyethylene glycol
PNS	peripheral nervous system
PPDO	poly(p-dioxanone)
PPF	poly (propylene fumarate)
PPP	poly(para-phenylene)
PPy/CNT-Gox	polypyrrole/CNTs-glucose oxidase
PRET	plasmonic resonance energy transfer
PSA	prostate specific antigen
PS–PB	polystyrene–polybutadiene

PSt	polystyrene
PT	photothermal
PTT	photothermal therapy
PTX	paclitaxel
PU	polyurethane
QDs	quantum dots
RBM	radical breathing mode
RdRP	RNA-dependent RNA polymerase gene
RF	radiofrequency
RI	refractive index
RNA	ribonucleic acid
RO	reverse osmosis
ROS	reactive oxygen species
rSCs	rabbit Schwann cells
SARS-CoV-2	severe acute respiratory syndrome coronavirus 2
SD	Sprague–Dawley
SEF	surface-enhanced fluorescence
SERS	surface enhanced Raman scattering
SFI	sciatic nerve functional index
SGM	scanning gate microscopy
shRNA	small hairpin RNA
siRNA	small interfering RNA
SPCE	screen-printed carbon electrode
SPECT	single photon emission computed tomography
SPIO	super paramagnetic iron oxide
SPION	super-paramagnetic iron oxide nano-particle
SPR	surface plasmon resonance
SPRF	surface plasmon resonance-assisted fluoroimmunoassay
SSA	specific surface area
ssDNA	single-stranded deoxyribonucleic acid
SWCNTs	single wall carbon nanotubes
SWIR	shortwave-infrared-red
SWV	square wave voltammetry
TAM	tamoxifen
TAT	thermoacoustic tomography
TE	thermionic emission
TEM	transmission electron microscope
TEVGs	tissue engineering vascular grafts

TNF	tumor necrosis factor
UF	ultra-filtration
US	ultrasound
VA	vertically aligned
VACNT	vertically aligned CNT
VACNT/PE	vertically aligned carbon nanotube/polyethylene
VEGF	vascular endothelial growth factor
VHSs	van Hoff singularities
VOCs	volatile organic compounds
WHO	World Health Organization

Preface

Carbon nanotubes with their small sizes have impressive properties with remarkable applications in pharmacy and medicine due to their high surface area. Nowadays, extensive applications of carbon nanotubes have been on the rise in the biomedical field and in the development of nano-medicines due to their use in bio-imaging, biosensing, and drug delivery.

Carbon nanotubes with drug loading capabilities and biocompatibility have been challenging for modified carbon-based nanomaterials, and in this new title, recent biomedical applications of carbon nanotubes are studied in the light of various advantages.

This new book reports the most recent studies in the development of carbon nanotubes and their applications in targeting drug delivery, cancer therapy, bioimaging, biosensors, and human health. In this new volume, the authors report the modern development of modified CNTs that contribute to emerging challenges in biomedical applications and human health.

The book is divided into three main parts. In the first part, we explain why the unique features of carbon nanotubes make them an ideal candidate for applications in biomedicine. In the second part of this book, we summarize the method of carbon nanotubes functionalization and their applications in medical diagnosis and therapy. In the last part of this volume, we show how the rapid growth in carbon nanotubes has influenced the medical sectors as sensing elements for biosensors, biomedical imaging, and human health.

PART I
Fundamentals

CHAPTER 1

Biomedical Applications of Carbon Nanotubes

MIR SAHANUR ALI,[1,2] SOUVIK MUKHERJEE,[3] ABHISEK MAJHI,[1] MIR INTAJ ALI,[4] MIR SAHIDUL ALI,[1] JONATHAN TERSUR ORASUGH,[5,6,7] and DIPANKAR CHATTOPADHYAY[1,2]

[1]*Department of Polymer Science and Technology, University of Calcutta, Kolkata, West Bengal, India*

[2]*Center for Research in Nanoscience and Nanotechnology, Acharya Prafulla Chandra Roy Sikhsha Prangan, University of Calcutta, JD-2, Saltlake City, Kolkata, West Bengal, India*

[3]*Department of Pharmacy, Guru Ghasidas Central University, Bilaspur, Chhattisgarh, India*

[4]*Central Institute of Petrochemicals Engineering and Technology (CIPET), Institute of Petrochemicals Technology (IPT), Bhubaneswar, Patia, Odisha, India*

[5]*Department of Chemical Sciences, University of Johannesburg, Doorfontein, Johannesburg, South Africa*

[6]*DST-CSIR National Center for Nanostructured Materials, Council for Scientific and Industrial Research, Pretoria, South Africa*

[7]*Department of Textile Technology, Kaduna Polytechnic, Tudun-Wada, Kaduna, Nigeria*

Carbon Nanotubes for Biomedical Applications and Healthcare.
Chin Hua Chia, Swati Gokul Talele, Ann Rose Abraham, and A. K. Haghi, (Eds.)

ABSTRACT

Recent advancements and extensive research in nanotechnology, biotechnology, materials engineering the applications of nanomaterial are evolving extensively and greatly. Due to the unique properties of carbon nanotubes (CNTs), the developed CNT-based device/systems enjoy exclusive chemical, physical, and biological properties which make them a good candidates in the biomedical applications, but they also have some inherent properties which arise great concern about their biosafety. Due to the excellent thermal and electrical conductivity, biocompatibility, corrosion resistance, and high surface area due to nano-dimension, it may be modified/designed and functionalized basis on our demand. The several distinctive features of CNT are reported for several biomedical applications. CNTs are suitable for diagnostic and therapeutic agents. Carbon nanotubes form various novel carrier systems which are also capable to site-specific targeting the delivery of therapeutic pharmaceutical drugs. In this chapter, we discuss the synthesis, properties, modification of CNT, and recent progress of carbon nanotubes and their application for bio-sensing, targeted drug delivery and toxicity.

1.1 INTRODUCTION

The development of science and changing lifestyles of human civilization has resulted in the prominence of various deadly diseases such as cancer, diabetes, hypertension, and other cardiovascular diseases, whose causes and conditions are still the focus of research for medical professionals [1–4]. Unique biological, chemical, and physical peculiarity makes them a good candidate for biomedical applications, CNTs in the field of medicine, biotechnology have in recent times started to arise, raising great courage. Therefore, to save society from all these diseases, in the 21st century with the support of nanotechnology scientists opened a new door of medical research. Nanotechnology is a type of engineering technology, where on an approximately 1 to 100-nanometer scale, the chemical and natural way in which molecules, the earthly matter created by atoms are synthesized and newly formed and regulated in a new way. The importance of new concepts has spread from medicine to industry today. Using this concept of nanotechnology, a new nanomaterial with a wide range of important electrical, chemical, thermal, mechanical, and structural characteristics, consist an extensive range of chemical bonding energies, has revolutionized biomedical research (Such as Drug delivery, cancer diagnosis, etc.). The carbon atom is formed in the outer cell with 4 electron valency which is capable of forming various forms.

CNTs enjoy all these properties of carbon. The fourth solid carbon allotropes is carbon nanotubes, which were first discovered by Japanese scientist Sumio Iijima in 1991 as a surprising byproduct of fullerenes synthesis in the soot of the arc-discharge method [5]. It is of two types such as: (i) single-wall carbon nanotubes (which looks like hollow cylinder type in which Bravis lattice vector exists); and (ii) Multiwall nanotubes (which looks like tree ring type in which Vander walls force exists). Nonetheless, we have analyzed several databases (such as Web of Science and Scopus) to determine just how much the biomedical field has improved using the concept of carbon nanotubes in the past 20 years [2, 4]. Our analysis of the data revealed that 3,630 articles have been published as a total article, proceeding paper, and early access, where 1.69% of articles were based on biomedical applications (*see* Figure 1.1) and the most work was done in 2016 and 2019.
As shown in Figure 1.2, the USA has taken the lead in research and India has come in fourth place based on country priority.

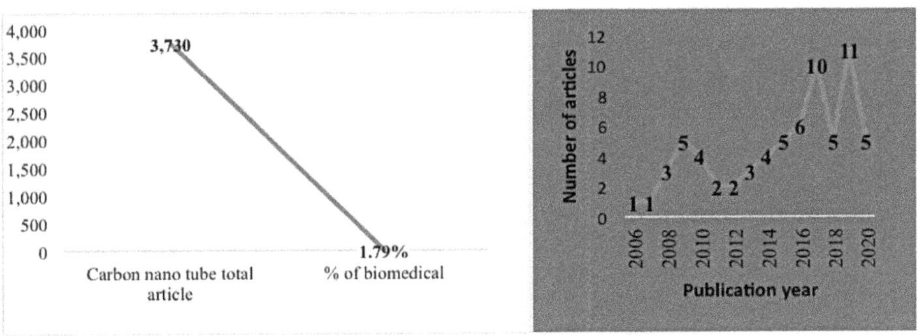

FIGURE 1.1 Total articles and number of published articles year wise.

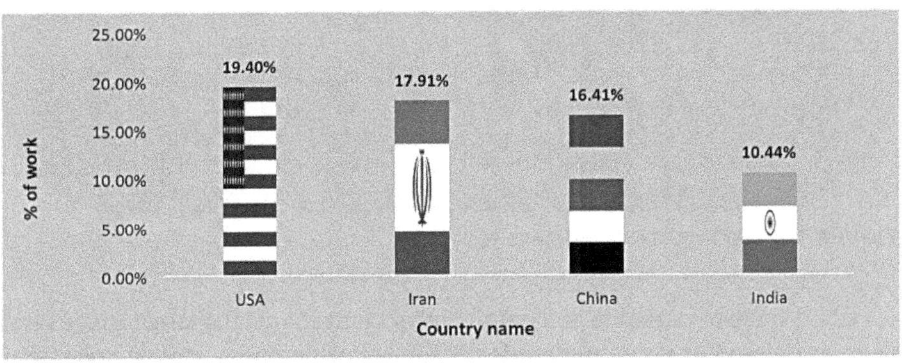

FIGURE 1.2 Priority country of CNT-based research.

1.2 FUNCTIONALIZATION OF CNT

The key obstacle with CNTs for the biomedical applications is the congenital difficulty to handle them for front line uses. Indeed CNTs have a tendency to aggregate into bundles from side to side robust attractive bonding interactions, which are very problematic to unsettle. As grown, pristine buckytubes have exceedingly hydrophobic surfaces and are insoluble in distilled water or any common organic/inorganic solvents. Incorporations of functional moieties onto the CNTs surface helps and facilitates to solubilize them and therefore analyze them. Surface functionalization of CNT shown in Figure 1.3.

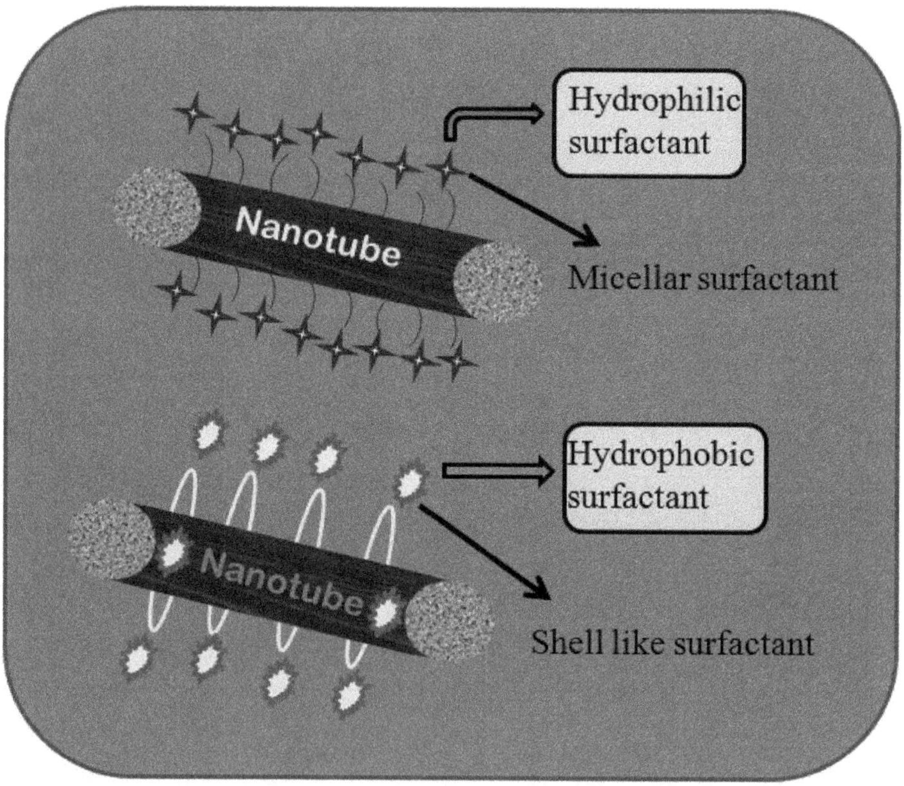

FIGURE 1.3 Surface functionalization of CNT.

CNTs have remarkable and unique physicomechanical characteristics and were acclaimed as novel materials for future technologies almost soon after their discovery. They are now widely acknowledged as key contributors to nanotechnology, which is concerned with the control and use of material on a nanometer to molecular scale and the production of nanoscale building blocks with fundamentally novel physical, chemical, and biological properties and activities. CNTs are poorly soluble and dispersible in organic and aqueous media, and they are exceedingly resistant to wetting in all of their forms. Making composites of these hydrophobic nanotubes with other materials and producing coordinated assemblies, which are essential for the development of photonic and electrical devices, are similarly difficult. Appropriate functionalization of CNTs, that is, the addition of chemical functional groups, is a solution for circumventing these limitations and has thus become a desirable objective for materials scientists and synthetic chemists. Functionalization can enhance solubility [6] and processability while also allowing nanotube characteristics to combine with those of other materials. Chemical bonding could be employed to modify the nanotube's interaction with other entities such as polymer, biopolymer matrices, solvents, and other nanotubes. Functionalized CNTs possess unique electrical and/or mechanical properties than nonfunctionalized nanotubes, and so may be used to fine-tune the chemistry and physics of CNTs. When it comes to CNT functionalization, it is consequential to distinguish between functionalization like covalent and noncovalent, single wall carbon nanotubes (SWCNTs) and multi-wall carbon nanotubes (MWCNT) functionalization, and the functionalization of individual tubes and tubes bundles. Covalent functionalization is the process that involves attaching functional entities to the carbon scaffold of a nanotube. Whereas in the other hand, supramolecular complexation employing various adsorption forces, such as van der Waals' and p-stacking interactions, is the most common non-covalent functionalization method. Before diving into the functionalization of CNT, let us discuss the reactivity of CNT.

Due to the lack of functional groups, a perfect SWCNT is a cylindrical aromatic macromolecule and chemically inert [7]. Local strain is caused by two main sources in nonplanar conjugated organic molecules: curvature-induced pyramidalization of both the conjugated carbon atoms and p-orbital misalignment between nearby pairs of conjugated carbon atoms. Even though CNT sidewalls and fullerene soccer ball-like surfaces are both instances of curved carbon, their chemistry differs significantly.

1.2.1 COVALENT FUNCTIONALIZATION

Addition chemistry has just begun to be used to covalently functionalize SWCNTs, a method that is thought to be particularly promising for nanotube modification and derivatization. However, controlling the chemo- and regioselectivity of such additions, which need very "hot" addends like arynes, carbenes, or halogens, as well as dramatic reaction conditions, is difficult. Furthermore, identifying functionalized SWCNTs as such, as well as the precise position and mechanism of addition, is extremely difficult [8].

The "oxidative purification" of nanotubes by liquid-phase or gas-phase oxidation, is a general functionalization procedures which introduces carboxylic groups and other oxygen-bearing functionalities including hydroxyl, carbonyl, ester, and nitro groups into the tubes. Boiling nitric acid, sulfuric acid, or mixtures of both "piranha" (sulfuric acid–hydrogen peroxide) and gaseous oxygen, ozone, or air as the oxidant at elevated temperatures, or combinations of nitric acid and air oxidation have all been used for oxidative treatment ("purification") [9–18]. The introduction of carboxylic groups and other oxygen-bearing groups at the tubes' ends and at defect sites is aided by oxidative treatment, which results in the tubes being decorated with an indeterminate number of oxygenated functions. However, due to the huge aspect ratio of CNTs, significant sidewall functionalization occurs as well (*see* Figure 1.4). Holzinger et al. [19] developed an innovative purification process for SWCNTs by using HNO_3-oxidation in combination with column chromatography and vacuum filtering.

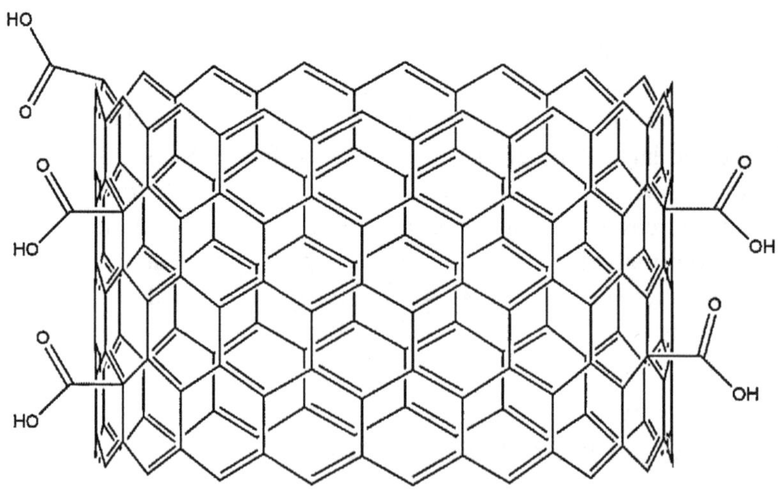

FIGURE 1.4 Depicting a section of oxidative purified SWCNT with functional groups at terminal and sidewall position.

The oxidative insertion of carboxylic groups to nanotubes opens up a wide range of functional possibilities through the alteration of carboxylic functionalities and provides anchor groups for subsequent modification. Carboxamides can be made from carboxylic acids using carboxylic acid chlorides, allowing for the decorating of oxidized tubes with nucleophiles like aliphatic amines, aryl amines, amino acids derivatives, peptides, amino-group-substituted dendrimers, and so on. The carboxylic groups can be triggered by converting them to acyl chloride groups employing thionyl chloride ($SOCl_2$), and then amidating the acyl chlorides to generate carboxamides (shown in Figure 1.5).

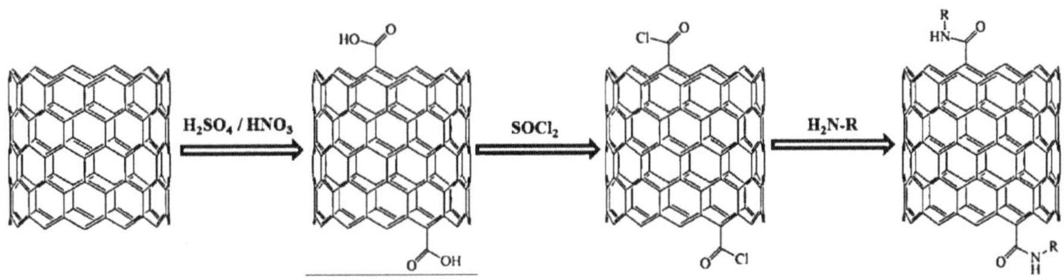

FIGURE 1.5 Representing the oxidative modification of SWCNTs, accompanied by thionyl chloride treatment and subsequent amidation.

By defect group functionalization, Newkome-type dendrons were connected to the SWCNT's and MWCNT's carbon frameworks and thus facilitated to the formation of first and second-generation ammine dendrimers by further treatment [20].

Fluorination of SWCNTs was achieved by reacting them with elemental fluorine at temperatures ranging from 150°C to 600°C. The chlorination on CNT can be achieved by means of electrochemical modification. On the other hand, the functionalization of CNT can be put into practice by hydrogenation of CNT, the addition of nitriles, radicals, nucleophilic carbene, etc.

1.3 BIOMEDICAL APPLICATIONS OF CNT

While comparing other bulk nanomaterials, CNTs possess some important characteristics due to their surface area to volume ratio, which make them for versatile applications in the biomedical field. Figure 1.6 shows some different biomedical applications of CNTs. CNTs are hydrophobic in nature and so it's suitable for various biomedical applications. Figure 1.6 shows different biomedical applications of CNTs.

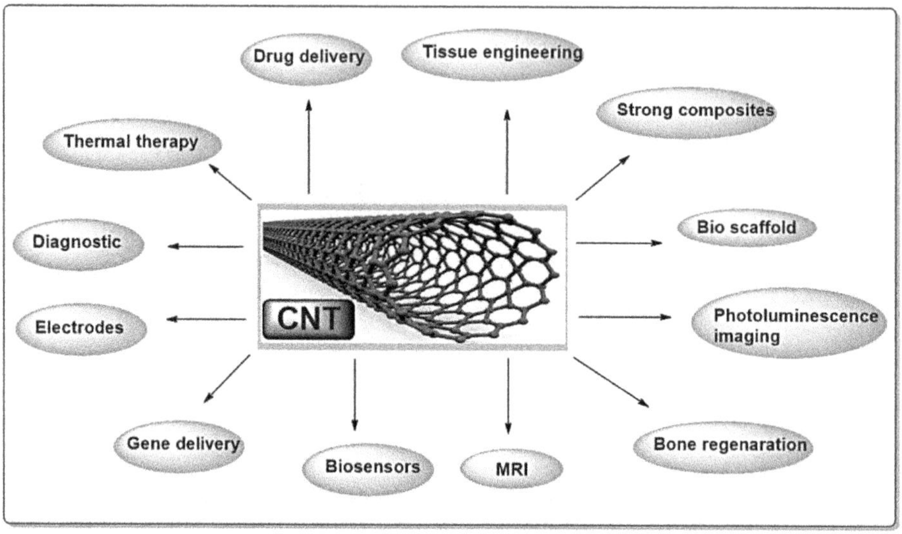

FIGURE 1.6 Different biomedical applications of CNT.

1.3.1 BIOSENSOR

Biosensors are vibrant among the recent tools discovered for the biomedical recognition for the bioactive molecules. Biosensors have superior electro-mechanical to sensation of the biomolecules or bio-based materials. The amplified surface reactive zone of CNTs matures them as a key vehicles for organic species detection at macro- to nano-level/range, this important properties of biosensors makes them further suitable as an ultra-level sensitive biosensor. The superior sensitivity, earlier action, greater lifecycle, longevity, and improved shelf life properties make them a good candidate for biosensor applications [21]. Nanobiosensors are useful for the detection of diverse disease and biomolecules.

By virtue of the remarkable structural, optical, electronic, and mechanical properties of CNTs have diverse features and acquire focus to new generation probes in CNTs-based biosensors. The first invention of biosensors appeared with the development of electrochemical strategies for detection of analytes in the 1950s. In 1956 Leland Clark Jr described the initial and most famous of electrochemical oxygen biosensor (Clark oxygen electrode), consisting of a Pt (platinum) cathode at which oxygen is reduced and a silver (Ag)/silver chloride (AgCl) corresponding reference electrode [22]. Rapid development of nanotechnologies and the discovery of emergence of nanomaterials with attractive physicochemical properties, a new cutting age of biosensors denoted to as nanobiosensors, which includes nanoparticles (NPs) and nanotubes (NTs), nanocomposites has been developed, that combines the benefits of nanomaterials, especially their small size and large surface/volume ratio. The fascinating nanomaterials have smart and attractive prospects for biosensing applications, to enhance sensitivity and lower detection limits [23]. By advantage of their exceptional structural, mechanical, electronic, and intrinsic optical properties such as photoluminescence in the near infrared (NIR). CNTs platform opening several interesting features of engineered new generation probes [24–26].

The enzymatic electrochemical biosensors, based on CNTs and their composites utilize bio-specificity of the enzymatic response to direct electrical transference among biomolecules, particularly enzymes and CNT/CNT composites bulk electrode materials [27]. Figure 1.7 shows different CNT-based biosensors. Protein grafted surface modified/functionalized CNTs are employed for the construction of a lab-on-a-chip (LOC) which is enable to detect lower concentration lipoprotein and could be useful for biomolecular detection [28, 29] Feng et al. stated a throwaway paper-oriented bipolar electrode (BPE) systems for the sense electrochemiluminescent revealing the prostate specific antigen (PSA) and displayed that its reaction was expressively improved after the modification of the BPE cathode with MWNTs [30]. The signal transducer of a dsDNA screen-printed carbon based electrode device/biosensor was improved by MWNTs and colloidal gold nanoparticles (GNPs) for sensing plant alkaloid (e.g., berberine, an isoquinoline) with enhanced antimicrobial and anticancer response [31].

Volatile organic compounds (VOCs) sensing present in human breath to detect lung cancer is fetching an important technique for widespread screening, due to its ability and low cost advantages. SWCNTs functionalized with tricosane ($C23H48$) based biosensor showed remarkable sensitivity toward polar type VOC molecules, which have the ability to donate electrons to the CNTs after being absorbed [32].

D-(+)-galactose contained conjugated SWCNTs were produced using molybdenum electrodes for the successful detection of cancer marker galactin-3 [33]. Fayazfar et al. stated a new platform founded on electrochemical growth of GNPs on structurally aligned MWCNTs for subtle label-free DNA detection of the TP53 gene mutation [34].

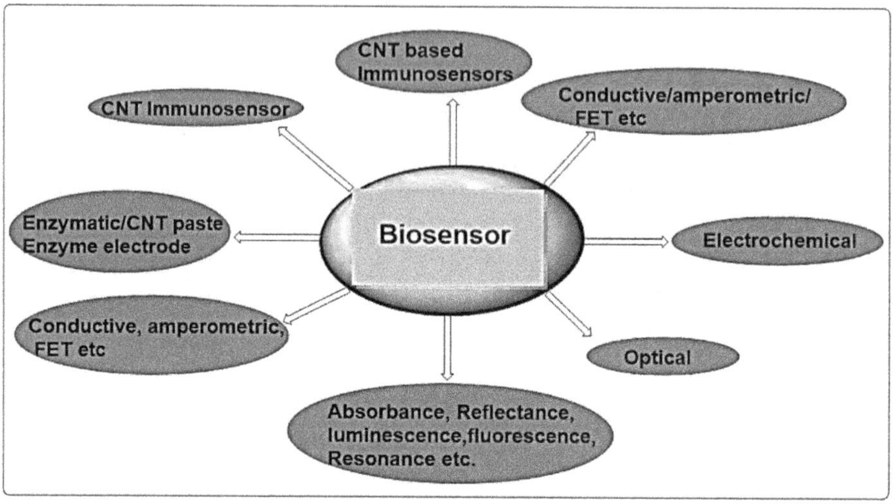

FIGURE 1.7 Different types of CNT-based biosensors.

1.3.2 DRUG DELIVERY

Due to excellent properties of CNTs, it has been applied for designing a wide range of drug delivery systems (DDS) for the treatment of many diseases. Some unique properties of CNTs (optical, adequate chemical stability and high drug loading and sustained releasing capacity,) make them superb nanocarriers for drug delivery applications [35]. Anticancer drug delivery systems based on CNT are established which involves selective targeting achieved through surface functionalization [36]. The advancement of peptide-modified SWCNTs has shown a high anti-tumor result and higher tumor-targeting [37]. The innovative cocoon-like nanoparticles constructed with polyethylene glycol and MWCNTs also have big future as nano-biomaterials and can conveniently be loaded with curcumin, a natural anticancer medication. Drug delivery through to the blood-brain barrier utilizing carbon nanotubes (BBB). Even though it is difficult to cross the BBB, medication delivery to the brain is impeded. Some modern data have proven that functionalized carbon nanotubes can be used to target the brain; they are appropriate nanocarriers of brain targeting [38, 39].

The brain targeted medication transportation was facilitated through doped multi-walled carbon nanotubes (f-MWNTs) with the brain targeting ligand moiety Angiopep-2 (ANG), which also has a good compatibility for the low-density lipoprotein receptor-related protein-1 (LRP1). The research also showed that ANG conjugated CNTs boosted BBB permeability and brain tumor targeting *in vitro* and *in vivo* [40]. A combination of oxidizing MWCNTs-PEG and angiopep-2 as a targeting ligand has already been found to show dual targeting capability in brain glioma [35, 41–44].

1.4 TOXICITY OF CNT

Safety is the major priority of any material used for biomedical turf. Together with developing number of CNTs applications in the medical field [26, 45], questions are elevated about the potential toxicity of CNTs. Toxicity can be explored by putting cell cultures to CNT suspensions formulated with or without surfactant ingredients and disseminated employing ultra/probe sonication. Surfactants, which seem to be ubiquitous in CNT suspensions, are documented to become very toxic to cells and may therefore lead to the detected toxicity of the CNT specimens [46]. If the metal-based particles/ catalyst content in CNTs is still not eradicated even during synthesis and refinement process, free radicals can form, caused by oxidative stress damage to cells and cell membranes [47]. This is exclusively vital since the annual manufacture of bucky tubes is now reaching thousands of tons per annum. Toxicological studies of CNTs have been scrutinized on animal models. Poland et al. in an experimental analysis, witnessed the structural likeness of CNTs with asbestos fibers [48]. Still now, there is no standardized proper way to know the physiological behavior in biological systems, and that's why the toxicity of nanomaterials is undetermined till now date. The determination of appropriate exposure protocols such as computational simulation of nanomaterials and cell interaction directs the dynamic of nanoparticles in multifaceted environment consist of those in organism [49–52].

1.5 CONCLUSION

Due to the increasing demands of our current civilization, in particular medical care issues related with aging of the people, next cutting age remedial diagnostics entail execution of swift, subtle, early detection and cost-effective substitutes to the more traditional immunological assays presently castoff. Similarly, diseases and hazardous substances in our environment bring severe hazards, prompting sensitive recognition procedures to discourse concerns about our farming and world stability.

Carbon nanotubes (CNTs) have a massive range of queerish parameters, spanning size range, biocompatibility, and physiochemical prowess, which make them a useful stage for biomedical endeavors. CNTs can be loaded with anticancer drugs entity. Although, CNTs-based biosensors are promising, it still has many obstacles in practical applications. The progress of CNT-based materials has multidimensional aspects in biomedical field which needs the cooperation between materials scientists, and engineers, who developed or fabricates the new CNT-based materials for biomedical applications.

ACKNOWLEDGMENT

The authors wish to thank the Center for Research in Nanoscience and Nanotechnology (CRNN), and the Department of Polymer Science and Technology, University of Calcutta for their technical support. Mir Intaj Ali thankfully acknowledge to CIPET (IPT) Bhubaneswar for the facility of lab and computer.

KEYWORDS

- **biomedical applications**
- **bio-sensing**
- **carbon nanotubes (CNT)**
- **drug delivery**
- **nano-carrier**
- **toxicity**

REFERENCES

1. Gao, W., & Kono, J., (2019). Science and applications of wafer-scale crystalline carbon nanotube films prepared through controlled vacuum filtration. *Royal Society Open Science, 6*(3), 181605.
2. Anzar, N., Hasan, R., Tyagi, M., Yadav, N., & Narang, J., (2020). Carbon nanotube–a review on synthesis, properties and plethora of applications in the field of biomedical science. *Sensors International, 1*, 100003.
3. Raphey, V. R., Henna, T. K., Nivitha, K. P., Mufeedha, P., Sabu, C., & Pramod, K., (2019). Advanced biomedical applications of carbon nanotube. *Materials Science and Engineering: C., 100*, 616–630.

4. Patil, A., Mishra, V., Thakur, S., Riyaz, B., Kaur, A., Khursheed, R., Patil, K., & Sathe, B., (2019). Nanotechnology derived nanotools in biomedical perspectives: An update. *Current Nanoscience, 15*(2), 137–146.
5. Iijima, S., (1991). Helical microtubules of graphitic carbon. *Nature, 354*(6348), 56–58.
6. Niyogi, S., Hamon, M. A., Hu, H., Zhao, B., Bhowmik, P., Sen, R., & Haddon, R. C., (2002). Chemistry of single-walled carbon nanotubes. *Accounts of Chemical Research, 35*(12), 1105–1113.
7. Bahr, J. L., & Tour, J. M., (2002). Covalent chemistry of single-wall carbon nanotubes. *Journal of Materials Chemistry, 12*(7), 1952–1958.
8. Hirsch, A., (2002). Functionalization of single-walled carbon nanotubes. *Angewandte Chemie International Edition, 41*(11), 1853–1859.
9. Rinzler, A. G., Liu, J., Dai, H., Nikolaev, P., Huffman, C. B., Rodriguez-Macias, F. J., & Smalley, R. E., (1998). Large-scale purification of single-wall carbon nanotubes: Process, product, and characterization. *Applied Physics A: Materials Science & Processing, 67*(1).
10. Dujardin, E., Ebbesen, T. W., Krishnan, A., & Treacy, M. M., (1998). Purification of single-shell nanotubes. *Advanced Materials, 10*(8), 611–613.
11. Vaccarini, L., Goze, C., Aznar, R., Micholet, V., Journet, C., & Dernier, P., (1999). Purification procedure of carbon nanotubes. *Synthetic Metals, 103*(1–3), 2492–2493.
12. Vaccarini, L., Goze, C., Aznar, R., Micholet, V., Journet, C., Bernier, P., & Loiseau, A., (1999). Purification des nanotubes de carbone monofeuillets. *Comptes Rendus de l'Académie des Sciences-Series IIB-Mechanics-Physics-Astronomy, 327*(9), 925–931.
13. Nagasawa, S., Yudasaka, M., Hirahara, K., Ichihashi, T., & Iijima, S., (2000). Effect of oxidation on single-wall carbon nanotubes. *Chemical Physics Letters, 328*(4–6), 374–380.
14. Holzinger, M., Hirsch, A., Bernier, P., Duesberg, G. S., & Burghard, M., (2000). A new purification method for single-wall carbon nanotubes (SWNTs). *Applied Physics A., 70*(5), 599–602.
15. Sumanasekera, G. U., Allen, J. L., Fang, S. L., Loper, A. L., Rao, A. M., & Eklund, P. C., (1999). Electrochemical oxidation of single wall carbon nanotube bundles in sulfuric acid. *The Journal of Physical Chemistry B., 103*(21), 4292–4297.
16. Liu, J., Rinzler, A. G., Dai, H., Hafner, J. H., Bradley, R. K., Boul, P. J., & Smalley, R. E., (1998). Fullerene pipes. *Science, 280*(5367), 1253–1256.
17. Morishita, K., & Takarada, T., (1999). Scanning electron microscope observation of the purification behavior of carbon nanotubes. *Journal of Materials Science, 34*(6), 1169–1174.
18. Tohji, K., Goto, T., Takahashi, H., Shinoda, Y., Shimizu, N., Jeyadevan, B., & Nishina, Y., (1996). Purifying single-walled nanotubes. *Nature, 383*(6602), 679–679.
19. Kuznetsova, A., Popova, I., Yates, Jr. J. T., Bronikowski, M. J., Huffman, C. B., Liu, J., & Chen, J. G., (2001). Oxygen-containing functional groups on single-wall carbon nanotubes: NEXAFS and vibrational spectroscopic studies. *Journal of the American Chemical Society, 123*(43), 10699–10704.
20. Hirsch, A., & Vostrowsky, O., (2005). Functionalization of carbon nanotubes. In: *Functional Molecular Nanostructures* (pp. 193–237). Springer, Berlin, Heidelberg.
21. Obite, F., (2017). Development of carbon nanotube-based biosensors development of carbon nanotube-based biosensors. In: Geoffrey, I., Felix, O., & Obaiduir, R., (eds.), *Int. J. Nano Biomater*. (Vol. 6, pp. 83–109). https://doi.org/10.1504/ IJNBM.2016.079682.

22. Clark, L. C. J., (1956). Monitor and control of blood and tissue oxygen tensions. *ASAIOJ., 2*, 41–48.
23. Dutta, K., De, S., Das, B., Bera, S., Guria, B., Ali, M. S., & Chattopadhyay, D., (2021). Development of an efficient immunosensing platform by exploring single-walled carbon nanohorns (SWCNHs) and nitrogen doped graphene quantum dot (N-GQD) Nanocomposite for early detection of cancer biomarker. *ACS Biomaterials Science & Engineering, 7*(12), 5541–5554.
24. Munzer, A. M., Heimgreiter, M., Melzer, K., Weise, A., Fabel, B., Abdellah, A., et al., (2013). Back-gated spray-deposited carbon nanotube thin film transistors operated in electrolytic solutions: An assessment towards future biosensing applications. *J. Mater. Chem. B, 1*, 3797–3802. doi: 10.1039/c3tb20170h.
25. Holzinger, M., Le Goff, A., & Cosnier, S., (2014). Nanomaterials for biosensing applications: A review. *Front. Chem., 2*, 63. doi: 10.3389/fchem.2014.00063.
26. Mundra, R. V., Wu, X., Sauer, J., Dordick, J. S., & Kane, R. S., (2014). Nano tubes in biological applications. *Curr. Opin. Biotechnol., 28*, 25–32. doi: 10.1016/j.copbio.2013.10.012.
27. Kurbanoglu, S., Ozkan, S. A., & Merkoci, A., (2017). Nanomaterials-based enzyme electrochemical biosensors operating through inhibition for biosensing applications. *Biosens. Bioelectron, 89*(Part 2), 886–898.
28. Choi, J. H., Nguyen, F. T., Barone, P. W., Heller, D. A., Moll, A. E., Patel, D., Boppart, S. A., & Strano, M. S., (2007). Multimodal biomedical imaging with asymmetric single-walled carbon nanotube/iron oxide nanoparticle complexes. *Nanoletters, 4*, 861–867. https://doi.org/10.1021/nl062306v.
29. Lin, Y., Taylor, S., Li, H., Fernando, K. A. S., Qu, L., Wang, W., Gu, L., et al., (2004). Advances toward bioapplications of carbon nanotubes. *J. Mater. Chem., 14*, 527–541. https://doi.org/10.1039/B314481J.
30. Feng, Q. M., Pan, J. B., Zhang, H. R., Xu, J. J., & Chen, H. Y., (2014). Disposable paper-based bipolar electrode for sensitive electrochemiluminescence detection of a cancer biomarker. *Chem. Commun. (Camb)., 50*, 10949–10951. doi: 10.1039/C4CC03102D.
31. Ovádeková, R., Jantová, S., Letasiová, S., Stepánek, I., & Labuda, J., (2006). Nanostructured electrochemical DNA biosensors for detection of the effect of berberine on DNA from cancer cells. *Anal. Bioanal. Chem., 386*, 2055–2062. doi: 10.1007/s00216-006-0830-6.
32. Liu, F. L., Xiao, P., Fang, H. L., Dai, H. F., Qiao, L., & Zhang, Y. H., (2011). Single-walled carbon nanotube-based biosensors for the detection of volatile organic compounds of lung cancer. *Phys. E Low Dimens. Syst. Nanostruct., 44*, 367–372. doi: 10.1016/j.physe.2011.08.033.
33. Park, Y. K., Bold, B., Lee, W. K., Jeon, M. H., An, K. H., Jeong, S. Y., et al., (2011). D-(+)-galactose-conjugated single-walled carbon nanotubes as new chemical probes for electrochemical biosensors for the cancer marker galectin-3. *Int. J. Mol. Sci., 12*, 2946–2957. doi: 10.3390/ijms12052946.
34. Fayazfar, H., Afshar, A., Dolati, M., & Dolati, A., (2014). DNA impedance biosensor for detection of cancer, TP53 gene mutation, based on gold nanoparticles/aligned carbon nanotubes modified electrode. *Anal. Chim. Acta, 836*, 34–44. doi: 10.1016/j.aca.2014.05.029.

35. Chou, C. C., Hsiao, H. Y., Hong, Q. S., Chen, C. H., Peng, Y. W., Chen, H. W., & Yang, P. C., (2008). Single-walled carbon nanotubes can induce pulmonary injury in mouse model. *Nano Lett., 8*, 437–445. https://doi.org/10.1021/nl0723634.
36. Ji, Z., Lin, G., Lu, Q., Meng, L., Shen, X., Dong, L., Fu, C., & Zhang, X., (2012). Targeted therapy of SMMC -7721 liver cancer *in vitro* and *in vivo* with carbon nanotubes-based drug delivery system. *J. Colloid Interface Sci., 365*, 143–149. https://doi.org/10. 1016/j. jcis.2011.09.013.
37. Chen, J., Chen, S., Zhao, X., Kuznetsova, L. V., Wong, S. S., & Ojima, I., (2008). Functionalized single-walled carbon nanotubes as rationally designed vehicles for tumor-targeted drug delivery. *J. Am. Chem. Soc., 130*, 16778–16785. https://doi.org/10. 1021/ja805570f.
38. Foldvari, M., & Bagonluri, M., (2008). Carbon nanotubes as functional excipients for nanomedicines: II. Drug delivery and biocompatibility issues, nanomedicine nanotechnology. *Biol. Med., 4*, 183–200. https://doi.org/10.1016/j.nano. 2008.04.003.
39. Zhou, J., Li, J., Wu, D., & Hong, C., (2017). CNT-based and MSN-based organic/ inorganic hybrid nanocomposites for biomedical. *Adv. Bioinspired Biomed. Mater.*, 169–192. https://doi.org/10.1021/bk-2017-1253.ch009.
40. Kafa, H., Wang, J. T., Rubio, N., Klippstein, R., Costa, P. M., Hassan, H. A. F. M., Sosabowski, J. K., et al., (2016). Translocation of LRP1 targeted carbon nanotubes of different diameters across the blood–brain barrier *in vitro* and *in vivo*. *J. Control. Release 225,* 217–229. https://doi.org/10.1016/j.jconrel.2016.01.031.
41. Ren, J., Shen, S., Wang, D., Xi, Z., Guo, L., Pang, Z., Qian, Y., et al., (2012). Biomaterials the targeted delivery of anticancer drugs to brain glioma by PEGylated oxidized multi-walled carbon nanotubes modified with angiopep-2. *Biomaterials, 33*, 3324–3333. https://doi.org/10.1016/j.biomaterials.2012. 01.025.
42. Flavio, F., Contreras-Torres, Daniel Salas-Treviño, Adolfo Soto-Domínguez, & Gerardo De Jesús García-Rivas. (2022). Carbon Nanotubes in Tumor-Targeted Chemotherapeutic Formulations: A Review of Opportunities and Challenges. *ACS Applied Nano Materials, 5*(7), 8649–8679. https://doi.org/10.1021/acsanm.2c01118.
43. Oskoueian, A., Amin, M. K., Bayat, S., Oskoueian, E., Ostovan, F., & Toozandehjani, M., (2018). Fabrication, characterization, and functionalization of single walled carbon nanotube conjugated with tamoxifen and its anticancer potential against human breast cancer cells. *J. Nanomater., 13*. https://doi. org/10.1155/2018/8417016.
44. Douradinha, B., & Doolan, D. L., (2018). Harnessing immune responses against plasmodium for rational vaccine design. *Trends Parasitol., 27*, 274–283. https://doi. org/10.1016/j.pt.2011.01.002.
45. Vardharajula, S., Ali, S. Z., Tiwari, P. M., Ero˘ glu, E., Vig, K., Dennis, V. A., et al., (2012). Functionalized carbon nanotubes: Biomedical applications. *Int. J. Nanomedicine, 7*, 5361–5374. doi: 10.2147/IJN. S35832.
46. Dong, L., Joseph, K. L., Witkowski, C. M., & Craig, M. M., (2008). Cytotoxicity of single-walled carbon nanotubes suspended in various surfactants. *Nanotechnology, 19*, 0957–4484. doi: 10.1088/0957-4484/19/25/255702.
47. Plata, D. L., Gschwend, P. M., & Reddy, C. M., (2008). Industrially synthesized single-walled carbon nanotubes: Compositional data for users, environmental risk assessments, and source apportionment. *Nanotechnology, 19*, 185706. doi: 10.1088/0957-4484/19/18/185706.

48. Poland, C. A., Duffin, R., Kinloch, I., Maynard, A., Wallace, W. A., Seaton, A., et al., (2008). Carbon nanotubes in traduced into the abdominal cavity of mice show asbestos-like pathogenicity in a pilot study. *Nat. Nanotechnol., 3*, 423–428. doi: 10.1038/nnano.2008.111.
49. Yang, S. T., Fernando, K. A., Liu, J. H., Wang, J., Sun, H. F., Liu, Y., et al., (2008). Covalently PEGylated carbon nanotubes with stealth character *in vivo. Small, 4*, 940–944. doi: 10.1002/smll.200700714.
50. Muller, J., Huaux, F., Moreau, N., Misson, P., Heilier, J. F., Delos, M., et al., (2005). Respiratory toxicity of multi-wall carbon nanotubes. *Toxicol. Appl. Pharmacol., 207*, 221–231. doi: 10.1016/j.taap.2005.01.008.
51. Shvedova, A. A., Kisin, E. R., Mercer, R., Murray, A. R., Johnson, V. J., Potapovich, A. I., et al., (2005). Unusual inflammatory and fibrogenic pulmonary responses to single-walled carbon nanotubes in mice. *Am. J. Physiol. Lung Cell. Mol. Physiol., 289*, 10. doi: 10.1152/ajplung.00084.2005.
52. Sayes, C. M., Liang, F., Hudson, J. L., Mendez, J., Guo, W., Beach, J. M., et al., (2006). Functionalization density dependence of single-walled carbon nanotubes cytotoxicity *in vitro. Toxicol. Lett., 161*, 135–142. doi: 10.1016/j.toxlet.2005.08.011.z

CHAPTER 2

Biotechnological and Biomedical Applications of CNTs

T. R. ANILKUMAR

Inter-University Center for Evolutionary and Integrative Biology, University of Kerala, Kariavattom, Trivandrum, Kerala, India

ABSTRACT

Carbon nanotubes (CNTs) are carbon-based nanomaterials in which graphene sheets composed of carbon atoms arranged in benzene rings, rolled up to form cylinders. CNTs have been classified into single-walled (SWCNTs) and multi-walled carbon nanotubes (MWCNTs) based on the number of graphene sheets involved in the formation of CNTs. CNTs have been reported to have versatile applications in the field of biomedicine and biotechnology. This is mainly due to the unique chemical, physical, and biological characteristics of CNTs. This chapter aims to describe some of the biotechnological and biomedical applications of carbon nanotubes such as bio-sensing, gene therapy and drug delivery, tissue engineering, etc. Even though CNTs have such a wide application, some of the disadvantages reported by various literatures are the non-compatibility of CNTs with biological systems. But this was being able to overcome by various functionalization approaches which have been shown to enhance chemical reactivity to reagents and leads to increased biocompatibility (Figure 2.1).

Carbon Nanotubes for Biomedical Applications and Healthcare.
Chin Hua Chia, Swati Gokul Talele, Ann Rose Abraham, and A. K. Haghi, (Eds.)

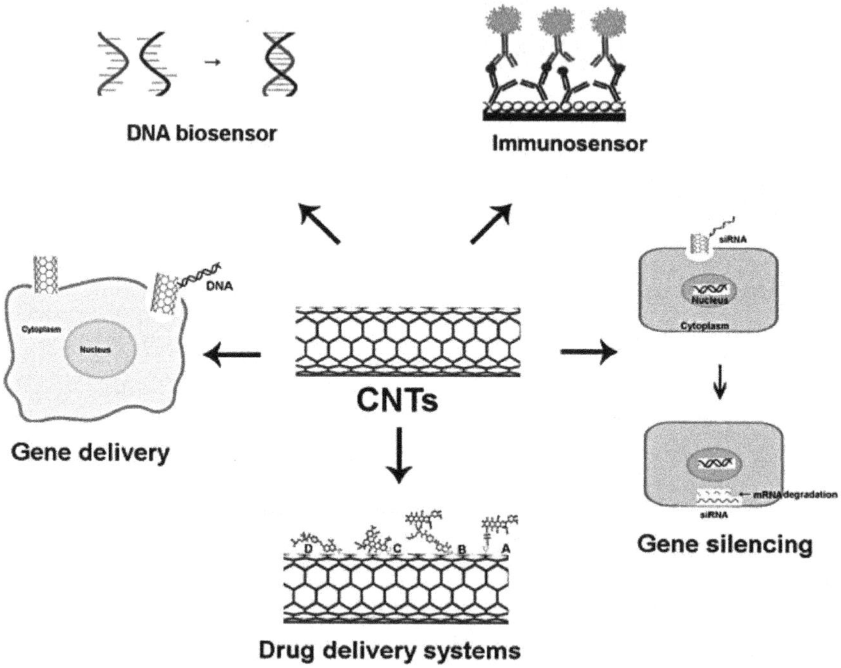

FIGURE 2.1 Graphical abstract.

2.1 INTRODUCTION

The field of nanotechnology has been showing an unprecedented growth over the years and nanomaterials, the end product of the technology is known to play an immense role in the field of biomedicine and biotechnology such as bio-sensing, gene therapy, drug delivery systems. The versatility of application of Nanomaterials is because of its unique properties [1, 2]. Carbon nanotubes are tubular structures composed of one or many layers of graphene sheets made of carbon atoms arranged in benzene rings. These tubes are capped at both the ends by one half of a fullerene-like molecule [3]. CNTs have been classified into single-walled (SWCNTs) and multi-walled carbon nanotubes (MWCNTs) based on the number of graphene sheets involved in the formation of CNTs. Single-walled carbon nanotubes (SWCNTs) consists of a single graphene sheet rolled into a cylinder of length in several microns and diameter ranges in 0.4–2 nm while multi-walled carbon nanotubes (MWCNTs) consists of two or more multiple layers of concentrically arranged graphene sheets with the layers are separated by 0.34 nm and diameter of the layers ranges between 2 and 100 nm [4] (Figure 2.2). Fullerenes, carbon nanotorous, carbon nanohorns, carbon nanopeapods, and carbon nanobuds are other known carbon-based nanomaterials [5]. Carbon nanotubes were mainly synthesized by laser-ablation technique, chemical vapor deposition (CVD) and carbon arc-discharge technique [6, 7]. There were reports on the improvisation of Chemical Vapor Deposition methods employing catalysts to increase the rate of the reaction [8]. One of the limitations of CNTs hindering the biomedical application is its lack of solubility. But many studies have shown that this incompatibility could be overcome by functionalization approach which is found to improve the solubility, enhance chemical reactivity to reagents and enhance biocompatibility. The functionalization of CNTs involves the covalent modification of π-conjugated skeleton of CNTs, noncovalent modification by adsorbing various biomolecules and endohedral filling of the inner cavity [9].

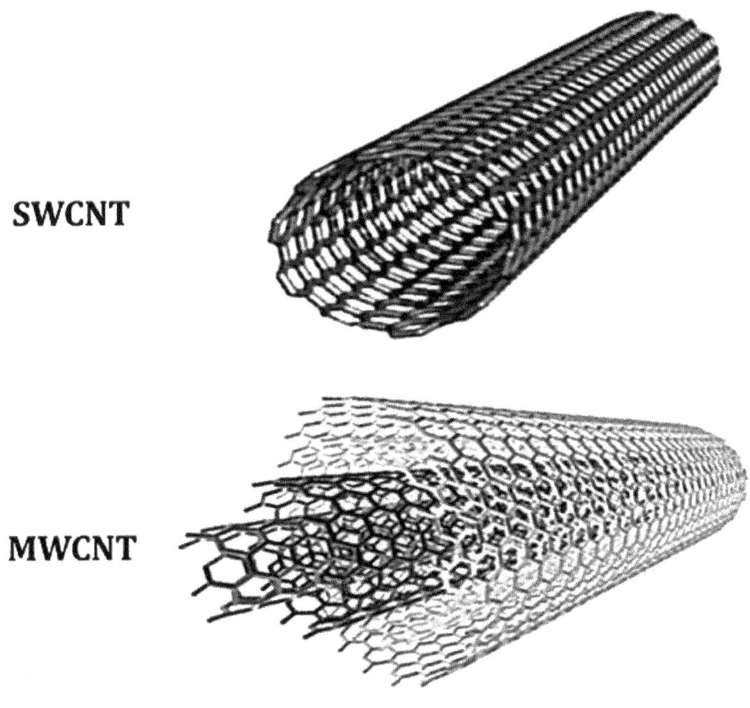

FIGURE 2.2 Single-walled carbon nanotubes and muti-walled carbon nanotubes.

Modern medicine has benefitted a lot with the merging of Nanotechnology with medicine. This has led to the advancement of many novel materials useful in medical diagnosis and treatment. It has also played a role in boosting the economy as the production of these materials in industrial scales will be the driving force for the emerging economies [10]. Carbon nanotubes (CNTs) plays an active role among nanomaterials in revolutionizing biomedical research owing to their chemical, thermal, mechanical, electrical, and structural properties. Elasticity and electron transport properties such as metallic, semiconducting, and superconducting are also reported in nanomaterials [11]. There has been a growing demand for CNTs in the past decade owing to its application in biomedical field which includes biosensors, probes [6], drug discovery and delivery systems associated with pharmaceutical industries, tools, and devices in radiation oncology, etc. [12, 13]. The most essential part of CNTs in clinical settings is its safety feature with biological, environmental, and safety profiles should have been characterized. CNTs vary significantly in size, structure, morphology, and purity and it mainly depends on synthesis part which includes preparation, purification, and functionalization [14, 15]. CNTs exhibit toxicity depending upon many factors. These factors include method of synthesis, size especially surface-to-volume ratio, concentration, shape, oxidation, composition, and functional group(s) [16–18]. One of the factors that reduces biocompatibility is its hydrophobicity [19]. One of the factors of toxicity of CNTs is its ability to induce damage on DNA and cell membrane, induce toxicity through oxidative stress and modification of mitochondrial activities and is found to alter the intracellular metabolic pathways. It is known to cause cytotoxicity through both necrosis and apoptosis [13].

2.2 CARBON NANOTUBES AS BIOSENSORS

One of the most important applications of CNTs is its role as Biosensors. CNTs adaptability to use as Biosensors is contributed by its ability to detect biomolecules employing biological recognition with chemical or physical transduction. High surface-to-volume ratio, electronic properties and edge-plane like defects of CNTs makes it a suitable candidate for its role as biosensors [11, 20]. The first carbon nanotubes (CNTs) based electrochemical sensor was reported by Britto et al. [21]. Since the development of this CNTs has gained enormous attention as electrochemical sensors in the subsequent years [22]. CNTs are the most prominent nanomaterials for biomedical applications because of its unique structure, which contributes to its mechanical, electrical, and optical properties [23]. Despite these advantageous features, in order to utilize CNTs as electrochemicalsensors, it must be biocompatible to use in the *in vitro* and *in vivo* systems. There should be efforts to minimize the van der Waals and π π stacking interactions by functionalizing it covalently or non-covalently [24–26]. Biomarkers are known to be used for diagnosis, prognosis, evaluation of therapy effectiveness and risk assessment. Electrochemical (bio)sensors must be of low cost, high sensitivity, specificity, and portability [27–29].

Ultrasensitive biosensing properties of CNTs are mainly due to their larger surface area-to-volume ratio, and this enables CNTs to detect biological molecules at low concentration. CNTs has got a fast response time due to high electron-transfer time which are measured employing NADH and hydrogen peroxide reaction CNTs are stable due to the less surface fouling and low redox potential [30]. CNTs-based biosensors are superior in quality than material based sensors such as silicon sensors with regard to sensitivity, high surface-to-volume ratio and hollow tubular structure. CNTs are also used as a substrate for immobilizing enzymes [31]. One such CNTs based Biosensor designed to detect phenolic compounds is Tyrosinase biosensor. There are also reports on novel tyrosinase-based biosensor developed for the detection of dopamine [32]. In one approach, this is synthesized on glassy carbon electrode functionalized with multi-walled carbon nanotubes, tyrosinase (Tyr) and 1-butyl-3-methylimidazolium chloride (IL) within a dihexadecyl phosphate (DHP) film. During its synthesis, 1-ethyl-3-(3-dimethylaminopropyl) carbodiimide/*N*-hydroxysuccinimide (EDC/NHS) was used as a cross linking agent to immobilize MWCNTs, IL, and Tyr. Characterization was done by cyclic voltammetry (CV) in presence of catechol as substrate in which IL-MWCNTs nanocomposite showed good biocompatibility and conductivity and it showed the biocatalytic activity in the oxidation of catechol to *o*-quinone [33]. Tyrosinase sensors is found to have a better response signal since it was designed to combine the electrocatalytic activity of MWCNTs with the conductivity and biocompatibility of 1-butyl-3-methylimidazolium chloride (IL).

Biosensor for detecting Androsterone in human serum samples is yet another example for a CNTs based sensors which are proved to be so fast in detection, highly sensitive and stable. It was designed for the electrochemical detection of NADH generated in the dehydrogenation of androsterone by the enzyme 3α-hydroxysteroid dehydrogenase. Here the enzyme is immobilized on to a composite electrode platform of MWCNTs, octylpyridinium hexafluorophosphate (OPPF) ionic liquid and NAD(+) cofactor [34]. CNTs based biosensors to measure glucose levels has been gaining momentum in medical diagnostics and food industries. In Glucose biosensors, glucose is detected by its catalytic oxidation into gluconic acid and hydrogen peroxide in the presence of oxygen. A single-wall carbon nanotube records gate voltage corresponds to the level of glucose concentration [35].

In DNA sensors, the main sensing element is either single stranded or double-stranded (dsDNA). It is also found that single stranded DNA is highly adsorptive to CNTs than double stranded dsDNA. It has been widely exploited in the identification of new strains and organisms by DNA sequencing. Genosensors are designed on the surface of physical transducer which enables the detection of gene sequence by DNA hybridization. This has got wide application like DNA chips for diagnosis and molecular diagnosis [36]. DNA biosensors are simple in setup and chemistry when compared to other biosensors such as optical DNA biosensors and electrochemical sensors [37]. DNA biosensors are mostly found to be modified with multi-walled carbon nano-tubes, gold nanoparticles and polydopamine (PDA) for detecting the DNA sequence.

2.2.1 CNT-BASED BIOSENSORS FOR PROTEIN BIOMARKERS

Carbon nanotubes-based electrochemical (bio)sensors has been extensively used for the detection of protein biomarkers:

1. **Carcinoembryonic Antigen (CEA):** These are glycoproteins of molecular weight of 200 kDa [38], produced by cells of the gastro-intestinal tract during embryonic development [39]. It is known that the concentration of CEA decreases after birth and the normal range of CEA in the blood in healthy adults is lower than 2.5 ng mL^{-1}) [40]. Elevated levels of CEA is associated with ovarian carcinoma, lung and breast cancer [41], and especially colorectal adenocarcinoma [42]. CEA is the most widely used tumor biomarkers and its level indicates effectiveness of cancer therapy, success of a tumor surgery and the progression of tumor. There are different ways for the quantification of CEA [43] in which anti-CEA primary antibody has been immobilized on various bioanalytical platforms and transduces the bioaffinity event.

2. **Prostate Specific Antigen (PSA):** It is reported to be a biomarker for prostate cancer. PSA is a 34 kDa protein consists of 240 amino acids.

PSA values above 1.5 ng mL^{-1} predicts the risk of malignancy [44]. CNTs based biosensors with biorecognition platform made by the incorporation of poly(dimethyldiallylammonium chloride), carboxylated MWC-NTs and ceria mesoporous nanospheres (CeO2NSs) and immobilizing anti-PSA primary antibody. Biorecognition was transduced by DPV which was detected by a decrease in the oxidation current of o-phenylenediamine catalyzed by CeO2NSs [45]. An immunosensor and DNA sensor are schematically represented in Figure 2.3.

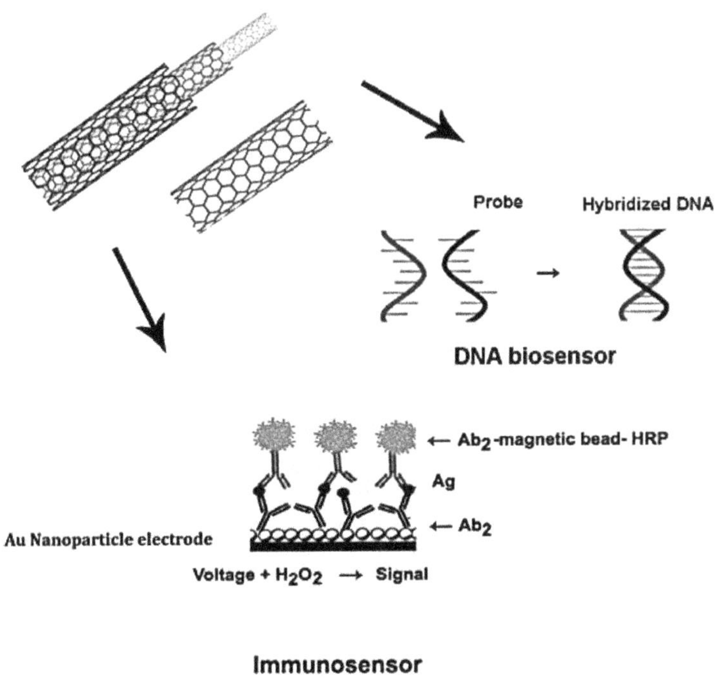

FIGURE 2.3 Immunosensor and DNA sensor. Ag-Ab binding and H_2O_2 conversion using horseraddish peroxide generates a signal.

3. **Alpha-Fetoprotein (AFP):** It is a glycoprotein of molecular weight 70 kDa, structurally similar to albumin in adult. It is normally found in plasma and shows similar physicochemical properties of albumin [46]. It is found to be secreted by the liver, gastrointestinal tract and yolk sac of a human fetus [47, 48]. The normal level of Alpha-fetoprotein in healthy adults is around 3.4 ng mL, while higher levels

were noted in newborns up to one year. It is known that in pregnant women, AFP is a biomarker of neural tube and ventral wall defects. It is also reported as a biomarker of malignancies such as yolk sac-derived germ cell tumors, hepatocellular carcinoma (HCC) and benign liver diseases (hepatitis and cirrhosis), and less frequently in patients with other tumors [49–51].

Many electrochemical biosensors have been designed to detect AFP and early detection of these biomarkers will be enable to analyze the progress of treatment and offer many advantages [20, 38]. A label-free glycobiosensor was developed to analyze the level of glycan expression of AFP (AFP N-glycan) in serum samples. The extent of glycosylation varies in cancer and normal cells, and hence this could be used in the diagnosis of malignancy. This sensor is designed by immobilizing wheat-germ agglutinin lectin at SPE modified with carboxylated SWCNTs [52]. Another biosensor employed with sensitive label-free detection of AFP was prepared by attaching cSWCNTs with anti-AFP primary antibody (Ab1) mesoporous silica (MSP) previously grafted with aminopropylethoxysilane [53]. Another label-free AFP biosensor is designed with immunosensor Prussian blue (PB) film modified GCE is coated with single walled carbon nanotubes. Here SWCNTs are functionalized with polylysine in which HRP conjugated antibody against AFP was immobilized. Here the concentration of AFP was measured as an electric current of H_2O_2 obtained by DPV which is linearly proportional to the concentration.

4. **Cytokines:** These are proteins involved in cell signaling and immune modulation their quantification plays an important role in early prognosis and diagnosis of many diseases [54]. There are many CNTs based electrochemical biosensors developed either in the primary biorecognition or as part the label conjugate. Tumor necrosis factor-alpha (TNF) is a well-known cytokine associated with many disorders such as diabetes, graft rejection, inflammatory diseases such as rheumatoid arthritis, neonatal listeriosis, HIV infection, endotoxic shock, systemic erythema nodosum leprosum and severe meningococcemia [55]. There are label-free immunosensors designed based on SPE, modified with MWCNTs and functionalized with fullerene and the ionic liquid 1-butyl-3-methylimidazolium-bis(trifluoromethylsulfonyl)imide ([C4mimi][NTf2]) (MWCNTs-C60-[C4mimi][NTf2]) [56] and bimetallic Ag@Pt core-shell NPs and Chit (MWCNTs-Ag@Pt-Chit) [57]. TNF leads to surface

blockage and hence a reduced oxidation current of catechol was obtained and recorded.

5. **Troponin:** Cardiovascular diseases (CVDs) are blood circulation disorders of the heart which includes coronary heart disease, congenital heart disease and stroke which causes 46.2% of deaths among non-communicable diseases as per World Health Organization (WHO) statistics [58]. Early and quick diagnosis plays an important role in the successful prognosis of any disease. CVDs are characterized by the increase in the level of biochemical markers especially Cardiac markers in blood caused by the leak out of from the damaged myocardial cells [59, 60]. There are four biomarkers known to be associated with the diagnosis of myocardial infarction which includes MB isoform of creatine kinase, cardiac troponin I and T, and myoglobin [61]. Myoglobin is a small protein cardiac biomarker ranges in size in the range 17.8 kDa, increases in the serum in high quantity after cardiac injury. This is one of the marker released as early as 1–3 h reaching maximum at the onset of symptoms at 6–12 h [62]. Normal range of Myoglobin is 50 to 200 ng mL^{-1} and its level increases up to ~600 ng mL^{-1} at the onset of symptoms. Another biomarker is muscle isoenzyme CK-MB specific for cardiac injury and the level shoots up in serum within 4–6 h after the onset of Myocardial Infarction peaks to 39–185 ng mL^{-1} at 18–24 h [63, 64]. Cardiac troponin I (cTnI) and T (cTnT) are known to be more sensitive and specific than Mb and CK-MB [65]. Cardiac troponins I and T are released from dead cells after 2–4 h and 3–4 h, respectively, after Myocardial infarction. These markers remain in the bloodstream for more than 10 days with the concentration peaks at 1–2 days after myocardial infarction. Normal range of Cardiac troponin is 0.001 μg L^{-1} and it shoot ups to 100 μg L^{-1} during MI patients [66] and an even a low concentration of 0.01 μg L^{-1} is associated with heart failure.

Detection of cardiac biomarkers was done by CNT-based electrochemical biosensors in which antitroponin antibodies are bound to CNTs at the electrode surface [67]. Redoxprobes $[Fe(CN)_6]^{3-/4-}$ and H_2O_2 are suitable for the detection of cTnT. Another CNT based immunosensor for cardiac Troponin T is a conductive polymer film in which carboxylated CNTs are bound covalently to the electrode surface through polyethyleneimine. This enables the detection of cardiac Troponin using anti-cTnT monoclonal antibodies [68].

MWCNTs embedded with SU-8 electrospun nanofibers are designed for the ultrasensitive detection of cardiac biomarkers employing Electrochemical Impedance spectroscopy. MWCNTs confer better electrical and transduction properties to composite nanofibers while SU-8 enables the functionalization and biocompatibility. These synthesized Nanofibers are useful for the detection of all MI biomarkers such as cardiac Troponin I, Myoglobin, and Creatine Kinase MB (CK-MB). These biomarkers were detected by nanotubes functionalized with their antibodies. The detection of these biomarkers was done by using Electrochemical Impedance Spectroscopy and a minimum detection limit is achievable [69].

2.2.2 CNT-BASED BIOSENSORS FOR NUCLEIC ACIDS BIOMARKERS

2.2.2.1 MICRORNA

microRNAs (miRNAs) are non-coding ribonucleic acid (RNA) molecules with length ranges between 19 and 25 nucleotides that regulate the expression of genes by repressing the translation of mRNA [70]. miRNA is found to regulate 60% of protein-coding genes in human [71] and a single miRNA molecule is known to regulate hundreds of mRNAs [72, 73]. Several pathologies have been associated with abnormal miRNAs including cardiovascular [74, 75] central nervous system injury and neurodegenerative diseases, and [76, 77], liver [78, 79], kidney [80] diseases, and even immune dysfunction [81, 82]. There are many reports on several miRNAs reported as markers for diagnosis and prognosis due to their occurrence in different body fluids in stable form which enable their extraction and analysis [83]. Thus the quantification of a set of miRNAs holds a clinical significance and impact on health care [84].

2.3 CARBON NANOTUBES IN BIOMEDICAL IMAGING

Biomedical imaging is a branch of science known to have received inputs from different disciplines and fields of science. Biomedical emerging is an emerging tool to capture high resolution images of cells, tissues, and organs. Imaging will help to study the behavior of cells, tissues, and organs. It is known that Carbon nanotubes are versatile and can be manipulated in different ways to use in various biomedical imaging to analyze and improve functionalities [85]. SWCNTs exhibit quasi 1-D nature and the optical properties of

SWCNTs enable their use as optical probes. They also exhibit high optical absorption, strong resonance Raman scattering, and photoluminescence in the NIR range enable its use in biological systems *in vitro* and *in vivo* [86].

2.3.1 IN VITRO PHOTOLUMINESCENCE IMAGING

SWNTs with band gaps of the order of ~1 eV, dependent on the diameter and chirality, exhibits photoluminescence near infrared (900–1,600 nm) enable biological imaging. This is due to the high transparency of biological tissue near 800–1,000 nm and low autofluorescence from tissue in the NIR range [87]. Another advantage of SWNTs is the large separation between the excitation (550–850 nm) and emission bands (900–1,600 nm) which will reduce background from Raman scattering and autofluorescence. It is known that NIR photoluminescence from micelle-encapsulated SWNTs, yields a quantum efficiency as low as 10^{-3} [88]. Cell surface receptors can be probed by bioinert PEGylated SWNTs conjugated with antibodies to these receptors as NIR fluorescent tags [89].

2.3.2 IN VITRO RAMAN IMAGING

Single-walled nanotubes show strong resonance Raman scattering due to quasi 1-D nature. It possesses both Raman scattering features such as radial breathing mode and tangential mode [90]. Raman microscopy are used to image SWNTs in liver cells, as well as tissue slices, using either the RBM peak or G-band peak of SWNTs [91–94]. Raman imaging helps in the imaging of Cancer cells by labeling with isotopic unique formulations of "colored" SWNTs, conjugated with various targeting ligands including Herceptin, Erbitux, and RGD peptide [91, 95]. The SWNT Raman excitation and scattering photons are in the NIR region, which is the most transparent optical window for biological systems *in vitro* and *in vivo.*

2.3.3 SWNTS FOR IN VIVO ANIMAL IMAGING

Biomedical imaging employing SWNT has been performed in a living animal with first such an imaging was performed by Weisman group in 2007 [96]. In this work NIR fluorescence microscopy was employed for observation when

Drosophila were fed by food containing SWNTs. *In vivo* tumor imaging of RGD-conjugated PEGylated SWNTs was done in live mice [97, 98].

CNTs with fluorescence emission near-infrared region enables the high-speed label-free detection in live cells. Single-walled carbon nanotubes and multi-walled carbon nanotubes exhibit fluorescence near infrared II (NIR-II) region with a good tissue penetration and resolution. Raman imaging employing Raman scattering of SWNTs by various groups enable *in vitro* and *in vivo* imaging. The strong absorption in the near infrared II (NIR-II) region is used for photoacoustic imaging which can be enhanced by adding organic dyes or coating with gold shells [99]. There are many reports of Raman [91, 95, 100] photoacoustic [101] and near-infrared photoluminescence imaging [102, 103] have been used to visualize nanotubes in biological environments [104].

Photoacoustic imaging allows imaging of deeper tissues with high contrast and spatial resolution. Tomographic imaging of skin and other superficial organs can be done using laser-induced photoacoustic microscopy. It also enables early detection of breast cancers by near-infrared light or radio-frequency-wave-induced photoacoustic imaging [105]. It is also known that photoacoustic signal can be enhanced by using single-walled carbon nanotubes conjugated with cyclic Arg-Gly-Asp (RGD) peptides as contrast agent for photoacoustic imaging of tumors and Intravenous administration of these nanotubes showed eight times efficacy in determining tumor in mice than non-targeted nanotubes [101]. Low temperature scanning gate microscopy (SGM) technique employing two coupled single wall carbon nanotube quantum dots in a multiple quantum dot system was performed at a temperature of 170 mK. Localization of single wall carbon nanotube quantum dots was achieved by conductance images contacted by two metallic electrodes. The single electron transport has been observed by varying the position or voltage bias of a conductive atomic force microscopy [106].

There are also reports on Inorganic nanoparticles being used as biomedical imaging agents which imparts high sensitivity, high spatial and temporal resolution. A major hurdle in the use of these nanomaterials is the toxicity of inorganic nanomaterials, which cause the release of ROS and chemical instability [107]. Modification of CNTs helps to bring new perspectives for the analysis of the behavior of nanomaterials. It is also known that assembling gold nanostructures would enhance fluorescence intensity and helps to achieve ferritin receptor-mediated targeting and biomedical imaging both *in vitro* and *in vivo* [106].

2.4 CARBON NANOTUBES IN DRUG AND GENE DELIVERY

CNTs have been extensively used as drug delivery systems for the treatment of many diseases. CNT-based anticancer drugs have gained much attention recently due to targeted delivery and controlled release of the drugs [108–110]. Such systems are known to improve the efficacy of the drug while minimizing the hazardous effects of the systemic toxicity of the drug in the whole body.

Single wall carbon nanotubes (SWCNTs) have gained much attention over the years owing to their ability to carry a high cargo loading, structural flexibility and intrinsic stability. This would also may lead to prolong the circulation time and bioavailability of the drug molecules. SWCNTs non-covalently modified with aspargine-glycine-arginine (NGR) is found to carry anticancer drug tamoxifen (TAM). Tamoxifen loaded aspargine-glycine-arginine has been exhibiting good optical properties and cytotoxicity and helps to selectively target tumors, facilitates the combination of chemotherapy with photothermal therapy [111]. Another single wall carbon nanotubes (SWCNTs) based targeted drug delivery system triggers the release of the drug with the change in pH in which SWCNTs derivatized with carboxylate groups, coated with a polysaccharide material are loaded with the anticancer drug doxorubicin. This is dug is known to bind at physiological pH (pH 7.4) and released at a lower pH, a characteristic of the tumor environments. It is also reported that loading and release of the drug doxorubicin can be controlled by modification of the the polysaccharide coating of the nanotubes. Folic acid can be used as an additional agent by tethering it to the SWCNTs to selectively deliver doxorubicin into the lysosomes of cells with a greater efficiency than free doxorubicin [112].

CNTs deliver drugs to specific tumor site which minimizes the systemic toxicity and undesirable side effects of anticancer drugs with a CNT-based anticancer drug is also known to overcome the problem of multidrug resistant cancer cells and effective in sensitizing cancer cells without affecting cell proliferation and cell cycle [113]. CNTs can be used as carrier of immunization against some antigens [18]. There are instances of immunizations against tumors through CNT-based vaccination [114]. SWCNTs can also be used to transport Acetylcholine (Ach) to the brain by traditional ways and this could be a treatment strategy for Alzheimer's disease where neurons are unable to synthesize acetylcholine (Figure 2.4) [115].

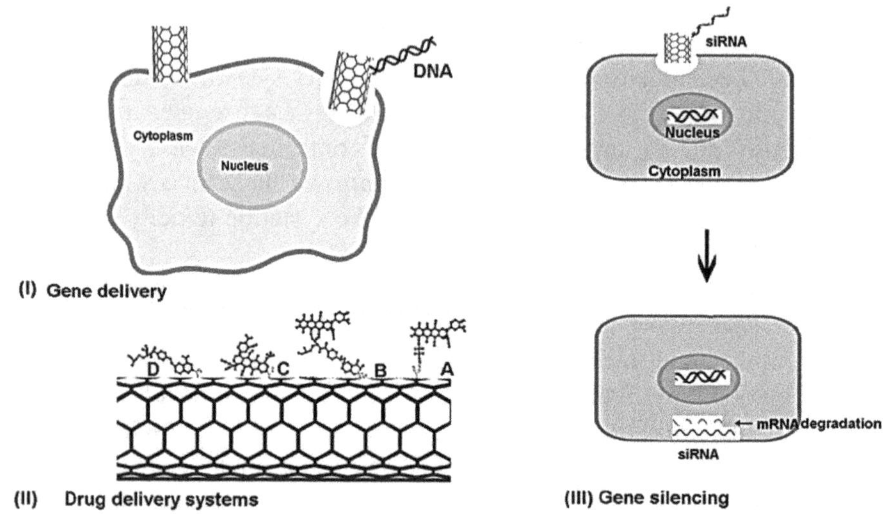

FIGURE 2.4 Schematic representation of **(I)** gene delivery systems; (II) drug delivery systems with: **(A)** covalent modification of carbon nanotubes with DOX by PEGylation of carboxylic acids; **(B)** attachment of DOX to polysaccharide coated carbon nanotubes; **(C)** π-π stacking of acid-treated carbon nanotubes with epirubicin; and **(D)** methotrexate attachment to amino functionalized carbon nanotubes.

2.5 TISSUE ENGINEERING AND REGENERATIVE MEDICINE

Modern approaches in medicine such as Tissue engineering and regenerative medicine mainly deals with the development of engineered artificial tissues, which has wide applications as replacement grafts and in drug delivery. It is known that delivering pro-angiogenic gene such as vascular endothelial growth factor-165 (VEGF) is a good therapeutic interruption in cardiovascular diseases. In an approach, It was found to be delivered along with a nanocomplex of graphene oxide (GO) employing an injectable and biocompatible hydrogel. This was found to be effective for transfection into myocardial tissues and induce favorable therapeutic effects without invoking cytotoxic effects [116]. In these approaches, cells are seeded or encapsulated in a suitable biomaterial for growing engineered tissues. Major tissue engineering vascular grafts (TEVGs) designed to replace the damaged arteries of various cardiovascular diseases are of different types including Scaffolds from decellularized tissue skeletons to biopolymers and biodegradable synthetic polymers. The major disadvantage of these TEVGs are inability to mimic the mechanical properties of native tissues, and the ability for long-term patency and growth required for *in vivo* function. Electrospinning is a popular technique used for the production of scaffolds to address these issues [117]. It is also known that electrospun nanofibers are also used as suitable scaffolds for neural tissue engineering. Multi-walled carbon nanotubes (MWCNTs)-coated electrospun poly(L-lactic acid-co-caprolactone) (PLCL) nanofibers improved the neurite outgrowth of rat dorsal root ganglia (DRG) neurons and focal adhesion kinase (FAK) expression of PC-12 cells. These findings suggest that MWCNTs-coated nanofibrous scaffolds may be alternative materials for nerve regeneration and functional recovery in neural tissue engineering [118].

CNTs are used as enhancer of electrical properties of the scaffold for neural and cardiac tissue growth while functionalization with groups attracting calcium cations would help in the enhancement of bone growth [119]. There are reports on the functionalization of MWCNTs with fibroblast growth factors used in scaffolds enables bone formation [120].

2.6 CONCLUSION

This chapter mainly discussed about the biotechnological and biomedical applications of Carbon nanotubes (CNTs) which includes biosensors, delivery of therapeutic drugs and genes, biomedical imaging and use as scaffolds in tissue engineering, etc. CNTs are amenable to functionalization using various groups or biomolecules either covalently or noncovalently to increase the biocompatibility and decrease the cytotoxicity. The functionalization is found to be essential for the delivery of drugs and gene delivery systems. However, cytotoxicity remains to be a major limiting factor of CNTs in biological systems. These cytotoxicities of various CNTs depend up on the parameters such as the method of preparation, functionalization, and the doses of CNTs.

There are reports on various metal impurities used in the synthesis of CNTs could have an impact on toxicity. It is known that different types of cell-viable indicator dyes used in combination with CNTs contributes to cytotoxicity profiles. The most common indicator dyes in use are alamar blue, neutral red, MTT (3-(4,5-dimethylthiazol-2-yl)-2,5-diphenyltetrazolium bromide), coomassie and WST-1 (a water-soluble tetrazolium salt) [121]. Cytotoxicity of CNTs is mostly contributed by the concentration and type of metal impurities, length, and type of carbon nanotubes, presence of functionalization groups, etc. [122]. In another study even though CNTs were able to enter macrophages and influence cell physiology and function, they did not show any toxicity on cell viability as measured by the quantitative analysis of inflammatory mediators such as NO, TNF-alpha, and IL-8. It is also found that the metal particles associated with the commercial nanotubes are responsible for the biological effects [123]. Other studies conducted to investigate the physicochemical features of multiwalled carbon nanotubes (MWCNTs) on toxicity and biocompatibility, found that increase in the concentration of CNTs affects cell viability and deduced an optimum concentration of 5–10 mug/mL ideal for design and development of artificial MWCNT nano-vectors for gene and drug therapy against cancer [124]. Many studies show that the contaminated tubes with impurities cause immunological toxicity and localized alopecia, whereas extremely pure implanted tubes showed good biocompatibility. Although many studies for toxicological characterization of carbon nanotubes in biological systems, detailed understanding of the uptake CNTs by the cells, internalization, and altered gene expression associated with the CNT toxicity has been elusive. This understanding will enable for the future development of biocompatible CNTs for biomedical applications.

KEYWORDS

- **biosensors**
- **CNTs**
- **drug delivery**
- **gene therapy**
- **microbial fuel cells**

REFERENCES

1. Zhang, A., & Lieber, C. M., (2016). Nano-Bioelectronics. *Chem Rev., 116*(1), 215–257. doi: 10.1021/acs.chemrev.5b00608.
2. Zhu, X., Li, J., He, H., Huang, M., Zhang, X., & Wang, S., (2015). Application of nanomaterials in the bioanalytical detection of disease-related genes. *Biosens. Bioelectron., 74*, 113–133. doi: 10.1016/j.bios.2015.04.069.

3. Dresselhaus, M. S., Dresselhaus, G., & Jorio, A., (2004). Unusual properties and structure of carbon nanotubes. *Annual Review of Materials Research, 34*(1), 247–278. doi: 10.1146/annurev.matsci.34.040203.114607.
4. Georgakilas, V., Perman, J. A., Tucek, J., & Zboril, R., (2015). Broad family of carbon nanoallotropes: Classification, chemistry, and applications of fullerenes, carbon dots, nanotubes, graphene, nanodiamonds, and combined superstructures. *Chem. Rev., 115*(11), 4744–4822. doi: 10.1021/cr500304f.
5. Mehra, N. K., Keerti, J., & Narendra, K. J., (2015). Pharmaceutical and biomedical applications of surface engineered carbon nanotubes. *Drug Discovery Today, 20*(6), 750–759. doi: https://doi.org/10.1016/j.drudis.2015.01.006.
6. Xue, Y., (2017). Chapter 11 – carbon nanotubes for biomedical applications. In: Huisheng, P., Qingwen, L., & Tao, C., (eds.), *Industrial Applications of Carbon Nanotubes* (pp. 323–346). Boston: Elsevier.
7. Iijima, S., (1991). Helical microtubules of graphitic carbon. *Nature, 354*(6348), 56–58. doi: 10.1038/354056a0.
8. José-Yacamán, M., Miki-Yoshida, M., Rendón, L., & Santiesteban, J. G., (1993). Catalytic growth of carbon microtubules with fullerene structure. *Applied Physics Letters, 62*(2), 202–204. doi: 10.1063/1.109315.
9. Tasis, D., Nikos, T., Alberto, B., & Maurizio, P., (2006). Chemistry of carbon nanotubes. *Chemical Reviews, 106*(3), 1105–1136. doi: 10.1021/cr050569o.
10. Alshehri, R., Asad, M. I., Anwarul, H., Adnan, A., Farid, A., & Adnan, M., (2016). Carbon nanotubes in biomedical applications: Factors, mechanisms, and remedies of toxicity. *Journal of Medicinal Chemistry, 59*(18), 8149–8167. doi: 10.1021/acs.jmedchem.5b01770.
11. Pumera, M., (2009). The electrochemistry of carbon nanotubes: Fundamentals and applications. *Chemistry, 15*(20), 4970–4978. doi: 10.1002/chem.200900421.
12. Beg, S., Rizwan, M., Sheikh, A. M., Hasnain, M. S., Anwer, K., & Kohli, K., (2011). Advancement in carbon nanotubes: Basics, biomedical applications and toxicity. *J. Pharm. Pharmacol., 63*(2), 141–163. doi: 10.1111/j.2042-7158.2010.01167.x.
13. Vardharajula, S., Ali, S. Z., Tiwari, P. M., Eroğlu, E., Vig, K., Dennis, V. A., & Singh, S. R., (2012). Functionalized carbon nanotubes: Biomedical applications. *Int. J. Nanomedicine, 7*, 5361–5374. doi: 10.2147/ijn.s35832.
14. Karousis, N., Rigini, M. P., Argiris, S., Paraskevi, V., Petros, G., Yiannis, S., Georgios, S., et al., (2009). Peptidomimetic–functionalized carbon nanotubes with antitrypsin activity. *Carbon, 47*(15), 3550–3558. doi: https://doi.org/10.1016/j.carbon.2009.08.025.
15. Pagona, G., & Tagmatarchis, N., (2006). Carbon nanotubes: Materials for medicinal chemistry and biotechnological applications. *Curr. Med. Chem., 13*(15), 1789–1798. doi: 10.2174/092986706777452524.
16. Lanone, S., & Boczkowski, J., (2006). Biomedical applications and potential health risks of nanomaterials: Molecular mechanisms. *Curr. Mol. Med., 6*(6), 651–663. doi: 10.2174/156652406778195026.
17. Bhirde, A. A., Patel, S., Sousa, A. A., Patel, V., Molinolo, A. A., Ji, Y., Leapman, R. D., et al., (2010). Distribution and clearance of PEG-single-walled carbon nanotube cancer drug delivery vehicles in mice. *Nanomedicine (Lond), 5*(10), 1535–1546. doi: 10.2217/nnm.10.90.

18. Foldvari, M., & Bagonluri, M., (2008). Carbon nanotubes as functional excipients for nanomedicines: II. Drug delivery and biocompatibility issues. *Nanomedicine, 4*(3), 183–200. doi: 10.1016/j.nano.2008.04.003.
19. Yan, L., Feng, Z., Shoujian, L., Zhongbo, H., & Yuliang, Z., (2011). Low-toxic and safe nanomaterials by surface-chemical design, carbon nanotubes, fullerenes, metallofullerenes, and graphenes. *Nanoscale, 3*(2), 362–382. doi: 10.1039/C0NR00647E.
20. Li, N., Ma, H., Cao, W., Wu, D., Yan, T., Du, B., & Wei, Q., (2015). Highly sensitive electrochemical immunosensor for the detection of alpha fetoprotein based on PdNi nanoparticles and N-doped graphene nanoribbons. *Biosens. Bioelectron., 74*, 786–791. doi: 10.1016/j.bios.2015.07.049.
21. Britto, P. J., Santhanam, K. S. V., & Ajayan, P. M., (1996). Carbon nanotube electrode for oxidation of dopamine. *Bioelectrochemistry and Bioenergetics, 41*(1), 121–125. doi: Https://doi.org/10.1016/0302-4598(96)05078-7.
22. Tiwari, J. N., Vij, V., Kemp, K. C., & Kim, K. S., (2016). Engineered carbon-nanomaterial-based electrochemical sensors for biomolecules. *ACS Nano, 10*(1), 46–80. doi: 10.1021/acsnano.5b05690.
23. Kunzmann, A., Britta, A., Tina, T., Harald, K., Annika, S., & Bengt, F., (2011). Toxicology of engineered nanomaterials: Focus on biocompatibility, biodistribution and biodegradation. *Biochimica et Biophysica Acta (BBA) – General Subjects, 1810*(3), 361–373. doi: https://doi.org/10.1016/j.bbagen.2010.04.007.
24. Gao, C., Zheng, G., Jin-Huai, L., & Xing-Jiu, H., (2012). The new age of carbon nanotubes: An updated review of functionalized carbon nanotubes in electrochemical sensors. *Nanoscale, 4*(6), 1948–1963. doi: 10.1039/C2NR11757F.
25. Kim, S. W., Taehoon, K., Yern, S. K., Hong, S. C., Hyeong, J. L., Seung, J. Y., & Chong, R. P., (2012). Surface modifications for the effective dispersion of carbon nanotubes in solvents and polymers. *Carbon, 50*(1), 3–33. doi: https://doi.org/10.1016/j.carbon.2011.08.011.
26. Primo, E. N., Gutierrez, F. A., Luque, G. L., Dalmasso, P. R., Gasnier, A., Jalit, Y., Moreno, M., et al., (2013). Comparative study of the electrochemical behavior and analytical applications of (bio)sensing platforms based on the use of multi-walled carbon nanotubes dispersed in different polymers. *Anal. Chim. Acta, 805*, 19–35. doi: 10.1016/j.aca.2013.10.039.
27. Sánchez, S., Martin, P., Enric, C., & Esteve, F., (2007). Carbon nanotube/polysulfone composite screen-printed electrochemical enzyme biosensors. *Analyst, 132*(2), 142–147. doi: 10.1039/B609137G.
28. Ronkainen, N. J., & Okon, S. L., (2014). Nanomaterial-based electrochemical immunosensors for clinically significant biomarkers. *Materials (Basel), 7*(6), 4669–4709. doi: 10.3390/ma7064669.
29. Campuzano, S., Yáñez-Sedeño, P., & Pingarrón, J. M., (2017). Electrochemical genosensing of circulating biomarkers. *Sensors (Basel), 17*(4). doi: 10.3390/s17040866.
30. Tîlmaciu, C. M., & Morris, M. C., (2015). Carbon nanotube biosensors. *Front Chem., 3*, 59. doi: 10.3389/fchem.2015.00059.
31. Jacobs, C. B., Jennifer, P. M., & Jill, V. B., (2010). Review: Carbon nanotube based electrochemical sensors for biomolecules. *Analytica Chimica Acta, 662*(2), 105–127. doi: https://doi.org/10.1016/j.aca.2010.01.009.

32. Florescu, M., & David, M., (2017). Tyrosinase-based biosensors for selective dopamine detection. *Sensors (Basel), 17*(6). doi: 10.3390/s17061314.
33. Vicentini, F. C., Bruno, C. J., Christopher, B. M. A., & Fatibello-Filho, O., (2013). Tyrosinase biosensor based on a glassy carbon electrode modified with multi-walled carbon nanotubes and 1-butyl-3-methylimidazolium chloride within a dihexadecyl phosphate film. *Sensors and Actuators B: Chemical, 188*, 1101–1108. doi: https://doi.org/10.1016/j.snb.2013.07.109.
34. Mundaca, R. A., Moreno-Guzmán, M., Eguílaz, M., Yáñez-Sedeño, P., & Pingarrón, J. M., (2012). Enzyme biosensor for androsterone based on 3α-hydroxysteroid dehydrogenase immobilized onto a carbon nanotubes/ionic liquid/NAD^+ composite electrode. *Talanta, 99*, 697–702. doi: 10.1016/j.talanta.2012.07.008.
35. Pourasl, A. H., Ahmadi, M. T., Rahmani, M., Chin, H. C., Lim, C. S., Ismail, R., & Tan, M. L., (2014). Analytical modeling of glucose biosensors based on carbon nanotubes. *Nanoscale Res. Lett., 9*(1), 33. doi: 10.1186/1556-276x-9-33.
36. Teles, F. R. R., & Fonseca, L. P., (2008). Trends in DNA biosensors. *Talanta, 77*(2), 606–623. doi: 10.1016/j.talanta.2008.07.024.
37. Huang, Y., Shi, M., Zhao, L., Zhao, S., Hu, K., Chen, Z. F., Chen, J., & Liang, H., (2014). Carbon nanotube signal amplification for ultrasensitive fluorescence polarization detection of DNA methyltransferase activity and inhibition. *Biosens. Bioelectron, 54*, 285–291. doi: 10.1016/j.bios.2013.10.065.
38. Wang, H., Li, H., Zhang, Y., Wei, Q., Ma, H., Wu, D., Li, Y., et al., (2014). Label-free immunosensor based on Pd nanoplates for amperometric immunoassay of alpha-fetoprotein. *Biosens. Bioelectron, 53*, 305–309. doi: 10.1016/j.bios.2013.10.010.
39. Hammarström, S., Engvall, E., Johansson, B. G., Svensson, S., Sundblad, G., & Goldstein, I. J., (1975). Nature of the tumor-associated determinant(s) of carcinoembryonic antigen. *Proc. Natl. Acad. Sci. U S A, 72*(4), 1528–1532. doi: 10.1073/pnas.72.4.1528.
40. Fakih, M. G., & Padmanabhan, A., (2006). CEA monitoring in colorectal cancer. What you should know. *Oncology (Williston Park), 20*(6), 579–587. discussion 588, 594, 596 passim.
41. Ballesta, A. M., Molina, R., Filella, X., Jo, J., & Giménez, N., (1995). Carcinoembryonic antigen in staging and follow-up of patients with solid tumors. *Tumor. Biol., 16*(1), 32–41. doi: 10.1159/000217926.
42. Naghibalhossaini, F., & Ebadi, P., (2006). Evidence for CEA release from human colon cancer cells by an endogenous GPI-PLD enzyme. *Cancer Lett., 234*(2), 158–167. doi: 10.1016/j.canlet.2005.03.028.
43. Hasanzadeh, M., & Nasrin, S., (2017). Advanced nanomaterials for use in electrochemical and optical immunoassays of carcinoembryonic antigen. A review. *Microchimica Acta, 184*(2), 389–414. doi: 10.1007/s00604-016-2066-2.
44. Ross, T., Ahmed, K., Raison, N., Challacombe, B., & Dasgupta, P., (2016). Clarifying the PSA grey zone: The management of patients with a borderline PSA. *Int. J. Clin. Pract., 70*(11), 950–959. doi: 10.1111/ijcp.12883.
45. Kavosi, B., Abdollah, S., Rahman, H., & Kamal, A., (2014). A highly sensitive prostate-specific antigen immunosensor based on gold nanoparticles/PAMAM dendrimer loaded on MWCNTS/chitosan/ionic liquid nanocomposite. *Biosensors and Bioelectronics, 52*, 20–28. doi: https://doi.org/10.1016/j.bios.2013.08.012.

46. Justino, Celine, I. L., Armando, C. D., & Rocha-Santos, A. P. T., (2016b). Critical overview on the application of sensors and biosensors for clinical analysis. *TrAC Trends in Analytical Chemistry, 85*, 36–60. doi: https://doi.org/10.1016/j.trac.2016.04.004.
47. Li, Z., Zheng, L., Haiyan, S., & Chao, G., (2015). Superstructured assembly of nanocarbons: Fullerenes, nanotubes, and graphene. *Chemical Reviews, 115*(15), 7046–7117. doi: 10.1021/acs.chemrev.5b00102.
48. Gao, Q., Han, J., & Ma, Z., (2013). Polyamidoamine dendrimers-capped carbon dots/Au nanocrystal nanocomposites and its application for electrochemical immunosensor. *Biosens Bioelectron, 49*, 323–328. doi: 10.1016/j.bios.2013.05.048.
49. Justino, C. I. L., Duarte, A. C., & Rocha-Santos, T. A. P., (2016a). Critical overview on the application of sensors and biosensors for clinical analysis. *Trends Analyt. Chem., 85*, 36–60. doi: 10.1016/j.trac.2016.04.004.
50. Guo, J., Han, X., Wang, J., Zhao, J., Guo, Z., & Zhang, Y., (2015). Horseradish peroxidase functionalized gold nanorods as a label for sensitive electrochemical detection of alpha-fetoprotein antigen. *Anal. Biochem., 491*, 58–64. doi: 10.1016/j.ab.2015.09.006.
51. Wang, Y., Li, X., Cao, W., Li, Y., Li, H., Du, B., & Wei, Q., (2014). Ultrasensitive sandwich-type electrochemical immunosensor based on a novel signal amplification strategy using highly loaded toluidine blue/gold nanoparticles decorated KIT-6/carboxymethyl chitosan/ionic liquids as signal labels. *Biosens. Bioelectron, 61*, 618–624. doi: 10.1016/j.bios.2014.05.059.
52. Yang, H., Zhejian, L., Xiaomin, W., Ru, H., Honglan, Q., Qiang, G., Chenzhong, L., & Chengxiao, Z., (2013). Detection and discrimination of alpha-fetoprotein with a label-free electrochemical impedance spectroscopy biosensor array based on lectin functionalized carbon nanotubes. *Talanta, 111*, 62–68. doi: https://doi.org/10.1016/j.talanta.2013.01.060.
53. Lin, J., Zhijing, W., Huihui, Z., & Meijia, S., (2013). Sensitive immunosensor for the label-free determination of tumor marker based on carbon nanotubes/mesoporous silica and graphene modified electrode. *Biosensors and Bioelectronics, 41*, 342–347. doi: https://doi.org/10.1016/j.bios.2012.08.051.
54. Raphael, I., Nalawade, S., Eagar, T. N., & Forsthuber, T. G., (2015). T cell subsets and their signature cytokines in autoimmune and inflammatory diseases. *Cytokine, 74*(1), 5–17. doi: 10.1016/j.cyto.2014.09.011.
55. Blandizzi, C., Gionchetti, P., Armuzzi, A., Caporali, R., Chimenti, S., Cimaz, R., Cimino, L., et al., (2014). The role of tumor necrosis factor in the pathogenesis of immune-mediated diseases. *Int. J. Immunopathol. Pharmacol., 27*(1 Suppl), 1–10. doi: 10.1177/03946320140270s101.
56. Mazloum-Ardakani, M., Laleh, H., & Alireza, K., (2015). Label-free electrochemical immunosensor for detection of tumor necrosis factor α based on fullerene-functionalized carbon nanotubes/ionic liquid. *Journal of Electroanalytical Chemistry, 757*, 58–64. doi: https://doi.org/10.1016/j.jelechem.2015.09.006.
57. Mazloum-Ardakani, M., & Laleh, H., (2015). Highly-sensitive label-free immunosensor for tumor necrosis factor α based on Ag@Pt core–shell nanoparticles supported on MWCNTs as an efficient electrocatalyst nanocomposite. *RSC Advances, 5*(87), 70781–70786. doi: 10.1039/C5RA08016A.
58. Roger, V. L., Go, A. S., Lloyd-Jones, D. M., Benjamin, E. J., Berry, J. D., Borden, W. B., Bravata, D. M., et al., (2012). Heart disease and stroke statistics–2012 update: A report

from the American Heart Association. *Circulation, 125*(1), e2–e220. doi: 10.1161/CIR.0b013e31823ac046.
59. Yang, Z., & Min, Z. D., (2006). Cardiac markers and their point-of-care testing for diagnosis of acute myocardial infarction. *Clin. Biochem., 39*(8), 771–780. doi: 10.1016/j.clinbiochem.2006.05.011.
60. Hasanzadeh, M., Nasrin, S., Morteza, E., Miguel De La, G., & Eskandar, O., (2013). Electrochemical nano-immunosensing of effective cardiac biomarkers for acute myocardial infarction. *Trends in Analytical Chemistry, 49*, 20–30.
61. Aldous, S. J., (2013). Cardiac biomarkers in acute myocardial infarction. *Int. J. Cardiol., 164*(3), 282–294. doi: 10.1016/j.ijcard.2012.01.081.
62. Singh, V., Martinezclark, P., Pascual, M., Shaw, E. S., & O'Neill, W. W., (2010). Cardiac biomarkers – the old and the new: A review. *Coron. Artery Dis., 21*(4), 244–256. doi: 10.1097/MCA.0b013e328338cd1f.
63. Gibler, W. B., Young, G. P., Hedges, J. R., Lewis, L. M., Smith, M. S., Carleton, S. C., Aghababian, R. V., Jorden, R. O., Allison, E. J. Jr., Otten, E. J., et al., (1992). Acute myocardial infarction in chest pain patients with nondiagnostic ECGs: Serial CK-MB sampling in the emergency department. The emergency medicine cardiac research group. *Ann. Emerg. Med., 21*(5), 504–512. doi: 10.1016/s0196-0644(05)82515-6.
64. Moreira, F. T., Dutra, R. A., Noronha, J. P., & Sales, M. G., (2014). Novel sensory surface for creatine kinase electrochemical detection. *Biosens. Bioelectron, 56*, 217–222. doi: 10.1016/j.bios.2013.12.052.
65. Garg, P., Morris, P., Fazlanie, A. L., Vijayan, S., Dancso, B., Dastidar, A. G., Plein, S., et al., (2017). Cardiac biomarkers of acute coronary syndrome: From history to high-sensitivity cardiac troponin. *Intern. Emerg. Med., 12*(2), 147–155. doi: 10.1007/s11739-017-1612-1.
66. Agewall, S., Giannitsis, E., Jernberg, T., & Katus, H., (2011). Troponin elevation in coronary vs. non-coronary disease. *Eur. Heart J., 32*(4), 404–411. doi: 10.1093/eurheartj/ehq456.
67. Silva, B. V., Cavalcanti, I. T., Silva, M. M., & Dutra, R. F., (2013). A carbon nanotube screen-printed electrode for label-free detection of the human cardiac troponin T. *Talanta, 117*, 431–437. doi: 10.1016/j.talanta.2013.08.059.
68. Gomes-Filho, S. L. R., Dias, A. C. M. S., Silva, M. M. S., Silva, B. V. M., & Dutra, R. F., (2013). A carbon nanotube-based electrochemical immunosensor for cardiac troponin T. *Microchemical Journal, 109*, 10–15. doi: https://doi.org/10.1016/j.microc.2012.05.033.
69. Prakash, M. D., Singh, S. G., Sharma, C. S., & Siva, R. K. V., (2017). Electrochemical detection of cardiac biomarkers utilizing electrospun multiwalled carbon nanotubes embedded su-8 nanofibers. *Electroanalysis, 29*(2), 380–386. doi: https://doi.org/10.1002/elan.201501163.
70. Jayaraj, G. G., Smita, N., & Souvik, M., (2015). Nonconventional chemical inhibitors of microRNA: Therapeutic scope. *Chemical Communications, 51*(5), 820–831. doi: 10.1039/C4CC04514A.
71. Friedman, R. C., Farh, K. K., Burge, C. B., & Bartel, D. P., (2009). Most mammalian mRNAs are conserved targets of microRNAs. *Genome Res., 19*(1), 92–105. doi: 10.1101/gr.082701.108.
72. Pritchard, C. C., Cheng, H. H., & Tewari, M., (2012). MicroRNA profiling: Approaches and considerations. *Nat. Rev. Genet., 13*(5), 358–369. doi: 10.1038/nrg3198.

73. Bartel, D. P., (2009). MicroRNAs: Target recognition and regulatory functions. *Cell, 136*(2), 215–233. doi: 10.1016/j.cell.2009.01.002.
74. Wang, H., & Cai, J., (2017). The role of microRNAs in heart failure. *Biochim. Biophys. Acta Mol. Basis Dis., 1863*(8), 2019–2030. doi: 10.1016/j.bbadis.2016.11.034.
75. Vegter, E. L., Ovchinnikova, E. S., Van, V. D. J., Jaarsma, T., Berezikov, E., Van, D. M. P., & Voors, A. A., (2017). Low circulating microRNA levels in heart failure patients are associated with atherosclerotic disease and cardiovascular-related rehospitalizations. *Clin Res Cardiol., 106*(8), 598–609. doi: 10.1007/s00392-017-1096-z.
76. Stoicea, N., Du, A., Lakis, D. C., Tipton, C., Arias-Morales, C. E., & Bergese, S. D., (2016). The MiRNA journey from theory to practice as a CNS biomarker. *Front Genet, 7*, 11. doi: 10.3389/fgene.2016.00011.
77. Faravelli, I., & Corti, S., (2018). *MicroRNA-Directed Neuronal Reprogramming as a Therapeutic Strategy for Neurological Diseases, 55*(5), 4428–4436. doi: 10.1007/s12035-017-0671-7.
78. Wang, S., Wang, J. Q., & Lv, X. W., (2017a). Exosomal miRNAs as biomarkers in the diagnosis of liver disease. *Biomark. Med., 11*(6), 491–501. doi: 10.2217/bmm-2017-0011.
79. Long, X. R., Zhang, Y. J., Zhang, M. Y., Chen, K., Zheng, X. F. S., & Wang, H. Y., (2017). Identification of an 88-microRNA signature in whole blood for diagnosis of hepatocellular carcinoma and other chronic liver diseases. *Aging (Albany NY), 9*(6), 1565–1584. doi: 10.18632/aging.101253.
80. Kashani, K., Cheungpasitporn, W., & Ronco, C., (2017). Biomarkers of acute kidney injury: The pathway from discovery to clinical adoption. *Clin. Chem. Lab. Med., 55*(8), 1074–1089. doi: 10.1515/cclm-2016-0973.
81. Jin, C., Cheng, L., Höxtermann, S., Xie, T., Lu, X., Wu, H., Skaletz-Rorowski, A., et al., (2017). MicroRNA-155 is a biomarker of T-cell activation and immune dysfunction in HIV-1-infected patients. *HIV Med., 18*(5), 354–362. doi: 10.1111/hiv.12470.
82. Le, X., Yu, X., & Shen, N., (2017). Novel insights of microRNAs in the development of systemic lupus erythematosus. *Curr. Opin. Rheumatol., 29*(5), 450–457. doi: 10.1097/bor.0000000000000420.
83. Wang, S., Jian-Qing, W., & Xiong-Wen, L., (2017b). Exosomal miRNAs as biomarkers in the diagnosis of liver disease. *Biomarkers in Medicine, 11*(6), 491–501. doi: 10.2217/bmm-2017-0011.
84. Mahasneh, A., Al-Shaheri, F., & Jamal, E., (2017). Molecular biomarkers for an early diagnosis, effective treatment and prognosis of colorectal cancer: Current updates. *Exp. Mol. Pathol., 102*(3), 475–483. doi: 10.1016/j.yexmp.2017.05.005.
85. Wu, Y., Phillips, J. A., Liu, H., Yang, R., & Tan, W., (2008). Carbon nanotubes protect DNA strands during cellular delivery. *ACS Nano, 2*(10), 2023–2028. doi: 10.1021/nn800325a.
86. Liu, Z., Tabakman, S., Welsher, K., & Dai, H., (2009a). Carbon nanotubes in biology and medicine: *In vitro* and *in vivo* detection, imaging and drug delivery. *Nano Res., 2*(2), 85–120. doi: 10.1007/s12274-009-9009-8.
87. Aubin, J. E., (1979). Autofluorescence of viable cultured mammalian cells. *J. Histochem. Cytochem., 27*(1), 36–43. doi: 10.1177/27.1.220325.
88. O'Connell, M. J., Bachilo, S. M., Huffman, C. B., Moore, V. C., Strano, M. S., Haroz, E. H., Rialon, K. L., et al., (2002). Band gap fluorescence from individual single-walled carbon nanotubes. *Science, 297*(5581), 593–596. doi: 10.1126/science.1072631.

89. Welsher, K., Liu, Z., Daranciang, D., & Dai, H., (2008). Selective probing and imaging of cells with single walled carbon nanotubes as near-infrared fluorescent molecules. *Nano Lett., 8*(2), 586–590. doi: 10.1021/nl072949q.
90. Rao, A. M., Richter, E., Bandow, S., Chase, B., Eklund, P. C., Williams, K. A., Fang, S., et al., (1997). Diameter-selective Raman scattering from vibrational modes in carbon nanotubes. *Science, 275*(5297), 187–191. doi: 10.1126/science.275.5297.187.
91. Heller, D. A., Baik, S., Eurell, T. E., &. Strano, M. S., (2005). Single-walled carbon nanotube spectroscopy in live cells: Towards long-term labels and optical sensors. *Advanced Materials, 17*(23), 2793–2799. doi: https://doi.org/10.1002/adma.200500477.
92. Liu, Z., Davis, C., Cai, W., He, L., Chen, X., & Dai, H., (2008). Circulation and long-term fate of functionalized, biocompatible single-walled carbon nanotubes in mice probed by Raman spectroscopy. *Proc. Natl. Acad. Sci. U S A, 105*(5), 1410–1415. doi: 10.1073/pnas.0707654105.
93. Liu, Z., Winters, M., Holodniy, M., & Dai, H., (2007). siRNA delivery into human T cells and primary cells with carbon-nanotube transporters. *Angew. Chem. Int. Ed. Engl., 46*(12), 2023–2027. doi: 10.1002/anie.200604295.
94. Schipper, M. L., Nakayama-Ratchford, N., Davis, C. R., Kam, N. W., Chu, P., Liu, Z., Sun, X., et al., (2008). A pilot toxicology study of single-walled carbon nanotubes in a small sample of mice. *Nat. Nanotechnol., 3*(4), 216–221. doi: 10.1038/nnano.2008.68.
95. Liu, Z., Xiaolin, L., Scott, M. T., Kaili, J., Shoushan, F., & Hongjie, D., (2008). Multiplexed multicolor Raman imaging of live cells with isotopically modified single walled carbon nanotubes. *Journal of the American Chemical Society, 130*(41), 13540, 13541. doi: 10.1021/ja806242t.
96. Leeuw, T. K., Reith, R. M., Simonette, R. A., Harden, M. E., Cherukuri, P., Tsyboulski, D. A., Beckingham, K. M., & Weisman, R. B., (2007). Single-walled carbon nanotubes in the intact organism: Near-IR imaging and biocompatibility studies in drosophila. *Nano Lett., 7*(9), 2650–2654. doi: 10.1021/nl0710452.
97. Keren, S., Zavaleta, C., Cheng, Z., De La Zerda, A., Gheysens, O., & Gambhir, S. S., (2008). Noninvasive molecular imaging of small living subjects using Raman spectroscopy. *Proc. Natl. Acad. Sci U S A, 105*(15), 5844–5849. doi: 10.1073/pnas.0710575105.
98. Zavaleta, C., De La Zerda, A., Liu, Z., Keren, S., Cheng, Z., Schipper, M., Chen, X., et al., (2008b). Noninvasive Raman spectroscopy in living mice for evaluation of tumor targeting with carbon nanotubes. *Nano Lett, 8*(9), 2800–2805. doi: 10.1021/nl801362a.
99. Gong, H., Peng, R., & Liu, Z., (2013). Carbon nanotubes for biomedical imaging: The recent advances. *Adv. Drug Deliv. Rev., 65*(15), 1951–1963. doi: 10.1016/j.addr.2013.10.002.
100. Zavaleta, C., De La Zerda, A., Liu, Z., Keren, S., Cheng, Z., Schipper, M., Chen, X., et al., (2008a). Noninvasive Raman spectroscopy in living mice for evaluation of tumor targeting with carbon nanotubes. *Nano Letters, 8*(9), 2800–2805. doi: 10.1021/nl801362a.
101. De La Zerda, A., Cristina, Z., Shay, K., Srikant, V., Sunil, B., Zhuang, L., Jelena, L., et al., (2008). Carbon nanotubes as photoacoustic molecular imaging agents in living mice. *Nature Nanotechnology, 3*(9), 557–562. doi: 10.1038/nnano.2008.231.
102. Cherukuri, P., Sergei, M. B., Silvio, H. L., & Bruce, W. R., (2004). Near-infrared fluorescence microscopy of single-walled carbon nanotubes in phagocytic cells. *Journal of the American Chemical Society, 126*(48), 15638–15639. doi: 10.1021/ja0466311.

103. Jin, H., Daniel, A. H., & Michael, S. S., (2008). Single-particle tracking of endocytosis and exocytosis of single-walled carbon nanotubes in NIH-3T3 cells. *Nano Letters, 8*(6), 1577–1585. doi: 10.1021/nl072969s.
104. Tong, L., Yuxiang, L., Bridget, D. D., Yookyung, J., Mikhail, N. S., Donald, E. B., & Ji-Xin, C., (2012). Label-free imaging of semiconducting and metallic carbon nanotubes in cells and mice using transient absorption microscopy. *Nature Nanotechnology, 7*(1), 56–61. doi: 10.1038/nnano.2011.210.
105. Xu, M., & Lihong, W. V., (2006). Photoacoustic imaging in biomedicine. *Review of Scientific Instruments, 77*(4), 041101. doi: 10.1063/1.2195024.
106. Zhou, X., James, H., Yoichi, M., Grutter, P., & Koji, I., (2014). Scanning gate imaging of two coupled quantum dots in single-walled carbon nanotubes. *Nanotechnology, 25*, 495703. doi: 10.1088/0957-4484/25/49/495703.
107. Li, J., Chang, X., Chen, X., Gu, Z., Zhao, F., Chai, Z., & Zhao, Y., (2014). Toxicity of inorganic nanomaterials in biomedical imaging. *Biotechnol. Adv., 32*(4), 727–743. doi: 10.1016/j.biotechadv.2013.12.009.
108. Zhang, X., Meng, L., Lu, Q., Fei, Z., & Dyson, P. J., (2009a). Targeted delivery and controlled release of doxorubicin to cancer cells using modified single wall carbon nanotubes. *Biomaterials, 30*(30), 6041–6047. doi: 10.1016/j.biomaterials.2009.07.025.
109. Huang, H., Yuan, Q., Shah, J. S., & Misra, R. D., (2011). A new family of folate-decorated and carbon nanotube-mediated drug delivery system: Synthesis and drug delivery response. *Adv. Drug Deliv. Rev., 63*(14, 15), 1332–1339. doi: 10.1016/j.addr.2011.04.001.
110. Chen, C., Xie, X. X., Zhou, Q., Zhang, F. Y., Wang, Q. L., Liu, Y. Q., Zou, Y., et al., (2012). EGF-functionalized single-walled carbon nanotubes for targeting delivery of etoposide. *Nanotechnology, 23*(4), 045104. doi: 10.1088/0957-4484/23/4/045104.
111. Chen, C., Hou, L., Zhang, H., Zhu, L., Zhang, H., Zhang, C., Shi, J., et al., (2013). Single-walled carbon nanotubes mediated targeted tamoxifen delivery system using aspargine-glycine-arginine peptide. *J. Drug Target, 21*(9), 809–821. doi: 10.3109/1061186x.2013.829071.
112. Zhang, X., Lingjie, M., Qinghua, L., Zhaofu, F., & Paul, J. D., (2009b). Targeted delivery and controlled release of doxorubicin to cancer cells using modified single wall carbon nanotubes. *Biomaterials, 30*(30), 6041–6047. doi: https://doi.org/10.1016/j.biomaterials.2009.07.025.
113. Cheng, J., Meziani, M. J., Sun, Y. P., & Cheng, S. H., (2011). Poly(ethylene glycol)-conjugated multi-walled carbon nanotubes as an efficient drug carrier for overcoming multidrug resistance. *Toxicol. Appl. Pharmacol., 250*(2), 184–193. doi: 10.1016/j.taap.2010.10.012.
114. Villa, C. H., Dao, T., Ahearn, I., Fehrenbacher, N., Casey, E., Rey, D. A., Korontsvit, T., et al., (2011). Single-walled carbon nanotubes deliver peptide antigen into dendritic cells and enhance IgG responses to tumor-associated antigens. *ACS Nano, 5*(7), 5300–5311. doi: 10.1021/nn200182x.
115. Yang, Z., Zhang, Y., Yang, Y., Sun, L., Han, D., Li, H., & Wang, C., (2010). Pharmacological and toxicological target organelles and safe use of single-walled carbon nanotubes as drug carriers in treating Alzheimer's disease. *Nanomedicine, 6*(3), 427–441. doi: 10.1016/j.nano.2009.11.007.
116. Paul, A., Anwarul, H., Hamood, A. K., Akhilesh, K. G., Vijayaraghava, R. T. S., Mehdi, N., Su, R. S., et al., (2014). Injectable graphene oxide/hydrogel-based angiogenic gene

delivery system for vasculogenesis and cardiac repair. *ACS Nano, 8*(8), 8050–8062. doi: 10.1021/nn5020787.
117. Hasan, A., Adnan, M., Nasim, A., Monowar, H., Arghya, P., Mehmet, R. D., Fariba, D., & Ali, K., (2014). Electrospun scaffolds for tissue engineering of vascular grafts. *Acta Biomaterialia, 10*(1), 11–25. doi: https://doi.org/10.1016/j.actbio.2013.08.022.
118. Jin, Guang-Zhen, Meeju, K., Ueon, S. S., & Hae-Won, K., (2011). Neurite outgrowth of dorsal root ganglia neurons is enhanced on aligned nanofibrous biopolymer scaffold with carbon nanotube coating. *Neuroscience Letters, 501*(1), 10–14. doi: https://doi.org/10.1016/j.neulet.2011.06.023.
119. Zhao, B., Hui, H., Swadhin, M. K., & Robert, H. C., (2005). A bone mimic based on the self-assembly of hydroxyapatite on chemically functionalized single-walled carbon nanotubes. *Chemistry of Materials, 17*(12), 3235–3241. doi: 10.1021/cm0500399.
120. Hirata, E., Ménard-Moyon, C., Venturelli, E., Takita, H., Watari, F., Bianco, A., & Yokoyama, A., (2013). Carbon nanotubes functionalized with fibroblast growth factor accelerate proliferation of bone marrow-derived stromal cells and bone formation. *Nanotechnology, 24*(43), 435101. doi: 10.1088/0957-4484/24/43/435101.
121. Cui, Hui-Fang, Sandeep, K. V., Al-Rubeaan, K., John L. H. T., & Fwu-Shan, S., (2010). Interfacing carbon nanotubes with living mammalian cells and cytotoxicity issues. *Chemical Research in Toxicology, 23*(7), 1131–1147. doi: 10.1021/tx100050h.
122. Liu, Z., Scott, T., Kevin, W., & Hongjie, D., (2009b). Carbon nanotubes in biology and medicine: *In vitro* and *in vivo* detection, imaging and drug delivery. *Nano Research, 2*(2), 85–120. doi: 10.1007/s12274-009-9009-8.
123. Pulskamp, K., Diabaté, S., & Krug, H. F., (2007). Carbon nanotubes show no sign of acute toxicity but induce intracellular reactive oxygen species in dependence on contaminants. *Toxicol. Lett., 168*(1), 58–74. doi: 10.1016/j.toxlet.2006.11.001.
124. Vittorio, O., Raffa, V., & Cuschieri, A., (2009). Influence of purity and surface oxidation on cytotoxicity of multiwalled carbon nanotubes with human neuroblastoma cells. *Nanomedicine, 5*(4), 424–431. doi: 10.1016/j.nano.2009.02.006.

CHAPTER 3

Functionalized Carbon Nanotubes: Biomedical Applications

SURENDRA AGRAWAL,[1] SHANAIKA DEVADIGA,[1]
ASHWINI SERMASEKARAN,[1] and PRAVINA N. GURJAR[2]

[1]*Shobhaben Pratapbhai Patel School of Pharmacy and Technology Management, SVKM'S NMIMS (Deemed to be University), Mumbai, Maharashtra, India*

[2]*Sharadchandra Pawar College of Pharmacy, Otur, Pune, Maharashtra, India*

ABSTRACT

Carbon nanotubes are carbon allotropes where the hexagonal sheets of graphite are structured in a way that resembles a hollow tube-like structure. These structures can be single-walled or multi-walled in nature. The walls of carbon nanotubes offer ease of conjugation to several drugs used in cancers and to proteins that assist in developing new drug delivery. The large surface area provided in these hollow tubes is a noteworthy feature to increase drug loading. The functionalization of carbon nanotubes enhances the binding and loading potential of different drugs and biomolecules. The problems associated with biomedical application of carbon nanotubes has been solved by modifying the surface of these carbon nanotubes by adding different functional groups that strengthen the binding of the target molecules. The advancement in the functionalization of carbon nanotubes explored the horizon of their application like drug targeting, cancer drug delivery, bioimaging, and biosensing. Additionally, the nanotubes are been explored recently for tissue regeneration, diagnostics, and genetic engineering. This chapter summarizes all biomedical applications of carbon nanotubes.

Carbon Nanotubes for Biomedical Applications and Healthcare.
Chin Hua Chia, Swati Gokul Talele, Ann Rose Abraham, and A. K. Haghi, (Eds.)

3.1 INTRODUCTION

In the recent years, the pharmaceutical industry has seen an increase in the pool of drug delivery alternatives for improving various aspects like targeting, efficacy, and bioavailability [1]. Nanotechnology bringing forward different types of delivery alternatives also gives an opportunity for the use of carbon nanotubes (CNT) with the properties that they possess allowing current carrying similar to semiconductors and metals [2]. Their thermal stability and conductivity, superior structural integrity like tensile strength and stiffness and electric properties can be utilized in the pharmaceutical industry for conjugation with different biomolecules like enzymes, proteins, genes, etc. [3]. They are hollow tube like structures with the diameter of the tube ranging in nanometers, this hollow nature of the carbon nanotubes differentiates them from carbon nanofibers as they are packed in nature [4]. CNT were first discovered by Iijima in 1991 when he was working on synthesis of fullerene, he observed the formation of cylindrical sheets of graphite which were hollow in nature, these were observed when carbon was evaporated at the pressure of 100 Torr in the presence of argon gas during arch discharge evaporation. On the negative electrode Iijima observed the presence of graphite sheets which he deduced to be 'rolled graphite sheets inserted into each other'. These sheets of graphite were in the form of concentric loops or rolls of around 2–50 woven into one another [5].

CNT are another allotrope of carbon where the graphene sheets that possess hexagonal lattice arrangement of carbon atoms are seen to form a cylindrical sheet like structure. The classification of different types of CNT is based upon their structure. There can be a single sheet of graphite rolled into a cylindrical tube this is called a single walled carbon nanotube (SWCNT). The diameter of the cylinder in SWCNT is about 20–1,000 nm with length ranging from 0.4–0.3 nm. When more than one graphite sheets are rolled into each other in the form of a cylinder they are called multi-walled carbon nanotubes (MWCNT) having a diameter of 2–100 nm and length ranging from 1–50 um [6]. The carbon atoms in SWCNTs experience covalent forces between them that hold the structure together, whereas due to multiple sheets of graphite there also exists weak Van der Waals forces exists between two sheets in MWCNTs. Ideally carbon nanotubes are supposed to be hexagonally arranged carbon molecules similar to the arrangement of carbon atoms seen in fullerene but during formation there are introduction of certain defects namely the Stone Wales defect. Here there is a defect in the pi bonds connecting two six membered rings where the carbon atoms rotate to 90° resulting in the formation of a five membered and seven membered ring at the site of the defect. This particular defect site observed in CNTs are sites susceptible to addition reaction. Based on the arrangement of the rings of carbon atoms SWCNTs can be classified into armchair, zig zag or chiral [7, 8]. It should also be noted the SWCNTs and MWCNTs have large surface area which can be utilized for loading of various pharmaceutical agents. But it is also known that there is aggregation of CNTs into bundles thereby reducing their free surface area, CNTs that show this type of bundle formation are SWCNTs and to a much lesser extent in MWCNTs, hence dispersing agents might be necessary when it comes to reducing the aggregation or bundle formation in SWCNTs [9].

The structure of carbon nanotubes being different from other common spherical nanomaterials opens up new opportunities for its biomedical application [10]. CNT have one dimensional structure that facilitates addition of different functional groups to better customize the desired physciochemical properties that are required of it. This is possible by the ease of stacking of different aromatic rings on the polyaromatic structure of the carbon nanotubes, this functionalization approach is facilitated by two specific areas in the structure of the CNT one being the tip and the other being the sidewalls, these two areas are responsible for the reactivity and are susceptible to different addition and substitution reactions. Therefore, the π-π stacking and the high surface area provided by carbon nanotubes make them a promising candidate to be used as delivery system for many biomolecules like enzymes, nucleic acids and proteins that themselves have large aromatic systems [11]. When it comes to the biomedical use of carbon nanotubes, its use is not only limited to delivery systems, the optical properties exhibited by it are also utilized in bio-imaging techniques as contrast agents or as CNT based bio-sensing [12]. To add to this carbon nanotubes are also used for their ability to support tissue regeneration and repair. To summarize, carbon nanotubes have varied biomedical application with the major focus being on biomolecules and gene delivery. However, the use of CNTs has been affected by certain roadblocks that arise due to some of the physicochemical properties of CNTs. The research based on derivatization/functionalization aids in achieving desirable targeting and efficacy [13, 14].

3.2 FUNCTIONALIZATION OF CARBON NANOTUBES

CNT that are without any defects have certain physicochemical attributes that can be a hindrance in delivery and targeting of various biomolecules [15]. As biomolecules are required to be delivered inside the cell, the delivery system should have good aqueous solubility which is not possessed by carbon nanotubes [16]. Pristine CNTs are those CNTs that do not possess any structural defects. The pristine CNTs may have impurities like residual reagents that are added during manufacturing, metal catalysts. The pristine CNTs are subjected to strong acid treatment, which solves the problem of poor aqueous solubility and metal impurities. However, this process also shortens the length of the resulting CNTs, thereby reducing the available surface area for loading of target biomolecule [17]. To avoid such drawbacks, methods like centrifugation, gel permeation chromatography, filtration, and derivatization is used for the purpose of purification [18]. The structural orientation of the carbon atoms in the CNTs may lead to poor aqueous solubility. The sidewalls of the CNTs are less reactive due to the flat orientation of carbons as opposed to the pyramidal arrangement of carbon atoms in fullerene, this structural feature of CNTs makes it difficult for them to solubilize in aqueous solvents [19]. To further approach this problem functionalization of CNTs are carried out as follows:

i. Non-covalent functionalization; and
ii. Covalent functionalization.

3.2.1 NON-COVALENT FUNCTIONALIZATION

Non-covalent functionalization of CNTs has been employed to reduce the issues with solubility and altered electrical properties of the CNTs. Non-covalent Functionalization includes the use of surfactants, polymers, and nano-encapsulation to reduce the destructive purification process [20]. Surfactants forming aggregates around SWCNTs have proven to be an effective strategy to non-destructively purify the SWCNTs and disperse them into the aqueous phase. This is possible as the amphiphilic surfactant molecules have a hydrophobic part that interacts with the SWCNTs that form the inner core of the micelle. This is possible due to the π-π stacking as the hydrophobic part of the surfactant usually has an aromatic group that can interact with the SWCNTs [21]. Along with the use of surfactants even polymers can be used to wrap around the CNTs and form a stable complex that disperses in water. Polymers like polystyrene and polyvinyl pyrrolidone that have polar groups in their side chains can easily bind to the side walls of SWCNTs. For increasing the solubility of CNTs, there needs to be the presence of polar groups like amines or anilines for effective complex formation even change of solvent to a non-polar one can disturb the stability of the complex and dissociate the tubes. Some complexes of CNTs formed with polymers like poly(m-phenylene-co-2,5-dioctoxy-p-phenylenevinylene) (PmPV) can lead to a total change in the electric and optical properties of CNTs. These complexes have conductivity 8 times higher than pristine CNTs and can be easily characterized using UV/Vis Spectrometry [22]. It is also possible to non-covalently functionalize the surface of CNTs by exposing them to vapors that contain moieties that can non-covalently bind to the CNT surface following which this functionalized CNT can now be subjected to another stream of vapors that contain moieties that can stabilize this functionalized layer [23]. Thus, the resulting completely stable functionalized CNT can further be used for the surface incorporation of different target biomolecules. Non-covalent functionalization can also be done without the use of polymers or surfactant by directly forming bonds with metals as seen when metallothionein proteins and streptavidin have utilized the hydrophobic region of the protein to adsorb itself on the MWCNTs [24, 25]. This kind of approach to use the hydrophobic regions of the molecule to interact with the CNTs has been an important basis for the delivery of many biomolecules discussed further.

3.2.2 COVALENT FUNCTIONALIZATION

Covalent functionalization is done by forming covalent bonds by addition reaction. Though carbenes, arynes, and halogens when subjected to extreme conditions add onto the surface of the CNTs it is very difficult to control their addition due to the stereo and regioselective nature of such nucleophilic additions [26]. Dyke et al. also noted the reluctance of MWCNTs to undergo covalent functionalization process to give appropriate yield as compared to SWCNTs, this is mainly due to the structure of MWCNTs which due to its inner carbon wall brings forth the issues regarding steric hindrance during addition process [27].

One of the strategies adopted by the researchers for the covalent functionalization process includes basic reactions where an acyl peroxide is used to form carbon centered free radical for an organic compound that contains a terminal carboxylic acid group. This intermediate then converted to acyl chloride subsequently converted to amines or amides thus providing a site for further addition of other polymers for functionalization. Similarly, Smalley et al. explored a way where polymers can be made compatible with CNTs by manufacturing rods of polymer dispersed in SWCNTs leading to a polymer coated SWCNT fibers on nanoscale that can be used in solid preparations. CNTs can also be dispersed in solvents to generate a salt form [28]. Tour et al. modified the CNTs with diazonium compounds to imbibe certain groups with the CNTs that upon blending with polymer monomers can themselves stimulate the process of polymerization between each other or when made to react with polymers they can covalently bond with the polymer themselves. On similar lines, there are many approaches to functionalize the surface of CNTs for improvement or customization of different physicochemical properties according to the requirement of the delivery system [29].

3.3 TOXICITY OF CNT

Safety is the first and foremost element in any material which is been utilized in medicine. The toxicity of CNT is influenced by their structure, shape, surface functional groups, and dose. Over the last few years, numerous research has been conducted to investigate the potential harmful effects of carbon nanotubes. The findings of these studies were wildly disparate, demonstrating a strong reliance on the type of nanotube materials used as well as the methods used to functionalize them [30]. The reports demonstrated the toxic effect of the raw CNT when breathed into the lungs. Secondly, long MWNT which is of unfunctionalized nature constitute the carcinogenic risk [31] (Table 3.1).

TABLE 3.1 Toxicity of CNT

Sl. No.	Toxicity	Factors	Outcome
1.	Cytotoxicity	i. Amount and nature of metal impurity; ii. Length and type of CNT; iii. Type of surface functionalization; iv. Presence of dispersant or surfactant in dispersant solution.	DNA damage, cell damage, cell apoptosis.
2.	Fibrosis	Retention of long CNTs.	Interstitial, bronchial, and pleural fibrosis.
3.	Genotoxic	Long MWCNTs.	DNA damage, plasma membrane damage and aberrant phagocytosis.
4.	Oxidative damage	Activation of the NADPH oxidase with resultant massive generation of ROS.	Activation of the lysosomal–mitochondrial axis with attendant cell death.

3.4 STRUCTURES

3.4.1 WEIGHT OF CNTS

Multi-walled nanotubes being very light and small, they are easily inhaled and reach within the subpleural macrophages after an inhalation exposure which led to aggregation of mononuclear cell aggregates on the surface of pleural tissues and ultimately lead to subpleural fibrosis [32].

3.4.2 NUMBER OF WALLS

Similarly, muti-walled nanotubes breathed had limited pulmonary effects, but they did inhibit systemic immune function. For all these effects, dose plays a critical role. If dose inhaled is limited then the consequence of the toxicity will also be prevented [33]. Single walled carbon nanotubes even cause the skin toxicity on exposure. This is mainly caused because of the oxidative stress created in the skin [34].

3.4.3 LENGTH AND DIAMETER OF CNT

The length and diameter of the nanotubes will determine the penetration within the membrane of macrophages or the impact over internalization inside the cell. Different length, diameter, and rigidity has a control over toxicity. The probability of flexible CNTs to retain in organs is more. The studies have shown that the shorter multi-walled CNTs have a lower incidence of cytotoxicity than longer multi-walled CNTs. Similarly large diameter CNTs will cause higher toxicity compared to shorter diameter [35].

3.4.4 EFFECT OF FUNCTIONALIZATION ON TOXICITY

The process of functionalizing carbon nanotubes entails altering their surface by introducing functional groups that may improve their solubility in aqueous conditions. The technique can be either a covalent or non-covalent alteration, and it can help achieve increased compatibility with biological systems by increasing solubility in aqueous fluids. Coccini et al. [36] found a link between CNT cytotoxicity reduction and chemical functionalization that increases solubility, promotes dispersibility, and minimizes CNT clumping

[36]. Functionalization will facilitate cell targeting and specific cellular process [37].

3.5 EXPLORING CARBON NANOTUBES FOR THEIR BIOMEDICAL APPLICATIONS

3.5.1 CARBON NANOTUBES IN TISSUE ENGINEERING

In recent years, breakthroughs in the fields of cell and organ transplantation, as well as CNT chemistry, have aided the further development of CNT-based tissue engineering and regenerative medicine. Because carbon nanotubes are nontoxic, resistant to biodegradation, and can be functionalized with proteins to enhance organ regeneration, they may be the greatest tissue-engineering candidate among various alternative materials such as natural and synthetic polymers for tissue scaffolds. CNTs can be employed as additives in this field to improve the mechanical strength and conductivity of tissue scaffolding by combining with the host's body [38, 39].

MacDonald et al. have successfully coupled carboxylated SWCNTs with a polymer or collagen (poly-l-lactide or poly-D,L-lactide-co-glycolide) to generate a composite nanomaterial that can be used as a tissue regeneration scaffold. Cell tracking and tagging, monitoring cellular behavior, and improving tissue matrices are some of the other tissue engineering uses of CNTs that have recently been investigated. CNTs, for example, have been shown to improve bone tissue regeneration in mice and embryonic stem cell differentiation into neurogenic cells *in vitro* [40].

Correa-Duarte et al. created CNT-based 3D networks as cell growth scaffolds. The 3D interconnecting resistive network of CNTs was created by applying chemically induced capillary forces to a vertically oriented CNT array. This three-dimensional network resembled a scaffold for cell growth. The majority of L929 cells had attached to the CNT surface as well as the cavity walls. The fibroblasts had nearly entirely covered the whole surface of the CNT-based 3D scaffolds after seven days [41].

3.5.2 CARBON NANOTUBES IN GENE THERAPY

Gene therapy involves inserting a DNA molecule into the cell nucleus to fix a faulty gene that causes some chronic or inherited disorders. Liposomes, cationic lipids, and nanoparticles such as carbon nanotubes (CNTs) are examples of DNA delivery systems [42].

In comparison to DNA employed alone, DNA probes coupled to SWCNTs are protected from enzymatic cleavage and interference from nucleic acid binding proteins. As a result, the DNA-SWCNT complex exhibits higher biostability and enhances the self-delivery potential of DNA. Indeed, compared to naked DNA, stable complexes of plasmid DNA and cationic CNTs have exhibited an increase in gene therapy ability. CNTs coupled with DNA were discovered to release DNA before it was destroyed by the cell's defense mechanism, resulting in a considerable increase in transfection [43].

The use of carbon nanotubes as gene therapy vectors has demonstrated that these manufactured structures may efficiently transport genes inside mammalian cells while maintaining their integrity, since the CNT-gene complex has preserved the ability to express proteins [44]. Pantarotto et al. created novel functionalized SWCNT-DNA complexes with enhanced DNA expression as compared to naked DNA. Pantarotto et al. employed ammonium-functionalized carbon nanotubes (f-CNTs) to electrostatically adsorb plasmid DNA. F-CNTs containing DNA can pass through cell membranes and enter cells. Then, f-CNT-associated plasmid DNA was successfully transported to cells, with gene expression profiles up to 10 times greater than with free DNA without CNTs [45]. Tonelli et al. used carboxyfunctionalized multiwalled carbon nanotubes (f-MWNTs) to make a DNA complex. They discovered that f-MWNTs complexed with DNA can improve gene transport to Nile tilapia spermatogonial stem cells, and that their transfection efficacy was significantly higher than that of cationic lipids or electroporation, resulting in less cell death [46, 47].

3.5.3 CARBON NANOTUBES IN PROTEIN DELIVERY

The hollow nature of CNTs act as potential tubular vectors that can be filled with biomolecules and delivered to the target site after specific external stimuli. In fact, because multiple elements come into play at the nanoscale, protein smart encapsulation and preservation in CNTs is everything but simple. The concept is more difficult to realize than one may believe from an experimental standpoint [48].

Only a few experimental investigations on the topic exist as proof, despite the fact that the issue has been extensively researched *in silico*. CNTs may encapsulate a variety of proteins with firm binding, according to an early investigation on open-ended CNTs with internal diameters of 3–5 nm. However, the protein was so tightly bound within the CNTs that it became an impediment to continued protein release. In fact, under varied pH and ionic strength settings, buffer washes were unable to remove the encapsulated proteins. However, the discovery that encapsulating protected the proteins from radiation damage was a huge plus.

An example of protein encapsulation is seen when gold nanoparticles (AuNPs) are included in the hierarchical order by encapsulation, a new level of complexity is achieved. To control the orderly self-assembly of AuNPs along the CNTs, peptides capable of self-organizing into virus-like cages or tiny amphiphilic adhesion proteins were utilized. One of the benefits of these methods is the bottom-up organization of AuNPs into ordered arrays, which would otherwise require significantly more time-consuming top-down procedures. In one scenario, helical peptides were created to have a surface that resembled an alanine-coil-like structure on one side and a surface that resembled a leucine-zipper on the other. Peptides might interlock into an antiparallel hexamer around a SWNT of adequate size in this way. Convergent gold-binding sites would appear in pairs along the hexamer surface at the peptide ends after an extra cysteine was inserted at the N-terminus. As a result of the subsequent reduction of Au(III), TEM imaging revealed 2–4 nm-wide AuNPs arrays, with order imparted by the underlying CNT-peptide hybrid. Controlled hybrid nanostructures through protein-mediated noncovalent functionalization of carbon nanotubes.

Another intriguing aspect of CNTs is their large surface area, which is beneficial for enzyme support, such as in industrial biocatalysis. Increased enzyme stability and the ability to recycle enzymes are two advantages. Number of higher enzyme activity is obviously obtained with good spatial regulation of protein attachment onto the CNT surface, ensuring small molecule accessibility to the active site, just as it is with any other solid support. In contrast, if the enzyme catalytic site is involved in CNT interaction, there will be a significant reduction in substrate conversion to product, if not a complete loss [49]. Antifouling, sporicidal, and antimicrobial characteristics have been established in protein-CNT composites for use in self-cleaning paints and active coatings. Enzymes play an active part in these composites as a catalysis and CNT dispersing agent, while CNTs serve as enzyme supports and provide important mechanical qualities to the final material [50].

CNTs that have been functionalized with laminin promote neuronal adhesion and growth, as well as neurite elongation and the establishment of neural networks. They can also control axonal growth on flexible polyimide polymers, which means they have a lot of potential for nerve conduits in neural implants and nerve tissue engineering. The neural differentiation-promoting effect of CNTs on mesenchymal stem cells is thought to be mediated by neural growth factors adsorbing onto the tubes, emphasizing the importance of protein-CNT interactions in tissue engineering applications. When employed as a coating over a collagen sponge for bone regeneration, FGF-conjugated CNTs encouraged the proliferation of bone marrow stromal cells; following two weeks of implantation *in vivo*, the biomaterials were integrated with newly generated bone tissue [51–53].

3.5.4 CARBON NANOTUBES AS BIOSENSORS

A biosensor is an analytical instrument that combines a biological component with a physicochemical detector for the detection of an analyte. CNTs are being used in biosensing nanotechnology, which is a very intriguing application field for therapeutic monitoring and *in vitro* and *in vivo* diagnostics. Many researchers, for example, have combined carbon nanotubes with glucose-oxidase biosensors to improve blood sugar control in diabetic patients with greater precision and ease of manipulation than biosensors alone. Other CNT-enzyme biosensors have been created for therapeutic monitoring and diagnostics, such as CNT-based dehydrogenase biosensors or peroxidase and catalase biosensors [54, 55].

The sensitivity of the test for electrical detection of DNA was better with the alkaline phosphatase (ALP) enzyme connected to CNTs than with ALP alone. The sensitivity of the SWCNT-DNA sensor, which was created by combining SWCNTs with single-strand DNA (ssDNA), was significantly greater than that of typical fluorescence and hybridization experiments. Antigen detection may be added to this CNT-biosensor-linked experiment by applying specific antibody-antigen recognition. As a result, in illnesses where molecular markers exist, such as DNA or protein, it might give a quick and straightforward answer for molecular diagnostics [42]. CNTs can potentially be used to detect live cells. Subidya et al. summarized that the functionalized CNT devices could interact biocompatibly with live cells and identify biomolecules from these cells in real time [56]. In another study a hybrid film was developed by functionalizing vertically aligned carbon nanotube/polyethylene (VACNT/PE) with DNA and $Mn_3(PO_4)_2$, resulting in a high-electroactivity material. MDA-MB-231/$Mn_3(PO_4)_2$/DNA/VACNT/PE hybrid film was created by growing living human breast cancer cells

(MDA-MB-231) directly on the DNA/$Mn_3(PO_4)_2$ modified VACNT/PE hybrid film. Because the diffusion distance between cells and reaction sites was so low, researchers were able to develop a very sensitive approach for detecting reactive oxygen species (ROS) generated by cancer cells in response to pharmacological stimulation. The ROS molecules generated by living cells on the hybrid film can be quickly absorbed by the smart structure and converted to an electrical signal, the detection sensitivity of this *in situ* cell-attached hybrid film was more than six times that of cells in a culture medium [57]. Optical sensors may also be made out of carbon nanotubes. Barone and coworkers designed and disclosed SWNT-based NIR optical sensors. They may be able to control SWNT emission in response to the adsorption of certain biomolecules [58]. Using fluorescent SWNTs, Jin et al. were able to detect single-molecule H_2O_2 signaling from the epidermal growth factor receptor. This technology offers a novel way of looking at ROS signaling at the cellular level [59].

3.5.5 CNT USED IN BIOMEDICAL IMAGING

Biomedical imaging is an area that is undergoing extensive research and involves several methodologies from various sectors of study. This new technology can image the behavior of cells, tissues, organs, or the entire body at high resolution [60]. CNTs may be altered to be subjected to various techniques of testing because of their unique physical characteristics biomedical imaging to better understand and improve their functions and responses to their surroundings [61]. Fluorescence emission in the near infrared area is one way of biomedical imaging that is label-free and can be done at fast speed, allowing researchers to monitor nanotubes in live cells. Due to their high absorbance and the impurities in the form of metallic nanoparticles they contain, photoacoustic imaging and magnetic resonance imaging are two additional methods that can be performed on CNTs [62]. Optical features are common in SWNTs. Semiconducting SWNTs, for example, exhibit NIR photoluminescence characteristics and minimal autofluorescence. In the NIR range, intrinsic photoluminescence may permeate deep tissue beyond 1 mm. SWNTs were an appropriate material for NIR photoluminescence imaging because of these features. Raman or photoacoustic imaging may also be done using CNTs. By sonicating SWNTs with sodium cholate and then surfactant exchange, Welshe et al. created phospholipid-polyethylene glycol (PL-PEG)-coated SWNTs. Because the exchange procedure caused less damage, they considered this strategy was superior to directly sonicating SWNTs with PL-PEG [63]. PEG5000 was used to functionalize SWNTs, which was then combined with RGD at the top of PEF5000. For photoacoustic imaging of malignancies, the SWNTRGD can be utilized as a contrast agent [64]. Plain SWNTs or SWNTRGD at a dose of 1.2 mM were injected into two sets of mice with U87MG tumor xenografts. Those animals injected with SWNT-RGD showed a considerable increase in photoacoustic signal in the tumor when compared to control mice treated with simple SWNTs. Raman microscopy was used to corroborate these findings *ex vivo*. In living individuals, photoacoustic imaging of targeted SWNTs might help with cancer imaging and therapy [65].

3.5.6 CNTS USED AS DELIVERY CARRIER FOR CANCER THERAPY

Doxorubicin (DOX) is an anthracycline antibiotic that acts as a DNA intercalating agent and has been used to treat a variety of malignancies. It's commonly given intravenously, which means it has a poor dispersion, limited selectivity, and can't pass cellular barriers. Due to their potential to immobilize therapeutic molecules on the surface or in their hollow space and transport them through mammalian cell membranes, CNTs can be used as a new drug transporter to overcome these constraints associated with standard DOX delivery. On the oxidized SWCNT sidewall, DOX, monoclonal antibody, and fluorescein were combined to create an anticancer DDS. The monoclonal antibody identifies the tumor marker, carcinoembryonic antigen (CEA), and aids DOX binding to the intended target areas on cancer cells. When drug SWCNT complexes are delivered to WiDr colon cancer cells, they penetrate completely into the cells, releasing DOX into the nucleus while SWCNTs stay in the cytoplasm.

DOX may also be loaded onto polysaccharide materials [sodium alginate (ALG) and CHI] coated carboxyl functionalized SWCNT in another method. DOX binds to CNT at pH 7.4 and releases at a lower pH, as shown in lisosomes used in some tumor treatments. The folic acid receptors are overexpressed on the surface of cancer cells and therefore FA modified SWCNTs liposome increase the selectivity of DOX. DOX loading is aided by the usage of ALG, whereas FA binding is improved. The amount of DOX that enters the cell is high and to effective amounts [66].

The water-soluble SWCNT are non-covalently functionalized by polyethylene glycol 5000 (PL-PEG5000-NH_2) or covalently modified by

PEGylation on SWCNT with high degrees of p stacking of DOX with an ultrahigh loading capacity. The changes in pH modifies the drug binding and release, whereas the diameter of SWCNT alters the strength of p stacking of medicines. The cyclic arginine–glycine–aspartic acid (RGD) peptide conjugated to soluble SWCNT works as a ligand for integrin avb3 receptors, imparting recognition moieties and improving drug administration to integrin avb3-positive U87MG cells. When integrin avb3-negative MCF-7 cells are employed, however, there is no discernible improvement in RGD–SWCNT–DOX delivery [67].

Cisplatin (CDDP) is a platinum-based anticancer medication that is widely used to treat a variety of cancers. CDDP can be encapsulated into SWCNTs that have been shortened, then treated with strong acid and annealed in a high vacuum environment. Prostate cancer cells (PC3 and DU145) are inhibited *in vivo* by SWCNT–CDDP. However, the effect of released CDDP from SWCNT is not as strong as bare CDDP, which might be due to CDDP activity being lost during encapsulation [68].

KEYWORDS

- **bio-imaging**
- **covalent functionalization**
- **increase in surface area**
- **non-covalent functionalization**
- **tissue regeneration scaffold**

REFERENCES

1. Ibrahim, Y. H., Regdon, G., Hamedelniel, E. I., & Sovány, T., (2020). Review of recently used techniques and materials to improve the efficiency of orally administered proteins/peptides. *DARU Journal of Pharmaceutical Sciences, 28*(1), 403–416.
2. Sireesha, M., Jagadeesh, B. V., Kranthi, K. A. S., & Ramakrishna, S., (2018). A review on carbon nanotubes in biosensor devices and their applications in medicine. *Nanocomposites, 4*(2), 36–57.
3. Gurjar, P. N., Chouksey, S., Patil, G., Naik, N., & Agrawal, S. S., (2013). Carbon nanotubes: Pharmaceutical applications. *Asian Journal of Biomedical and Pharmaceutical Sciences, 3*(23), 8.

4. Lehman, J. H., Terrones, M., Mansfield, E., Hurst, K. E., & Meunier, V., (2011). Evaluating the characteristics of multiwall carbon nanotubes. *Carbon, 49*(8), 2581–2602.
5. Prasek, J., Drbohlavova, J., Chomoucka, J., Hubalek, J., Jasek, O., Adam, V., & Kizek, R., (2011). Methods for carbon nanotubes synthesis. *Journal of Materials Chemistry, 21*(40), 15872–15884.
6. Gupta, N., Gupta, S. M., & Sharma, S., (2019). Carbon nanotubes: Synthesis, properties and engineering applications. *Carbon Letters, 29*(5), 419–447.
7. Burghard, M., (2005). Electronic and vibrational properties of chemically modified single-wall carbon nanotubes. *Surface Science Reports, 58*(1–4), 1–109.
8. Merlen, A., Buijnsters, J. G., & Pardanaud, C., (2017). A guide to and review of the use of multiwavelength Raman spectroscopy for characterizing defective aromatic carbon solids: From graphene to amorphous carbons. *Coatings, 7*(10), 153.
9. Bianco, A., (2004). Carbon nanotubes for the delivery of therapeutic molecules. *Expert Opinion on Drug Delivery, 1*(1), 57–65.
10. Gandhi, S. N., Agrawal, S., Nagendran, S., & Gurjar, P., (2020). Iron oxide nanoparticles: Tuning to advanced nano drug delivery. *Nanoscience & Nanotechnology-Asia, 10*(6), 734–747.
11. Zhuang, W. R., Wang, Y., Cui, P. F., Xing, L., Lee, J., Kim, D., Jiang, H. L., & Oh, Y. K., (2019). Applications of π-π stacking interactions in the design of drug-delivery systems. *Journal of Controlled Release, 294*, 311–326.
12. Liu, Z., Tabakman, S., Welsher, K., & Dai, H., (2009). Carbon nanotubes in biology and medicine: *In vitro* and *in vivo* detection, imaging and drug delivery. *Nano Research, 2*(2), 85–120.
13. John, A. A., Subramanian, A. P., Vellayappan, M. V., Balaji, A., Mohandas, H., & Jaganathan, S. K., (2015). Carbon nanotubes and graphene as emerging candidates in neuroregeneration and neurodrug delivery. *International Journal of Nanomedicine, 10*, 4267.
14. Ma, P. C., Siddiqui, N. A., Marom, G., & Kim, J. K., (2010). Dispersion and functionalization of carbon nanotubes for polymer-based nanocomposites: A review. *Composites Part A: Applied Science and Manufacturing, 41*(10), 1345–1367.
15. Negri, V., Pacheco-Torres, J., Calle, D., & López-Larrubia, P., (2020). Carbon nanotubes in biomedicine. *Surface-modified Nanobiomaterials for Electrochemical and Biomedicine Applications*, 177–217.
16. He, H., Xiao, D., Pham-Huy, L. A., Dramou, P., & Pham-Huy, C., (2017). Carbon nanotubes used as nanocarriers in drug and biomolecule delivery. *Drug Delivery Approaches and Nanosystems*, 163–212.
17. Balasubramanian, K., & Burghard, M., (2005). Chemically functionalized carbon nanotubes. *Small, 1*(2), 180–192.
18. Hou, P. X., Liu, C., & Cheng, H. M., (2008). Purification of carbon nanotubes. *Carbon, 46*(15), 2003–2025.
19. Karousis, N., Suarez-Martinez, I., Ewels, C. P., & Tagmatarchis, N., (2016). Structure, properties, functionalization, and applications of carbon nanohorns. *Chemical Reviews, 116*(8), 4850–4883.
20. Lee, J., Kim, M., Hong, C. K., & Shim, S. E., (2007). Measurement of the dispersion stability of pristine and surface-modified multiwalled carbon nanotubes in various nonpolar and polar solvents. *Measurement Science and Technology, 18*(12), 3707.

21. Naqvi, S. T. R., Rasheed, T., Hussain, D., Ul Haq, M. N., Majeed, S., Ahmed, N., & Nawaz, R., (2020). Modification strategies for improving the solubility/dispersion of carbon nanotubes. *Journal of Molecular Liquids, 297*, 111919.
22. Choudhary, V., & Gupta, A., (2011). Polymer/carbon nanotube nanocomposites. *Carbon Nanotubes-Polymer Nanocomposites, 2011*, 65–90.
23. Gatti, T., Vicentini, N., Mba, M., & Menna, E., (2016). Organic functionalized carbon nanostructures for functional polymer-based nanocomposites. *European Journal of Organic Chemistry, 2016*(6), 1071–1090.
24. Dubey, R., Dutta, D., Sarkar, A., & Chattopadhyay, P., (2021). Functionalized carbon nanotubes: Synthesis, properties and applications in water purification, drug delivery, and material and biomedical sciences. *Nanoscale Advances, 3*(20), 5722–5744.
25. Zhao, Y. L., & Stoddart, J. F., (2009). Noncovalent functionalization of single-walled carbon nanotubes. *Accounts of Chemical Research, 42*(8), 1161–1171.
26. Fang, M., Wang, K., Lu, H., Yang, Y., & Nutt, S., (2009). Covalent polymer functionalization of graphene nanosheets and mechanical properties of composites. *Journal of Materials Chemistry, 19*(38), 7098–7105.
27. Dyke, C. A., & Tour, J. M., (2004). Overcoming the insolubility of carbon nanotubes through high degrees of sidewall functionalization. *Chemistry–A European Journal, 10*(4), 812–817.
28. Akbar, S., & Taimoor, A. A., (2009). Functionalization of carbon nanotubes: Manufacturing techniques and properties of customized nanocomponents for molecular-level technology. *Recent Patents on Nanotechnology, 3*(2), 154–161.
29. Zhang, W., Zhang, Z., & Zhang, Y., (2011). The application of carbon nanotubes in target drug delivery systems for cancer therapies. *Nanoscale Research Letters, 6*(1), 1–22.
30. Jha, R., Singh, A., Sharma, P., & Fuloria, N. K., (2020). Smart carbon nanotubes for drug delivery system: A comprehensive study. *Journal of Drug Delivery Science and Technology, 58*, 101811.
31. Stueckle, T. A., Sargent, L., Rojanasakul, Y., & Wang, L., (2016). Genotoxicity and carcinogenic potential of carbon nanomaterials. *Biomedical Applications and Toxicology of Carbon Nanomaterials*, 267–332.
32. Ryman-Rasmussen, J. P., Cesta, M. F., Brody, A. R., Shipley-Phillips, J. K., Everitt, J. I., Tewksbury, E. W., Moss, O. R., et al., (2009). Inhaled carbon nanotubes reach the subpleural tissue in mice. *Nature Nanotechnology, 4*(11), 747–751.
33. Mitchell, L., Lauer, F., Burchiel, S., & McDonald, J., (2009). Mechanisms for how inhaled multiwalled carbon nanotubes suppress systemic immune function in mice. *Nature Nanotechnology, 4*(7), 451–456.
34. Palmer, B. C., Phelan-Dickenson, S. J., & DeLouise, L. A., (2019). Multi-walled carbon nanotube oxidation dependent keratinocyte cytotoxicity and skin inflammation. *Particle and Fiber Toxicology, 16*(1), 1–15.
35. Budhathoki-Uprety, J., Harvey, J. D., Isaac, E., Williams, R. M., Galassi, T. V., Langenbacher, R. E., & Heller, D. A., (2017). Polymer cloaking modulates the carbon nanotube protein corona and delivery into cancer cells. *Journal of Materials Chemistry B, 5*(32), 6637–6644.
36. Coccini, T., Roda, E., Sarigiannis, D., Mustarelli, P., Quartarone, E., Profumo, A., & Manzo, L., (2010). Effects of water-soluble functionalized multi-walled carbon

nanotubes examined by different cytotoxicity methods in human astrocyte D384 and lung A549 cells. *Toxicology, 269*(1), 41–53.
37. Ursini, C. L., Cavallo, D., Fresegna, A. M., Ciervo, A., Maiello, R., Buresti, G., Casciardi, S., et al., (2012). Comparative cyto-genotoxicity assessment of functionalized and pristine multiwalled carbon nanotubes on human lung epithelial cells. *Toxicology in Vitro, 26*(6), 831–840.
38. Huang, B., (2020). Carbon nanotubes and their polymeric composites: The applications in tissue engineering. *Biomanufacturing Reviews, 5*(1), 1–26.
39. Patel, D. K., Dutta, S. D., Ganguly, K., Kim, J. W., & Lim, K. T., (2021). Enhanced osteogenic potential of unzipped carbon nanotubes for tissue engineering. *Journal of Biomedical Materials Research Part A, 109*(10), 1869–1880.
40. MacDonald, R. A., Laurenzi, B. F., Viswanathan, G., Ajayan, P. M., & Stegemann, J. P., (2005). Collagen–carbon nanotube composite materials as scaffolds in tissue engineering. *Journal of Biomedical Materials Research Part A: An Official Journal of The Society for Biomaterials, The Japanese Society for Biomaterials, and The Australian Society for Biomaterials and the Korean Society for Biomaterials, 74*(3), 489–496.
41. Correa-Duarte, M. A., Wagner, N., Rojas-Chapana, J., Morsczeck, C., Thie, M., & Giersig, M., (2004). Fabrication and biocompatibility of carbon nanotube-based 3D networks as scaffolds for cell seeding and growth. *Nano Letters, 4*(11), 2233–2236.
42. Liao, H., Paratala, B., Sitharaman, B., & Wang, Y., (2011). Applications of carbon nanotubes in biomedical studies. In: *Biomedical Nanotechnology* (pp. 223–241). Springer.
43. Stan, M. S., Strugari, A. F., Balas, M., & Nica, I. C., (2018). Biomedical applications of carbon nanotubes with improved properties. In: *Fullerens, Graphenes and Nanotubes* (pp. 31–65). Elsevier.
44. Ansari, S. Y., Ansari, S. A., Alshammari, F., & Anwar, S., (2022). CNT-based nano medicine from synthesis to therapeutic application. In: *Innovative Approaches for Nanobiotechnology in Healthcare Systems* (pp. 175–211). IGI Global.
45. Pantarotto, D., Singh, R., McCarthy, D., Erhardt, M., Briand, J. P., Prato, M., Kostarelos, K., & Bianco, A., (2004). Functionalized carbon nanotubes for plasmid DNA gene delivery. *Angewandte Chemie International Edition, 43*(39), 5242–5246.
46. Kam, N. W. S., & Dai, H., (2005). Carbon nanotubes as intracellular protein transporters: Generality and biological functionality. *Journal of the American Chemical Society, 127*(16), 6021–6026.
47. Tonelli, F., Lacerda, S., Silva, M., Avila, E., Ladeira, L., Franca, L., & Resende, R., (2014). Gene delivery to *Nile tilapia* spermatogonial stem cells using carboxi-functionalized multiwall carbon nanotubes. *RSC Advances, 4*(72), 37985–37987.
48. Grigoryan, G., Kim, Y. H., Acharya, R., Axelrod, K., Jain, R. M., Willis, L., Drndic, M., et al., (2011). Computational design of virus-like protein assemblies on carbon nanotube surfaces. *Science, 332*(6033), 1071–1076.
49. Karajanagi, S. S., Vertegel, A. A., Kane, R. S., & Dordick, J. S., (2004). Structure and function of enzymes adsorbed onto single-walled carbon nanotubes. *Langmuir, 20*(26), 11594–11599.
50. Dinu, C. Z., Zhu, G., Bale, S. S., Anand, G., Reeder, P. J., Sanford, K., Whited, G., et al., (2010). Enzyme-based nanoscale composites for use as active decontamination surfaces. *Advanced Functional Materials, 20*(3), 392–398.

51. Chen, Y. S., & Hsiue, G. H., (2013). Directing neural differentiation of mesenchymal stem cells by carboxylated multiwalled carbon nanotubes. *Biomaterials, 34*(21), 4936–4944.
52. Fabbro, A., Bosi, S., Ballerini, L., & Prato, M., (2012). Carbon nanotubes: Artificial nanomaterials to engineer single neurons and neuronal networks. *ACS Chemical Neuroscience, 3*(8), 611–618.
53. Park, S. Y., Choi, D. S., Jin, H. J., Park, J., Byun, K. E., Lee, K. B., & Hong, S., (2011). Polarization-controlled differentiation of human neural stem cells using synergistic cues from the patterns of carbon nanotube monolayer coating. *ACS Nano, 5*(6), 4704–4711.
54. Du, F., Zhu, L., & Dai, L., (2017). Carbon nanotube-based electrochemical biosensors. *Biosensors Based on Nanomaterials and Nanodevices, 19*, 273–294.
55. Zhu, Y., Wang, L., & Xu, C., (2011). *Carbon Nanotubes in Biomedicine and Biosensing.* Intech Open.
56. Sudibya, H. G., Ma, J., Dong, X., Ng, S., Li, L. J., Liu, X. W., & Chen, P., (2009). Interfacing glycosylated carbon-nanotube-network devices with living cells to detect dynamic secretion of biomolecules. *Angewandte Chemie International Edition, 48*(15), 2723–2726.
57. Hu, F. X., Kang, Y. J., Du, F., Zhu, L., Xue, Y. H., Chen, T., Dai, L. M., & Li, C. M., (2015). Living cells directly growing on a DNA/$Mn_3(PO_4)_2$-immobilized and vertically aligned CNT array as a free-standing hybrid film for highly sensitive in situ detection of released superoxide anions. *Advanced Functional Materials, 25*(37), 5924–5932.
58. Barone, P. W., Baik, S., Heller, D. A., & Strano, M. S., (2005). Near-infrared optical sensors based on single-walled carbon nanotubes. *Nature Materials, 4*(1), 86–92.
59. Jin, H., Heller, D. A., Kalbacova, M., Kim, J. H., Zhang, J., Boghossian, A. A., Maheshri, N., & Strano, M. S., (2010). Detection of single-molecule H_2O_2 signaling from epidermal growth factor receptor using fluorescent single-walled carbon nanotubes. *Nature Nanotechnology, 5*(4), 302–309.
60. Gong, H., Peng, R., & Liu, Z., (2013). Carbon nanotubes for biomedical imaging: The recent advances. *Advanced Drug Delivery Reviews, 65*(15), 1951–1963.
61. Tong, L., Liu, Y., Dolash, B. D., Jung, Y., Slipchenko, M. N., Bergstrom, D. E., & Cheng, J. X., (2012). Label-free imaging of semiconducting and metallic carbon nanotubes in cells and mice using transient absorption microscopy. *Nature Nanotechnology, 7*(1), 56–61.
62. De La Zerda, A., Zavaleta, C., Keren, S., Vaithilingam, S., Bodapati, S., Liu, Z., Levi, J., et al., (2008). Carbon nanotubes as photoacoustic molecular imaging agents in living mice. *Nature Nanotechnology, 3*(9), 557–562.
63. Welsher, K., Liu, Z., Sherlock, S. P., Robinson, J. T., Chen, Z., Daranciang, D., & Dai, H., (2009). A route to brightly fluorescent carbon nanotubes for near-infrared imaging in mice. *Nature Nanotechnology, 4*(11), 773–780.
64. Xue, Y., (2017). Carbon nanotubes for biomedical applications. In: *Industrial Applications of Carbon Nanotubes* (pp. 323–346). Elsevier.
65. Wu, D., Huang, L., Jiang, M. S., & Jiang, H., (2014). Contrast agents for photoacoustic and thermoacoustic imaging: A review. *International Journal of Molecular Sciences, 15*(12), 23616–23639.
66. Heister, E., Neves, V., Tîlmaciu, C., Lipert, K., Beltrán, V. S., Coley, H. M., Silva, S. R. P., & McFadden, J., (2009). Triple functionalization of single-walled carbon nanotubes

with doxorubicin, a monoclonal antibody, and a fluorescent marker for targeted cancer therapy. *Carbon, 47*(9), 2152–2160.

67. Zhang, X., Meng, L., Lu, Q., Fei, Z., & Dyson, P. J., (2009). Targeted delivery and controlled release of doxorubicin to cancer cells using modified single wall carbon nanotubes. *Biomaterials, 30*(30), 6041–6047.
68. Tripisciano, C., Kraemer, K., Taylor, A., & Borowiak-Palen, E., (2009). Single-wall carbon nanotubes based anticancer drug delivery system. *Chemical Physics Letters, 478*(4–6), 200–205.

CHAPTER 4

Application of Carbon Nanotubes for Targeted Drug Delivery

SANJANA SUBRAMANIAN[1,2] and SARA JONES[1]

[1]*Rajiv Gandhi Center for Biotechnology, Thiruvananthapuram, Kerala, India*

[2]*Vellore Institute of Technology (VIT), Vellore, Tamil Nadu, India*

ABSTRACT

Carbon nanotubes (CNTs) are carbon tubes on the scale of 1 to 100 nanometers, at which they acquire molecular properties such as surface curvature, pi orbital mismatch, orbital hybridization, and an increase in surface area, which are not observed at the macro-level. These properties make them suitable for the use of targeted drug delivery. Artificially produced through the electric arc discharge and laser ablation methods, CNTs had long been considered impractical until recently. Administered orally or through injections, CNTs interact directly with the body's cells. Mainly utilized in cancer therapy, they offer specialized treatment. Besides cancer therapy, they have found uses as nano-carriers as well in targeted medicine delivery, gene therapy, and CNS disease treatments. Although expensive, the solutions they bring to the biomedical industry are promising. This chapter explores methods of CNT production, types of CNTs and their roles in customized medical treatment, their advantages over conventional medicines, as well as their drawbacks.

4.1 INTRODUCTION

Nanotechnology is the study of atoms on an extremely small scale of 1 to 100 nanometers. At the quantum level, these atoms acquire different properties

Carbon Nanotubes for Biomedical Applications and Healthcare.
Chin Hua Chia, Swati Gokul Talele, Ann Rose Abraham, and A. K. Haghi, (Eds.)

than they do at the macro level. Such properties in carbon nanotubes include great tensile strength, high thermal conductivity, the ability to function as both metals and semiconductors, and chirality. These properties can be exploited to great effect in diverse fields such as medicine, electronics, and green energy. One such application, which we will discuss here, is the use of carbon nanotubes in targeted drug delivery.

4.2 CARBON NANOTUBES: AN OVERVIEW

Carbon nanotubes (CNTs) were invented in 1991 by Sumio Iijima, with light-weight properties and great versatility; however, due to prohibitive costs and high production temperatures of over 500°C, they were until recently considered impractical. Currently, with the advent of cheap production techniques and low temperatures, they have found major use in the biomedical industry.

On the macro-level, carbon atoms in graphite bond to each other, both with strong covalent bonds and with weak van der Waals' forces, forming honeycomb lattice structures. However, in the case of CNTs, carbon atoms roll themselves into cylindrical shapes. The covalent sp^2 bonds between each carbon atom result in high axial strength and Young's modulus, making CNTs the most widely used nanotechnology [1, 2].

CNTs have a tensile strength 100 times greater than that of steel, greater electrical conductivity than copper, and greater thermal conductivity than diamond (also known as ballistic conduction). CNTs are as versatile in form as they are in application. Several types of CNTs include:

- single-walled nanotubes (SWNTs);
- multi-walled nanotubes (MWNTs);
- double-walled nanotubes (DWNTs);
- long nanotubes;
- short nanotubes;
- open nanotubes;
- closed nanotubes;
- spiral nanotubes.

Of all these types, SWNTs and MWNTs are the most widely used. SWNTs are essentially single cylinders of graphene with approximate diameters of 1 nm and are one-dimensional in nature, giving them excellent electrical conductivity properties and making them a viable replacement for conventional electric wires. MWNTs consist of multiple layers of graphite wrapped over each other to form tubular structures, with diameters of 4 to 100 nm. Structurally, they are not sound, but have alternating amounts of flexibility and rigidity, with great stress resistance and superconductivity, making them viable in electronics as well [3].

DWNTs have similar properties as SWNTs, consisting of two CNTs, forming a double-layer configuration of two folding graphene sheets. They have greater strength, thermal stability, and chemical resistance than SWNTs [1].

Carbon nanotubes are an artificial construction and cannot naturally be found on earth. CNTs are mainly produced with two methods: electric arc discharge and laser ablation.

Electric arc discharge works on the principle of the sublimation of carbon. In this method, two graphite electrodes are placed in a water-cooled chamber, immersed in an inert atmosphere of a noble gas such as helium or argon. The cathode is fixed and the anode is mobile. The anode is moved towards the cathode such that a small current of 100A and an intense heat of 4,000 K are generated between the two electrodes. This sublimates the carbon and produces CNTs.

In the case of electric arc discharge, two kinds of CNT synthesis methods can be performed:

1. **Evaporation of Pure Graphite:** Producing CNT deposits on the cathode and soot on the chamber walls.
2. **Co-Evaporation of Graphite and Metal:** A transition metal catalyst is introduced into the chamber, producing CNTs along with transition metal deposits and collarets on the deposits.

Laser ablation is the process of carbon vaporization. This occurs by exposing the surface of a graphite disk to a pulsed laser in a quartz tube. The vaporized graphite produces carbon species, which are then channeled into a high-density helium/argon flow and deposited in a copper collector. Here too, it is possible to add metallic catalysts to the graphite surface (Table 4.1) [4, 5].

TABLE 4.1 Methods of CNT Production

Method	Mechanism	Medium	Temperature	Inert Gas	Products
Electric arc discharge	Electricity passed through electrodes	Inert water-cooled reaction chamber	4,000 K	Helium, argon	Polyhedral graphitic nanoparticles, MWNTs, SWNTs
Laser ablation	Laser beam scans the surface of the graphite disk	Quartz tube in temperature-controlled furnace	1473.15 K (1,200°C)	Helium, argon	Empty or filled graphitic nanoparticles, spherical metallic particles, MWNTs, SWNTs

4.3 CARBON NANOTUBES AS DRUG DELIVERY SYSTEM

The vast majority of CNTs in medicinal treatment have been employed in cancer therapy [6]. Conventional treatments for cancer include surgery and chemotherapy. Surgery is effective on detectable tumors, but not against individual cancer cells that circulate through the bloodstream and are responsible for metastasis. Chemotherapy is effective but has deleterious side-effects on healthy cells as well as cancerous cells, and many patients cannot withstand the treatment. In light of these limitations on mainstream treatments, CNTs are rapidly emerging as a viable option which targets highly specific cells and avoid damage to surrounding tissues and organs, unlike both conventional surgery and chemotherapy.

CNTs have unique physiochemical properties which allow them to be used in cutting-edge drug delivery systems. They exhibit surface curvature, leading to pi orbital mismatch, orbital hybridization, and an increase in surface area, making them ideal in targeted drug delivery. Surface curvature causes an increase in their solubility and therefore a corresponding increase in cellular absorption. Though the mechanisms are unclear, it is known that CNTs interact both directly with blood and with antigen-presenting cells, gaining entry into mammalian cells. This feature is especially important in cancer treatment, as with their entry into the bloodstream, CNTs can be absorbed into cancer cells via their selectively permeable membrane, cause DNA damage, and induce apoptosis. In this case, CNTs directly function as drugs as graphene is a cytotoxin which affects cell metabolism.

They can be administered orally and through injections. CNTs are commonly administered through abdominal, subcutaneous, and intravenous injections and circulate through the blood and lymphatic systems until they reach their target. CNTs tend to accumulate in the lymph node when they are injected and f-SWCNTs appear to be easily metabolized by the body [7].

These same qualities which make CNTs so effective in drug delivery and medicine are also responsible for potential problems such as poor target delivery and cytotoxicity. To prevent such issues from occurring, CNTs have been subject to biocompatibility tests and have undergone biomodification so as to prevent bioaccumulation in the bloodstream (Table 4.2).

TABLE 4.2 Advantages and Disadvantages of Cancer Treatments

Cancer Treatments	Benefits	Drawbacks
Surgery	• Useful in removing large tumors. • Keyhole surgery can be employed for small tumors.	• Not very effective against inoperable tumors. • Not effective against individual cancer cells. • Narrow in scope.
Chemotherapy	• Has wider reach than surgery. • Effective against metastatic cells.	• Destroys healthy cells, tissues, and organs. • Serious side-effects. • Many patients cannot withstand it.
CNTs	• Highly specific, customized treatment. • Does not affect healthy cells, tissues, and organs.	• Poor target delivery. • Potential cytotoxicity. • Possible bioaccumulation in bloodstream.

To be truly effective in drug delivery, CNTs need to have high solubility and absorption in the gastrointestinal tract and even dispersion throughout the body.

To increase the efficiency of CNT dispersion, several methods of modification have been proposed: covalent and non-covalent modifications. Subgroups of CNTs that are particularly well-suited for drug delivery methods include functional CNTs (f-CNTs). These have functional groups attached to the outer surface of the nanotubes, thereby increasing solubility and making them viable drug carriers, in the form of covalent modification. Functional modification of CNTs allows them to act as nano-carriers of drugs as they can store the relevant medicine on their surface. Anti-cancer drugs such as cis-platin and doxorubicin have been attached to CNTs in this manner, and CNTs are capable of acting as nano-carriers to anti-cancer proteins such as ricin A chain protein toxins, IgY antibodies, and mAbs as well.

Covalent functionalization gives great stability to the functional groups which are attached to the CNTs. Commonly attached functional groups include hydrophilic ones such as OH and COOH, which are attached to CNTs by oxidation treatment, including by dousing the CNTs in acid solution and creating small gaps or defects in the tubes in which COOH groups sit. These functional groups aid in cutting CNTs into short tubes, altering the nanotubes' electronic properties and lengths and thereby allowing them to be used in versatile drug delivery systems. The functional groups can also interact with other compounds such as SOCl to form other functional groups which can be used in drug delivery systems. Although covalent functionalization has potential future uses in CNT modification, it is difficult to control for specificity in location when the functional groups attach to the CNTS.

Besides functional groups, it is also possible to attach polymers to CNTs, which form colloidal dispersions in a three-step method:

- Disperse the functionalized CNTs to form a colloidal dispersion;
- Join the f-CNTs with a polymer matrix to form a composite; and
- Modify the composite with radiation.

In contrast, non-covalent modifications involve enveloping the CNTs in polymers, which increases their solubility. Non-covalent modifications depend on hydrophobic and π-π bonding between the carbon atoms and the atoms they interact with.

Other forms of dispersion used are surfactant-assisted dispersion, solvent dispersion, and biomolecular dispersion.

CNTs are not the only carbon nanomaterials to be used for medicinal purposes. Other than CNTs, other carbon-based nanomaterials (CBNs) can be divided into:

- graphenes;
- fullerenes;
- nanodiamonds; and
- mesoporous carbon.

Similar to CNTs, these other CBNs have large amounts of surface area, enabling them to function as effective drug carriers.

Due to their large surface area, great thermal conductivity properties, optical transparency, and strength, graphene nanoribbons (GNRs) and graphene quantum dots (GQDs) are also used in drug delivery, undergoing functional modification just like CNTs.

GNRs are created by cutting graphene sheets into thin tiles with increased width. They gain semimetal properties at the quantum level and have increased mammalian cell uptake. GNRs are planar in nature, quasi-one-dimensional with high thermal and electrical conductivity. They are non-toxic and show promise in drug delivery and cancer treatment.

GQDs are produced by slicing graphene into small pieces 2–20 nm in length. These are non-toxic and zero-dimensional, currently used in bioimaging.

Nano-diamonds (NDs) are tetrahedrally bonded carbon atoms in the form of a three-dimensional cubic lattice. They can be grouped into fluorescent nano-diamonds (FNDs) and detonation nano-diamonds (DNDs). DNDs are manufactured with explosive shocks, whereas FNDs are formed in settings of high pressure and temperature. NDs are versatile in nature: besides drug delivery, NDs are now being used in gene therapy, bone surgery, and scaffold, tissue engineering.

Fullerenes are an allotrope of carbon, comprising carbon atoms stacked in a spherical shape. As they do not have any toxic effects in humans, research is undergoing regarding their potential role in drug delivery.

Porous carbon can be grouped according to the size of their pores:

- microporous (<2 nm);
- mesoporous (2–50 nm);
- macroporous (<50 nm).

Mixed porous carbon is a combination of all three and has the greatest surface area of all, and mesoporous carbons are used in drug delivery [5].

4.4 SUMMARY

CNTs are witnessing a surge in research, development, and use in therapy. For long were out of reach of conventional cancer treatments due to impracticality and expense, they are fast emerging as a viable alternative to conventional surgery and chemotherapy. Possessing extraordinary properties such as increased strength and surface area and curvature at the quantum level, they provide optimum treatment while avoiding the typical pitfalls associated with the older cancer therapies. While they are not without their own disadvantages, CBNs in general and CNTs in particular are a promising new avenue in smart, optimized treatment, providing a new solution to old problems.

KEYWORDS

- **cancer**
- **disease**
- **drug delivery**
- **graphene**
- **nano-carrier**
- **nanotubes**

REFERENCES

1. Debnath, S. K., & Srivastava, R., (2021). Drug delivery with carbon-based nanomaterials as versatile nanocarriers: Progress and prospects. *Frontiers in Nanotechnology, 3*, 15.
2. Journet, C., & Bernier, P., (1998). Production of carbon nanotubes. *Applied Physics A: Materials Science & Processing, 67*(1).
3. Kantamneni, H., & Gollakota, A., (2013). Carbon nanotubes-based systems for targeted drug delivery: A review. *Int. J. Eng. Res. Technol., 2*, 1–8.
4. Pitroda, J., Jethwa, B., & Dave, S. K., (2016). A critical review on carbon nanotubes. *Int. J. Constr. Res. Civ. Eng., 2*(5), 36–42.
5. Raval, J. P., Joshi, P., & Chejara, D. R., (2018). Carbon nanotube for targeted drug delivery. In: *Applications of Nanocomposite Materials in Drug Delivery* (pp. 203–216). Woodhead Publishing.
6. Wong, B. S., Yoong, S. L., Jagusiak, A., Panczyk, T., Ho, H. K., Ang, W. H., & Pastorin, G., (2013). Carbon nanotubes for delivery of small molecule drugs. *Advanced Drug Delivery Reviews, 65*(15), 1964–2015.
7. Zhang, W., Zhang, Z., & Zhang, Y., (2011). The application of carbon nanotubes in target drug delivery systems for cancer therapies. *Nanoscale Research Letters, 6*(1), 1–22.

PART II

Carbon Nanotubes for Medical Diagnosis and Therapy

CHAPTER 5

Carbon Nanotubes in Cancer Diagnosis and Therapy

RONY RAJAN PAUL and MARIA MATHEW

Department of Chemistry, CMS College, Kottayam, Kerala

ABSTRACT

During the past few years, the field of nanomaterials has gained great progress due to their great potential in biomedical applications. Among the various nanomaterials, carbon nanotubes (CNTs), due to their unique physical and chemical properties have gained significant interest in the field of cancer diagnosis and therapy. Versatile functionalization, bio-compatibility, and unique electronic properties are some important features that make CNTs popular in this field. CNTs are capable of detecting the cancerous cells as well as acts as the tool for the targeted delivery of drugs or small therapeutic molecules to these cells.

5.1 INTRODUCTION

Nanotechnology has received much attention in recent years as an important tool for improving the safety of life and for promoting the health of society. As a branch of engineering, it deals with the understanding and control of matter in the nanometer scale. Recently, nanomaterials have demonstrated great applications in the biomedical field, for the effective delivery of biologically active cargo into the required sites for the cancer diagnosis and therapy [1–3]. Among the various nanomaterials developed till date, it was the CNTs that revolutionized the biomedical research due to their superior performance over other nanomaterials. Their unique electrical, optical,

Carbon Nanotubes for Biomedical Applications and Healthcare.
Chin Hua Chia, Swati Gokul Talele, Ann Rose Abraham, and A. K. Haghi, (Eds.)

magnetic, and bio-chemical properties [4] make them an efficient tool for the diagnosis and for transporting and translocating therapeutic molecules. Also their ability to cross the cell membrane is noteworthy. Recent researches are mainly focused on the use of functionalized CNTs for targeted drug delivery in the sites of interest [5–7].

Cancer is a disease in which abnormal cells divide uncontrollably with the potential to invade or spread to other parts of the body and thus eventually destroy the tissues. Among all the cancer treatment options, chemotherapy continues to be the most important one for killing free cancer cells and removing undetectable tumors. Despite its importance in cancer treatment, the drawbacks of chemotherapy such as toxicity, lack of selectivity of drugs for cancer tissues and cells, insolubility, and inability to exceed blood-tissue barrier [8, 9] forced the researchers to work for a drug that is capable of targeting the cancerous mass with broad therapeutic properties. The unusual properties of CNTs offer an opportunity to overcome chemotherapeutic limitations. CNTs are mainly used for cancer cell imaging, and their ability to enter into the cells are independent of the cell type and the functional groups present at their surface. Based on the *in-vitro* and *in-vivo* results obtained from various research works, it has been proved that CNTs are biocompatible. In addition to their biocompatibility, their transportability in biological fluids makes them a useful tool for all kinds of diagnosis and therapeutic as well as drug delivery applications [10]. In this chapter, we have summarized the properties of CNTs, methods of their functionalization and their applications in cancer diagnosis and treatment.

5.2 CARBON NANOTUBES

Carbon nanotubes, first discovered by Iijima in 1991 [11], are composed of graphite sheets rolled up into a cylinder like structure with the appearance of latticework fence (Figure 5.1). Mainly there are two types of CNTs – multi-walled carbon nanotubes (MWCNTs) composed of multiple layers graphene sheets and single walled carbon nanotubes (SWCNTs) consisting of a single graphene sheet. CNTs are produced mainly by three methods: laser ablation, electric arc discharge method and thermal or plasma enhanced chemical vapor deposition (CVD) [12]. CNTs possess peculiar physiochemical properties such as high aspect ratio, high surface area, high mechanical strength, high electrical and thermal conductivity, and are ultra-lightweighted [13]. Additionally, functionalized or modified CNTs have enhanced solubility in watery solutions [14]: solubility is one of the main properties that ensures biocompatibility under physiological conditions [15]. All these are some of the major advantages that make CNTs a hopeful candidate for enormous biomedical applications [16].

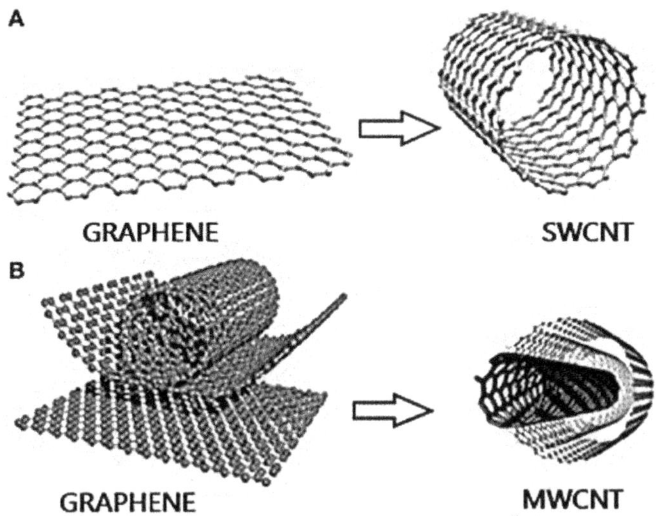

FIGURE 5.1 Structural representation of (A) MWCNT; and (B) SWCNT.

5.3 CNT FUNCTIONALIZATION

As mentioned earlier that, the solubility of CNTs in aqueous medium is the main factor that limits their applications in the biomedical field. However, this limitation can be addressed through functionalization [17]. Their bio-solubility can be enhanced *via* two main techniques such as non-covalent and covalent functionalization. CNTs can be divided into two zones depending upon their reactivity towards various functional groups, known as tips and side walls. Tips have stronger functional group bonding capabilities than side walls.

5.3.1 NON-COVALENT FUNCTIONALIZATION

Non-covalent functionalization can be achieved *via* various non-covalent interactions like π-stacking, hydrophobic, and van-der Waals interactions of CNTs with a wide range of molecules. According to some reports, these non-covalent interactions helps to preserve the atomic structure and electronic properties of CNTs. The charge developed on the CNT surface during chemical treatment can adsorb molecules *via* ionic interactions. However, non-covalent bonds provide weak strength to CNTs which makes them unsuitable for tumor-targeted drug delivery [18].

5.3.2 COVALENT FUNCTIONALIZATION

It is the chemical grafting of molecules on to the sp^2 hybridized carbon atoms of π-conjugated skeleton of CNTs. Covalent functionalization can be achieved through surface oxidation under strongly acidic conditions [19]. There are two main approaches for covalent functionalization of carbon nanotubes; (i) "ends and defect" modification; and (ii) "sidewall" modification:

1. **Ends and Defects:** Ends of CNTs are more reactive than side walls. Treating CNTs with oxidizing agents introduces functional groups like carboxylic acid, ketone, alcohol, and ester at CNT's end and defect sites, thus leaving the ends open and possibly cutting and shortening CNTs.
2. **Side Wall Functionalization:** Here CNTs can be cut and oxidized to produce a certain number of carboxylic acid groups and are subsequently derivatized with different types of molecules.

Thus, surface functionalization enhanced the water solubility of CNTs and their biocompatibility profile is completely transformed. Carboxyl groups introduced at the CNT surface can produce high negative charges which enhance the hydrophilicity of these materials [19, 20]. Binding with hydrophilic polymers such as polyethylene glycol (PEG) will form CNT-polymer conjugates and make oxidized CNTs more biostable [21]. A major drawback of this method is that it will lead to the partial loss of electronic and optical properties of CNTs [18, 23]. Therefore, functionalization could not be used in certain applications like imaging. On the other hand, the positive side is that these issues are of less importance in drug-delivery applications (Figure 5.2).

5.4 CARBON NANOTUBES IN CANCER DIAGNOSIS

Since radical resection of tumor at the early stage itself is the only cure to the disease, early screening and detection is very important in cancer treatment.

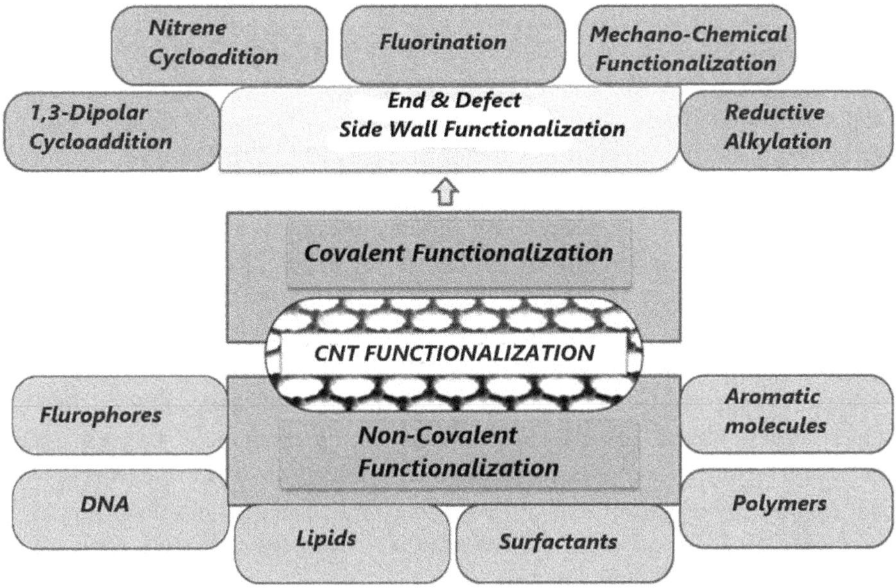

FIGURE 5.2 CNT functionalization.

However, certain factors act as a barrier for the timely detection. One is the conventional clinical cancer imaging techniques like X-ray, CT, and MRI, which don't have enough resolution for the early stage detection. As there is no distinct morphological changes at the initial stage, detection using these traditional techniques become impossible. Thus, the need of a reliable method for the early detection of biological changes led to the development of an advanced imaging technique called Positron emission tomography (PET). It has better sensitivity and accuracy than the conventional imaging technologies. PET is based on the changes in tissue biochemistry and metabolism. One of the most commonly used PET tracer is Fluorodeoxyglucose (FDG), which is being used by more than 95% of imaging technologies at present, due to its increased metabolism [24–27]. However, it is not a specific tracer for malignant diseases like cancer. This urges the need to find out new methods for the early detection and treatment of cancer.

Certain characteristic protein biomarkers that have the ability for early cancer detection are usually overexpressed in cancer cells. Some of the clinically significant tumor biomarkers include alpha-fetoprotein (AFP), carcinoembyronic antigen (CEA), carbohydrate antigen 19-9 (CA-19-9), carcinoma antigen 125 (CA125), prostate specific antigen (PSA), etc. All these biomarkers are widely used for the diagnosis of colorectal cancer, hepatocellular carcinoma, pancreatic cancer, prostate cancer, etc. However, due to the low sensitivity and specificity of these tumor markers, they are often excluded from the early detection of diseases, instead they are used in determining prognosis for the prediction of therapeutic responses and for tracking the therapy for advanced diseases [28, 29]. Due to the unique electrical, mechanical, and thermal properties of CNTs, they are considered to be an efficient tool for detecting the expression of indicative biological molecules at the early stage of cancer. Also, it has been reported that the analysis time as well as the expense for CNT-based diagnosis is very less compared to the ELISA commercial test kits with similar level of selectivity [30, 31].

As most types of cancer do not show observable symptoms during the initial stages, traditional clinical cancer imaging techniques are not useful for the early stage diagnosis and assessment of prognosis. Hence, it is crucial to look into the development of new imaging techniques that helps in early stage detection. In subsections, we are discussing the principle of some of the carbon nanotube-based diagnosis.

5.4.1 PHOTOACOUSTIC IMAGING (PAI)

Photoacoustic imaging (PAI) is a new imaging technique that is widely used in different biomedical fields [32–34]. In this technique pulsed laser is assimilated by molecules in the biological samples *via* absorptiometry to produce heat that can induce short-lived thermoelastic inflation resulting in broadband ultrasonic emission and ultrasound microphone to investigate these alterations and the detected signals can be converted into 2D and 3D images [35]. The main advantage of PAI over other optical imaging techniques are its high spatial resolution and its ability to image deeper tissues, which can be achieved with the help of external photoacoustic contrast-mediums. Single-walled and multi-walled carbon nanotubes are excellent photoacoustic-medium for PAI due to its strong capability to absorb light at near IR region (NIR) [36–38]. It has been reported that SWCNTs can provide more than two-fold signal amplification in thermoacoustic tomography (TAT) and more than six-fold signal amplification in photoacoustic tomography (PAT) [39, 40]. Thus CNTs with powerful NIR absorbance have become hopeful photoacoustic contrast agents in PAI that can help in the diagnosis of cancer.

5.4.2 *RAMAN IMAGING*

Raman scattering is a kind of photon scattering process in which photons are emitted with a shift in wavelength under light stimulation. Due to the absence of inherent enhancement mechanisms such as surface enhanced Raman scattering (SERS), the inherent Raman scattering by molecules are weak. SWCNTs are characterized by number of Raman peaks and the two most important are the radical breathing mode (RBM, 100–300 cm^{-1}) and tangential G-band (1,580 cm^{-1}). These peaks result from the vibration of carbon atoms in the radical direction and the tangential direction, respectively. Since Raman spectroscopy can provide valuable information regarding the chemical composition of biological cells and tissues, it find a lot of applications in biomedical diagnosis. Scattered photons of SWCNTs can reach to the NIR region and are hence useful for *in-vivo* imaging. Dai and coworkers have done the Raman imaging of live cells using isotopically modified SWCNTs [41] and they obtained distinct Raman G-band peaks.

5.5 CARBON NANOTUBES IN CANCER THERAPY

Among the various cancer treatment options, such as surgery, chemotherapy, thermotherapy, radiotherapy, and immunotherapy, surgery continues to be the effective method for removing cancerous cells. However, all these treatments will cause damage to the healthy cells as well [42, 43]. The new cancer treatment methods employing biotechnology also have many limitations [44, 45]. Amidst these, CNTs due to their unique properties, such as cellular uptake, high drug loading capability, thermal conductivity, large surface area-to-volume ratio, and excellent biocompatibility make them suitable carriers for target specific drug delivery to tumor cells. Figure 5.3 illustrates the various functions of CNTs in cancer therapy.

5.5.1 *CNTS IN CANCER CHEMOTHERAPY*

There are various factors that seriously influence the efficiency of chemotherapeutic drugs, such as their poor solubility, low stability and high toxicity over normal healthy cells and tissues. However, some studies demonstrated that, CNTs when administrated through veins can directly get into blood circulation and distribute in many internal organs, such as liver, spleen, heart, and kidney. This helps to increase the pharmaceutical

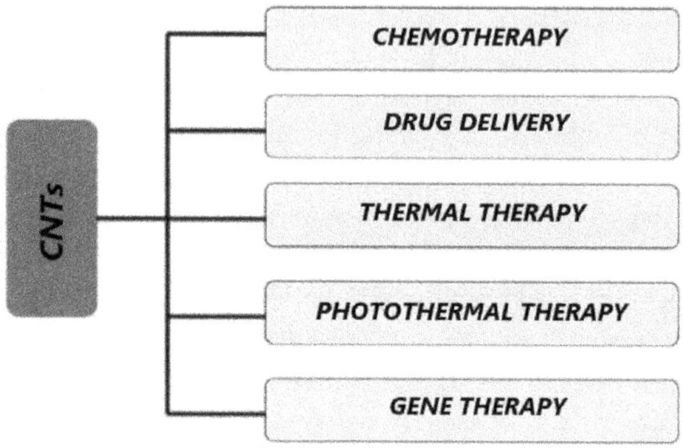

FIGURE 5.3 Multifunctional CNTs in cancer therapy.

efficacy and at the same time, the usage dose can be minimized. Making use of the biocompatibility of SWCNT, Liu et al. [46] made doxorubicin (DOX), an important chemo drug, loaded onto PEG functionalized SWCNT (PEG-poly-ethylene glycol) in order to prolong blood circulation time. To test this, SWCNT-DOX complex was injected to tumor mice. It was found that DOX can be delivered to tumor cells and SWCNT can be cleared from systematic blood circulation *via* renal excretion. Similarly, another important chemo drug named paclitaxel (PTX) can also be efficiently delivered to tumor cells using CNTs. Compared to DOX, the physical loading of PTX is quite difficult due to its poor solubility in aqueous medium. To overcome this, Lay et al. produced both PEG-graft single-walled (PEG-gSWCNT) and multiwalled (PEG-gMWCNT) carbon nanotubes to enhance the loading ability [47]. With the advancement of technology, researchers have modified SWCNT-based carriers to improve their efficiency of delivery. Epidermal growth factor (EGF) mediated SWCNT for the delivery of an anticancer agent called cisplatin is an example of this modification [48].

5.5.2 CNTS IN TARGETED DRUG DELIVERY

As mentioned above, conventional administration of chemotherapeutic agents is often neglected by their systemic toxicity due to lack of selectivity. In addition, their poor solubility, inability to cross cellular barriers [6] and especially the lack of clinical procedures to overcome multi-drug resistant cancer (MDR) [49], all these limits the administration of chemotherapeutic agents. So, in order to overcome these issues, researchers all over the world were in continuous search for a better drug delivery system. Among the several targeted therapies discovered, CNTs based drug delivery received much attention due to their unique physiochemical properties. Due to their large surface area, many biomolecules such as drugs, polypeptides, and nucleic acids can be integrated into CNT surface. Many researchers have found out that functionalized CNTs can pass through mammalian cell membrane *via* endocytosis or other mechanisms [50, 51]. This novel capability to penetrate into cell membranes makes them effective for the delivery of drug molecules to cytoplasm and nucleus. Then, the major question was how this drug loaded CNT recognize and enter into the target site for the desired action of the anticancer drug. This was achieved with the help of specific peptides or ligands integrated to their surface that can recognize cancer-specific receptors on the cell surface [52].

SWCNT and MWCNT are extensively used for the delivery of drug molecules to cancerous cells. SWCNT-based tumor-targeted drug delivery systems (DDS) generally consists of three parts: functionalized CNTs, tumor-targeting ligands and anticancer drugs. On interaction with cancer cells, DDS can recognize cancer-specific receptors which can result in receptor-mediated endocytosis. Now the tumor cells can efficiently and specifically absorb CNT complex with subsequent intracellular release of chemotherapeutic agents which will suppress the proliferation of cancerous cells (Figure 5.4).

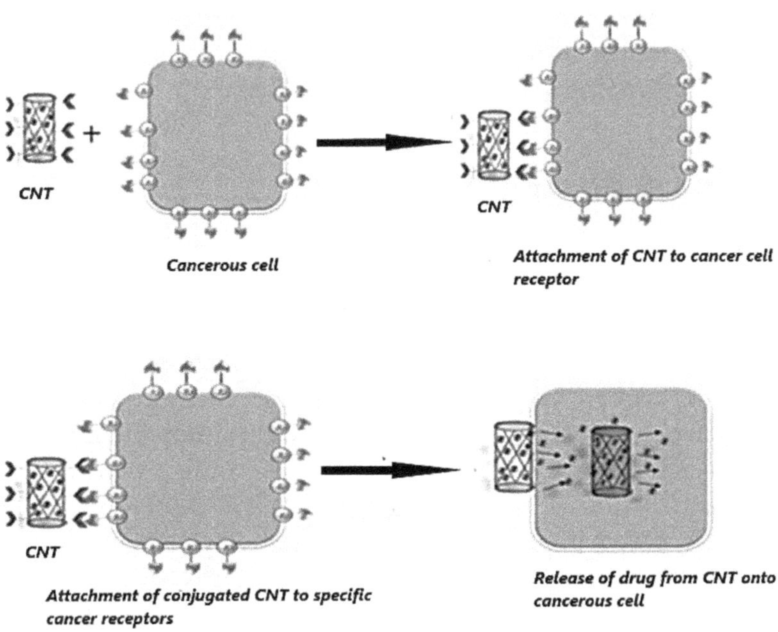

FIGURE 5.4 Action of CNTs in targeted drug delivery.

Conjugation of drug molecules with suitable conjugating agents together with the coating of polymers avoid the random bioavailability of relatively low molecular weight drugs and enhances its target specificity. Researchers from various fields concluded that CNTs modified with folic acid (FA) improve site-related responses for cancer targeting. Thus, targeted-cum-pH responsive FA conjugated MWCNTs have been developed for the delivery of DOX to tumor cells. This conjugated CNTs were then modified with fluorescein isothiocyanate (FITC), triethylamine and acetic anhydride to obtain FA-bound multifunctional CNTs, which exhibited excellent colloidal stability and biocompatibility. These CNT-based novel nanocarriers not only suppress the growth of cancer cells but significantly reduce the side effects caused by free DOX [53].

Lobaplatin (LBP), a chemotherapeutic drug used against lung cancer exhibited adverse toxic effects on body tissues during therapy. Yu et al. was successful in conjugating PEG-CNTs (PEG-polyethylene glycol) with LBP [54]. Fluorescein isothiocyanate (FITC) labeled PEG-CNTs showed targeted cell penetration, enhanced stability, biocompatibility, and excellent pH control. LBP-PEG-CNTs are very effective to suppress HepG2 (human liver cancer cell line) cell growth [55, 56]. In addition to these features, the intrinsic stability and structural flexibility of CNTs may prolong the circulation time as well as enhance the bioavailability of drugs conjugated to them [5]. All these results clearly indicated that CNTs can be used as an efficient tool for the tumor-targeted drug delivery in future.

5.5.3 CNTS IN THERMAL THERAPY

Thermal therapy applications of CNTs are considered to be a non-invasive, safe, and highly efficient technique in cancer treatment. Gannon et al. [57] found out that, heat released by the exposure of radiofrequency (RF) field on SWCNTs can cause the thermal destruction of cancer cells. In addition, the ability of carbon nanotubes to absorb near infrared radiations (NIR; 700–1,100 nm) and convert it into heat put forward an opportunity to develop new methods for cancer thermal therapy [53]. According to Biris et al. [58] infrared photothermal (PT) radiometry together with time-resolved imaging techniques is a very useful method to determine the temperature dynamics in scattered individual cancer cells which in turn helps in determining the appropriate dosing interval for laser PT therapy using relatively long laser pulses. This treatment approach is suitable for small tumors, tumor margins and micrometastases. Later, Moon and his group [59] developed a new method of treatment by combining the applications of SWCNTs and NIR radiation in nude mice bearing human epidermoid mouth carcinoma KB tumor cells on their backs. Intratumoral injection of PEG-SWCNTs solution followed by exposure to NIR radiation with a power density of 76 W/cm^3 for 3 min resulted in the complete destruction of tumors after 20 days of post treatments. The greatest achievement was most of the injected SWCNTs were excreted from their body. Similarly, MWCNT based treatment on kidney-tumor bearing mice was also very successful with low laser powers in short time period [60]. In order to enhance the selectivity of treatment and to decrease the CNT toxicity to normal cells, targeted CNTs can be achieved *via* covalent or non-covalent coating of cell-binding ligands such as peptides or monoclonal antibodies (MAbs) [21, 61–63].

5.5.4 CNTS IN PHOTOTHERMAL THERAPY

Although thermal therapy has been widely used for a long time in cancer treatment, photothermal therapy is still considered as the best method due to its improved selectivity and less harmful effects on non-tumor cells. Hyaluronic acid modified SWCNTs are excellent biocompatible water-soluble carriers for targeted therapy of tumors. This modified SWCNT has the ability to generate heat due to its photothermal sensitivity and hence it can be used for combined drug therapy and photothermal therapy and also for delivering photothermal therapeutic agents [64].

5.5.5 CNTS IN GENE THERAPY

Gene therapy is considered as one of the most promising and hopeful method in cancer treatment and an alternative to the conventional chemotherapy [65]. Generally, it is believed that tumor results from the alterations in gene and gene therapy aims to correct them. Initially, viral vectors were widely used for gene delivery as it can achieve a high level of gene expression. However, there are lot of concerns regarding their safety such as, viral vectors can be immunogenic, oncogenic, and sometimes may cause inflammation [66–68]. Their packaging capacity is also too limited [69]. Due to these limitations, viral vectors were replaced by non-viral vectors.

The two main approaches used in gene therapy are the introduction of gene into host cells or the delivery of molecules that silence pathogenic genes, for example, small interfering RNA (siRNA). Several non-viral delivery systems have been developed for the effective delivery of siRNA, including chemical modification using cationic polymers, cell penetrating peptides, cationic lipids and so on [70, 71]. However, compared with viral vectors, non-viral vectors are not much efficient in crossing the nuclear membrane [72], due to this reason the gene expression mediated by these vectors are lowered. All these drawbacks can be addressed by developing an effective delivery system. For the development of a new vector for gene delivery, certain conditions have to be fulfilled, such as protection of DNA from degradation, high membrane penetration, and low immunogenicity [72]. Thus, CNTs seems to be the best candidate for the therapeutic gene delivery due to their excellent efficiency in crossing the mammalian cell membrane. It was found out that functionalized CNTs can act as safer no-viral vectors for the delivery of DNA molecules into the cell membrane [73]. The transfection efficiency of non-covalently pegylated SWCNTs conjugated to siRNA *via* a disulfide spacer was studied *in vitro* [74]. SWCNTs successfully targeted siRNA and once it enter the tumor cells the disulfide bonds are broken releasing siRNA.

In a recent study on gene therapy, it was found out that the iC9 gene used to induce apoptosis in human breast cancer line MCF-7 was successfully delivered through pyridine functionalized MWCNTs. For the targeted gene expression in tumor cells, a new and innovative photoactivatable RNAi system was developed. It consists of polyetherimide-modified SWCNTs (PEI-SWCNTs) as the nanocarrier and Hsp 70B'-promoter-driven RNAi vector (Phsp-shT). Heating PEI-SWCNTs in MCF-7 cells activate gene knockdown that target human telomerase reverse transcriptase *via* RNAi in the near infrared field (NIR). Combining the effect of gene therapy and photothermal therapy of photoactiveatable RNAi system showed significant antitumor activity [75]. Thus, we are expecting a huge revolution in cancer treatment using CNT-based gene transfer vector systems.

5.6 TOXICITY OF CNTS

Even though CNTs possess excellent physiochemical characteristics suitable for their application in cancer treatment, their asbestos-like structure and needle-like appearance causes severe problems on lungs and respiratory tract [76, 77]. Asbestos is a very hazardous substance, inhaling asbestos can cause lung cancer and scars on the lungs. CNT toxicity is not only dependent on their structure [78] alone but on various factors like concentration of impurities present in them [79], their degree of functionalization [80] and agglomeration state [22]. Although no one can reject the promising features and wide range of applications offered by CNTs, the failure in reaching at a conclusion on their toxic effects and health related issues limits easy and rapid industrial transition and clinical translation.

5.7 CONCLUSION

The emergence of nanotechnology as the foremost and innovative branches of science have brought about remarkable impressions in various streams of research such as medicine, biology, industrial manufacturing process, electronics, and so on. Carbon nanotubes (CNTs), one among the various novel nanomaterials developed have received much attention in the recent years, due to their unique physical, chemical, biological, and mechanical properties. In this chapter, we have discussed the biomedical applications of CNTs in cancer diagnosis and therapy. Their excellence in target-specific drug delivery, high biocompatibility, high drug-loading capacity, inherent diagnostic capability, all these have contributed to their applications in cancer diagnosis and therapy. Despite all these advantages, the non-biodegradability and cytotoxicity of CNTs limits their applications to an extent. However, these limitations are found to be reduced through new methods of CNTs functionalization. Thus, in the near future, we are expecting more and more safe and effective applications of CNTs in cancer treatment.

KEYWORDS

- **cancer**
- **carbon nanotubes**
- **diagnosis**
- **functionalization**
- **therapy**
- **toxicity**

REFERENCES

1. Fukumori, Y., & Ichikawa, H., (2006). Nanoparticles for cancer therapy and diagnosis. *Adv. Powder Tecnnol., 17*(1), 1–28.
2. Vasir, J. K., & Labhasetwar, V., (2007). Biodegradable nanoparticles for cytosolic delivery of therapeutics. *Adv. Drug Deliv. Rev., 59*(8), 718–728.
3. Faraji, A. H., & Wipf, P., (2009). Nanoparticles in cellular drug delivery. *Bioorg. Med. Chem., 17*(8), 2950–2962.
4. Sahoo, N. G., Bao, H., Pan, Y., Pal, M., Kakran, M., Cheng, H. K. F., & Tan, L. P., (2011). Functionalized carbon nanomaterials as nanocarriers for loading and delivery of a poorly water-soluble anticancer drug: A comparative study. *Chem. Commun., 47*, 5235–5237.
5. Chen, J. Y., Chen, S. Y., Zhao, X. R., Kuznetsova, L. V., Wong, S. S., & Ojima, I., (2008). Functionalized single-walled carbon nanotubes as rationally designed vehicles for tumor-targeted drug delivery. *J. Am. Chem. Soc., 130*(49), 2950–2962.
6. Heister, E., Neves, V., Carmen, T., Lipert, K., Beltran, V. S., Coley, H. M., Silva, S. R. P., & Mcfadden, J. J., (2009). Triple functionalization of single-walled carbon nanotubes with doxorubicin, a monoclonal antibody, and a fluorescent marker for targeted cancer therapy. *Carbon, 47*, 2152–2160.
7. Bhirde, A. A., Patel, V., Gavarad, J., Zhang, G., Sousa, A. A., Masedunskas, A., Leapman, R. D., et al., (2009). Targeted killing of cancer cells *in vivo* and *in vitro* with EGF-directed carbon nanotube-based drug delivery. *ACS Nano, 3*(2), 307–316.
8. Alfarouk, K. O., Stock, C. M., Taylor, S., Walsh, M., Muddathir, A. K., Verduzco, D., Bashir, A. H. H., et al., (2015). Resistance to cancer chemotherapy: Failure in drug response from ADME to P-gp. *Cancer Cell Int., 15*, 71.
9. Wang, X., Zhang, H., & Chen, X., (2019). Drug resistance and combating drug resistance in cancer. *Cancer Drug Resist., 2*, 141–160.
10. Faria, P. C. B. D., Santos, L. I. D., Coelho, J. P., Ribeiro, H. P., Pimenta, M. A., Ladeira, L. O., Gomes, D. A., et al., (2014). Oxidized multiwalled carbon nanotubes as antigen delivery system to promote superior $CD8^+$ T cell response and protection against cancer. *Nano Lett., 14*(9), 5458–5470.
11. Iijima, S., (1991). Helical microtubules of graphitic carbon. *Nature, 354*, 56–58.
12. Yan, Y., Chan-Park, M. B., & Zhang, Q., (2007). Advances in carbon-nanotube assembly. *Small, 3*(1), 24–42.
13. Chen, Z., Wu, W., Chen, Z., Cong, X., & Qiu, J., (2012). Microstructural characterization on ZrC doped carbon/carbon composites. *Ceramics Int., 38*(1), 761–767.
14. Liu, J., Rinzler, A. G., & Daietal, H., (1998). Fullerene pipes. *Science, 280*(5367), 1253–1256.
15. Bianco, A., Kostarelos, K., & Prato, M., (2005). Applications of carbon nanotubes in drug delivery. *Curr. Opin. Chem. Biol., 9*(6), 674–679.
16. Bianco, A., Kostarelos, K., Partidos, C. D., & Prato, M., (2005). Biomedical applications of functionalized carbon nanotubes. *Chem. Commun., 7*(5), 571–577.
17. Kesharwani, P., Ghanghoria, R., & Jain, N. K., (2012). Carbon nanotube exploration in cancer cell lines. *Drug Discovery Today, 17*, 1023–1030.
18. Liu, Z., Sun, X., Nakayama-Ratchford, N., & Dai, H., (2007). Supramolecular chemistry on water-soluble carbon nanotubes for drug loading and delivery. *ACS Nano, 1*(1), 50–56.

19. Klumpp, C., Kostarelos, K., Prato, M., & Bianco, A., (2006). Functionalized carbon nanotubes as emerging nanovectors for the delivery of therapeutics. *Biochimi. Biophysica Acta—Biomembranes, 1758*(3), 404–412.
20. Bekyarova, E., Ni, Y., Malarkey, E. B., et al., (2005). Applications of carbon nanotubes in biotechnology and biomedicine. *J. Biomed. Nanotechnol., 1*(1), 3–17.
21. Kam, N. W. S., O'Connell, M., Wisdom, J. A., & Dai, H., (2005). Carbon nanotubes as multifunctional biological transporters and near infrared agents for selective cancer cell destruction. *Proc. Natl. Acad. Sci. U.S.A., 102*(33), 11600–11605.
22. Ebrahimi, N., & Mansoori, G. A. (2014). Reliability for Drug Targeting in Cancer Treatment through Nanotechnology (A Psychometric Approach). *Int. J. Med. Nano. Res., 1,* 1.
23. Niyogi, S., Hamon, M. A., Hu, H., Zhao, B., Bhowmik, P., Sen, R., Itkis, M. E., & Haddon, R. C., (2002). Chemistry of single walled carbon nanotubes. *Acc. Chem. Res., 35*(12), 1105–1113.
24. Ji, J. R., Liu, C., Zhang, B., Yang, F., Xu, J., Long, Y., Jin, C., et al. (2010). Carbon nanotubes in cancer diagnosis and therapy. *Biochim. Biophysica Acta—Reviews on Cancer, 1806*(1), 29–35.
25. Levy, R. P., (2007). PET-CT: Evolving role in hadron therapy. *Nuclear Instruments and Methods in Physics Research, Section B: Beam Interactions with Materials and Atoms, 261*(1, 2), 782–785.
26. Papathanassiou, D., Bruna-Muraille, C., Liehn, J. C., Nguyen, T. D., & Cur´e, H., (2009). Positron emission tomography in oncology: Present and future of PET and PET/CT. *Critical Reviews in Oncology/Hematology, 72*(3), 239–254.
27. Delbeke, D., Sch¨oder, H., Martin, W. H., & Wahl, R. L., (2009). Hybrid imaging (SPECT/CT and PET/CT): Improving therapeutic decisions. *Seminars in Nuclear Medicine, 39*(5), 308–340.
28. Duffy, M. J., (2007). Role of tumor markers in patients with solid cancers: A critical review. *Eur. J. Intern. Med., 18*(3), 175–184.
29. Rogers, L. K., Robbins, M., & Dakhlallahetal, D., (2015). Attenuation of MIR-17~92 cluster in bronchopulmonary dysplasia. *Ann. Am. Thorac. Soc., 12*(10), 1506–1513.
30. Panini, N. V., Messina, G. A., Salinas, E., Fern´andez, H., & Raba, J., (2008). Integrated microfluidic systems with an immune sensor modified with carbon nanotubes for detection of prostate specific antigen (PSA) in human serum samples. *Biosensors and Bioelectronics, 23*(7), 1145–1151.
31. Ho, J. A. A., Lin, Y. C., Wang, L. S., Hwang, K. C., & Chou, P. T., (2009). Carbon nanoparticle-enhanced immune electrochemical detection for protein tumor marker with cadmium sulfide biotracers. *Anal. Chem., 81*(4), 1340–1346.
32. Gong, H., Peng, R., & Liu, Z., (2013). Carbon nanotubes for biomedical imaging: The recent advances. *Adv. Drug Deliv. Rev., 65*(13), 1951–1963.
33. Wang, X., Pang, Y., Ku, G., Xie, X., Stoica, G., & Wang, L. V., (2003). Noninvasive laser-induced photoacoustic tomography for structural and functional *in vivo* imaging of the brain. *Nat. Biotechnol., 21*, 803–806.
34. Ku, G., & Wang, L. V., (2005). Deeply penetrating photoacoustic tomography in biological tissues enhanced with an optical contrast agent. *Opt. Lett., 30*(5), 507–509.
35. Hoelen, C. G. A., De Mul, F. F. M., Pongers, R., & Dekker, A., (1998). Three-dimensional photoacoustic imaging of blood vessels in tissue. *Opt. Lett., 23*(8), 648–650.

36. Robinson, J. T., Welsher, K., Tabakman, S. M., Sherlock, S. P., Wang, H., Luong, R., & Dai, H., (2010). High performance *in vivo* near-IR (>1 μm) imaging and photothermal cancer therapy with carbon nanotubes. *Nano Res., 3*(11), 779–793.
37. Liu, X., Tao, H., Yang, K., Zhang, S., Lee, S. T., & Liu, Z., (2011). Optimization of surface chemistry on single-walled carbon nanotubes for *in vivo* photothermal ablation of tumors. *Biomaterials, 32*(1), 144–151.
38. Moon, H. K., Lee, S. H., & Choi, H. C., (2009). *In vivo* near-infrared mediated tumor destruction by photothermal effect of carbon nanotubes. *ACS Nano, 3*(11), 3707–3713.
39. Avti, P. K., Hu, S., Favazza, C., Mikos, A. G., Jansen, J. A., Shroyer, K. R., Wang, L. V., & Sitharaman, B., (2012). Detection, mapping, and quantification of single walled carbon nanotubes in histological specimens with photoacoustic microscopy. *PLoS One, 7*(4).
40. Wu, L., Cai, X., Nelson, K., Xing, W., Xia, J., Zhang, R., Stacy, A. J., et al., (2013). A green synthesis of carbon nanoparticles from honey and their use in real-time photoacoustic imaging. *Nano Res., 6*(5), 312–325.
41. Liu, Z., Li, X., Tabakman, S. M., Jiang, K., Fan, S., & Dai, H., (2008). Multiplexed multicolor Raman imaging of live cells with isotopically modified single walled carbon nanotubes. *J. Am. Chem. Soc., 130*(41), 13540–13541.
42. Luo, J., Solimini, N. L., & Elledge, S. J., (2009). Principles of cancer therapy: Oncogene and non-oncogene addiction. *Cell, 136*(5), 823–837.
43. Sinha, R., Kim, G. J., Nie, S., & Shin, D. M., (2006). Nanotechnology in cancer therapeutics: Bioconjugated nanoparticles for drug delivery. *Mol. Cancer Ther., 5*(8), 1909–1917.
44. Haley, B., & Frenkel, E., (2008). Nanoparticles for drug delivery in cancer treatment. *Urol. Oncol., 26*(1), 57–64.
45. Webster, D. M., Sundaram, P., & Byrne, M. E., (2013). Injectable nanomaterials for drug delivery: Carriers, targeting moieties, and therapeutics. *Eur. J. Pharm. Biopharm., 84*(1), 1–20.
46. Liu, Z., Fan, A. C., & Rakhraetal, K., (2009). Supramolecular stacking of doxorubicin on carbon nanotubes for *in vivo* cancer therapy. *Angew. Chem. Int. Ed. Engl., 48*(41), 7668–7672.
47. Lay, C. L., Liu, H. Q., Tan, H. R., & Liu, Y., (2010). Delivery of paclitaxel by physically loading onto poly(ethylene glycol) (PEG)-graft carbon nanotubes for potent cancer therapeutics. *Nanotechnology, 21*(6).
48. Bhirde, A. A., Patel, V., & Gavardetal, J., (2009). Targeted killing of cancer cells *in vivo* and *in vitro* with EGF-directed carbon nanotube-based drug delivery. *ACS Nano, 3*(2), 307–316.
49. Lara, S. J. M., Van, V. L. E., & Yadav, S., (2009). Multifunctional-nanocarriers to overcome tumor drug resistance. *Cancer Treat. Rev., 34*(7), 592–602.
50. Sinha, N., & Yeow, J. T. W., (2005). Carbon nanotubes for biomedical applications. *IEEE Transactions on Nanobioscience, 4*(2), 180–195.
51. Zhang, X., Meng, L., Lu, Q., Fei, Z., & Dyson, P. J., (2009). Targeted delivery and controlled release of doxorubicin to cancer cells using modified single wall carbon nanotubes. *Biomaterials, 30*(30), 6041–6047.
52. Madani, S. Y., Naderi, N., Dissanayake, O., Tan, A., & Seifalian, A. M., (2011). A new era of cancer treatment: Carbon nanotubes as drug delivery tools. *Int. J. Nanomed., 6*, 2963–2979.

53. Yan, Y., Wang, R., Hu, Y., Sun, R., Song, T., Shi, X., & Yin, S., (2018). Stacking of doxorubicin on folic acid-targeted multiwalled carbon nanotubes for *in vivo* chemotherapy of tumors. *Drug Deliv., 25*(1), 1607–1616.
54. Yu, S., Li, Q., Wang, J., Du, J., Gao, Y., Zhang, L., Yang, Y., & Lu, Y., (2018). A targeted drug delivery system based on carbon nanotubes loaded with lobaplatin toward liver cancer cells. *J. Mater. Res., 33*(17), 2565–2575.
55. Yu, S., Zhang, Y., Chen, L., Li, Q., Du, J., Gao, Y., Zhang, L., & Yang, Y., (2018). Antitumor effects of carbon nanotube-drug complex against human breast cancer cells. *Exp. Ther. Med., 16*(2), 1103–1110.
56. Gannon, C. J., Cherukuri, P., Yakobson, B. I., Cognet, L., Kazius, J. S., Kittrell, C., Weisman, R. B., et al., (2007). Carbon nanotube-enhanced thermal destruction of cancer cells in a noninvasive radiofrequency field. *Cancer, 110*(12), 2654–2665.
57. Kam, N. W. S., O'Connell, M., Wisdom, J. A., & Dai, H., (2005). Carbon nanotubes as multifunctional biological transporters and near-infrared agents for selective cancer cell destruction. *Proc. Natl. Acad. Sci., 102*(3), 11600–11605.
58. Biris, A. S., Boldor, D., Palmer, J., Monroe, W. T., Mahmood, M., Dervishi, E., Xu, Y., et al., (2009). Nanophotothermolysis of multiple scattered cancer cells with carbon nanotubes guided by time-resolved infrared thermal imaging. *J. Biomed. Opt., 14*(2).
59. Moon, H. K., Lee, S. H., & Choi, H. C., (2009). *In vivo* near-infrared mediated tumor destruction by photothermal effects of carbon nanotubes. *ACS Nano, 3*(11), 3707–3713.
60. Burkea, A., Ding, X. F., Singha, R., Polyachenko, N. L., Rylander, M. N., Szot, C., Buchanan, C., & Whitney, J., (2009). Long-term survival following a single treatment of kidney tumors with multiwalled carbon nanotubes and near infrared radiation. *Proc. Natl. Acad. Sci., 106*(31), 12897–12902.
61. Marches, R., Chakravarty, P., Musselman, I. H., Bajaj, P., Azad, R. N., Pantano, P., Draper, R. K., & Vitetta, E. S., (2009). Specific thermal ablation of tumor cells using single-walled carbon nanotubes targeted by covalently-coupled monoclonal antibodies. *Int. Cancer J., 125*(12), 2970–2977.
62. Chakravarty, P., Marches, R., & Zimmermanetal, N. S., (2008). Thermal ablation of tumor cells with antibody-functionalized single walled carbon nanotubes. *Proc. Natl. Acad. Sci. U.S.A., 105*(5), 8697–8702.
63. Shao, N., Lu, S., Wickstrom, E., & Panchapakesan, B., (2007). Integrated molecular targeting of IGF1R and HER2 surface receptors and destruction of breast cancer cells using single wall carbon nanotubes. *Nanotechnology, 18*(31).
64. Hou, L., Yuan, Y., Ren, J., Zhang, Y., Wang, Y., Shan, X., Liu, Q., & Zhang, Z., (2017). *In vitro* and *in vivo* comparative study of the phototherapy anticancer activity of hyaluronic acid-modified single-walled carbon nanotubes, graphene oxide, and fullerene. *J. Nanopart. Res., 19*(8), 286.
65. Yang, Z. R., Wang, H. F., Zhao, J., et al., (2007). Recent developments in the use of adenoviruses and immunotoxins in cancer gene therapy. *Cancer Gene Ther., 14*(7), 599–615.
66. Mintzer, M. A., & Simanek, E. E., (2009). Nonviral vectors for gene delivery. *Chem. Rev., 109*(2), 259–302.
67. Gao, K., & Huang, L., (2009). Nonviral methods for siRNA delivery. *Mol. Pharm., 6*(3), 651–658.
68. Seow, Y., & Wood, M. J., (2009). Biological gene delivery vehicles: Beyond viral vectors. *Mol. Ther., 17*(5), 767–777.

69. Ragusa, A., Garcia, I., & Penades, S., (2007). Nnonparticles as nonviral gene delivery vectors. *IEEE Trans. Nanobiosci., 6*(4), 319–330.
70. Kim, W. J., & Kim, S. W., (2009). Efficient siRNA delivery with non-viral polymeric vehicles. *Pharm. Res., 26*(3), 657–666.
71. Reisscl, D., & Zimmer, A., (*2009*). Drug delivery of siRNA therapeutics: Potentials and limits of nanosystems. *Nanomed.: Nanotechnol. Biol. Med., 5*(1), 8–20.
72. Klumpp, C., Kostarelos, K., Patro, M., et al., (2006). Functionalized carbon nanotubes as emerging nanovectors for the delivery of therapeutics. *Biochim. Biophys. Acta, 1758*(3), 404–412.
73. Singh, R., Pantarotto, D., & McCarthy, D., (2005). Binding and condensation of plasmid DNA onto functionalized carbon nanotubes: Toward the construction of nanotube-based gene delivery vectors. *J. Am. Chem. Soc., 127*(12), 4388–4396.
74. Chen, H., Ma, X., Li, Z., Shi, Q., Zheng, W., Liu, Y., & Wang, P., (2012). *Biomed. Pharmacother., 66*, 334–338.
75. Ren, X., Lin, J., Wang, X., Liu, X., Meng, E., Zhang, R., Sang, Y., & Zhang, Z., (2017). Photoactivatable RNAi for cancer gene therapy triggered by near-infrared-irradiated single-walled carbon nanotubes. *Int. J. Nanomed., 12*, 7885–7896.
76. Poland, C. A., Duffin, R., Kinloch, I., et al., (2008). Carbon nanotubes introduced into the abdominal cavity of mice show asbestos-like pathogenicity in a pilot study. *Nat. Nanotech., 3*(7), 423.
77. Jaurand, M. C. F., Renier, A., & Daubriac, J., (2009). Mesothelioma: Do asbestos and carbon nanotubes pose the same health risk? *Part. Fiber Toxicol., 6*(16), 16.
78. Bottini, M., Bruckner, S., & Nilka, K., (2006). Multi-walled carbon nanotubes induce T lymphocyte apoptosis. *Toxicol. Lett., 160*(2), 121–126.
79. Prylutskaa, S. V., Grynyuka, I. I., Matyshevska, O. P., Yaschchak, V. M., Yu Prylutskyy, I., Ritter, U., & Scharff, P., (2008). Estimation of multi-walled carbon nanotubes toxicity *in vitro. Physica E, 40*(7), 2565–2569.
80. Sayes, C. M., Liang, F., & Hudsona, J. L., (2006). Functionalization density dependence of single-walled carbon nanotubes cytotoxicity. *Toxicol. Lett., 161*(2), 135–142.
81. Wick, P., Manser, P., & Imbach, L. K., (2007). The degree and kind of agglomeration affect carbon nanotube cytotoxicity. *Toxicol. Lett., 168*, 121–131.

CHAPTER 6

Carbon Nanotubes: As an Effective Opportunity for Diagnosis and Treatment of Cancer

SHWETA S. GEDAM, SWATI K. VETAL, SWATI G. TALELE, and ANIL G. JADHAV

Sandip Institute of Pharmaceutical Sciences, Mahiravani, Nashik, Maharashtra, India

ABSTRACT

Cancer is a wide term that encompasses a variety of diseases marked by excessive cell proliferation. Stopping the progression of cancer as soon as possible is one of the goals of cancer treatment. Despite current medical advancements, the resistance of malignant tumors to conventional medical therapies highlights the need for innovative therapeutic techniques. Carbon nanotubes (CNTs) have attracted a lot of interest in recent years since their discovery. Nanomaterials have progressed significantly., owing to their enormous potential in biomedical applications. They have become a prominent tool in cancer detection and therapy owing to their distinct physicochemical characteristics. They are regarded to be amongst the more potential nanomaterials since they can detect malignant cells as well as transport medications or tiny therapeutic compounds to them. CNTs are nanometer-sized tubular materials with axial symmetry, which gives them unique features that can be utilized to diagnose and treat cancer. CNTs can potentially deliver drugs to specific cells and tissues. Along with the rapid advancements in the production of nanotechnology-based materials, it is equally critical to understand

Carbon Nanotubes for Biomedical Applications and Healthcare.
Chin Hua Chia, Swati Gokul Talele, Ann Rose Abraham, and A. K. Haghi, (Eds.)

the toxicity of nanoparticles. As a result, the study's objective is to look into the medicinal uses of carbon nanotubes, with a focus on their use as therapeutic platforms in oncology.

6.1 INTRODUCTION

Surgery, chemotherapy, and/or nowadays, radiation is one among the most popular prevalent cancer treatments. Tumor cells are more susceptible to the consequences of chemotherapy and radiation; thus, they are utilized to remove them. However, the well-known negative effects significantly reduce their effectiveness, actual benefits, as well as a reduction in the number of potential candidates. Nanotechnology is a cutting-edge technology. Offering intriguing alternatives to current tumor-fighting techniques [1]. Carbon nanotubes (CNTs) have gotten a lot of press. And interest in nanotechnology over the last 20 years as a result of their distinctness in mechanical properties as well as very fascinating values of thermal and electrical conductivity. Furthermore, the ability to functionalize their surface with a variety of bio/chemical species opens the door to a slew of therapeutic and medication delivery possibilities. As a result, they stand out among the latest cancer "theranostics" treatments, which integrate diagnostic and therapy inside the similar nanostructure. The purpose of this content is to provide an outline of carbon nanotubes' potential influence on cancer research and treatment [2–4]. The value of carbon nanotubes for biosensing will be discussed in Section 6.2, followed by a detailed review of their usage in cancer detection and therapy in Section 6.3.

6.2 WHAT ARE CARBON NANOTUBES (CNTS) AND WHY DO THEY MATTER IN SENSING?

CNTs are a kind of carbon. A carbon nanotube is made up of a single coiled graphene sheet. As seen in Figure 6.1, the A graphene sheets can be coiled in a number of different ways. Varied varieties of CNTs with different characteristics are represented by different imaginary cut lines [5, 6]. In essence, three cut lines, known as chiral vectors, may be used to represent three varieties of CNTs structures: zigzag, armchair, and chiral.

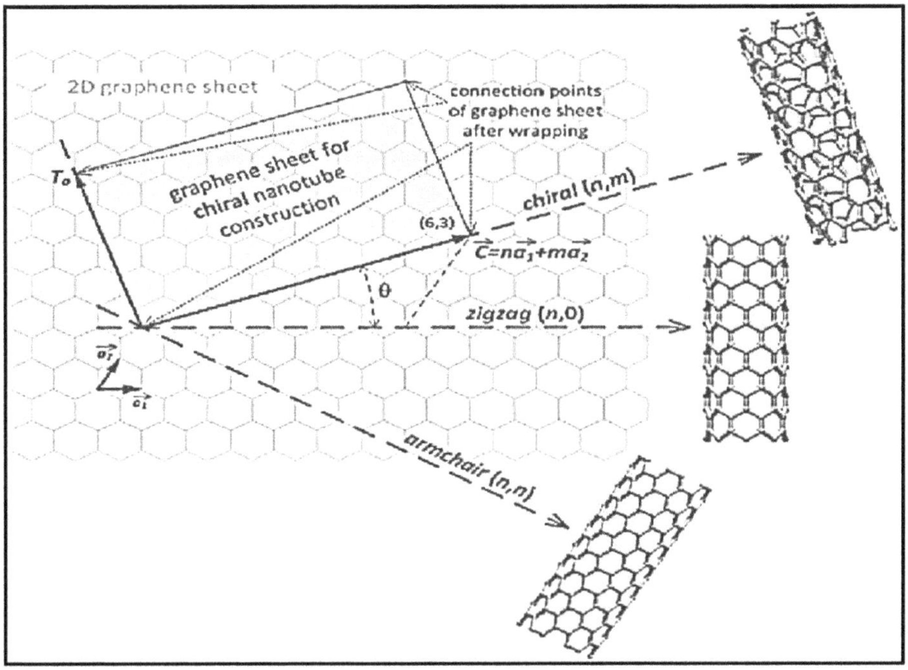

FIGURE 6.1 The production of a carbon nanotube from a single graphene sheet.

The number of a chiral vector's two integer components determines the structural type (n, m). If they're the same, the armchair's structure is investigated. If the two coefficients vary, the zigzag type is identified if m = 0, otherwise the chiral structure is present in all other situations [7]. Single-walled carbon nanotubes (SWCNTs) and multi-walled carbon nanotubes (MWCNTs) are two types of carbon nanotubes, which are made up of several graphene sheets wrapped in a concentric pattern. Diameters can range from just a few nano-meter range to hundreds of nanometers [8].

6.2.1 SYNTHESIS AND CHARACTERISTIC PROPERTIES OF CNTS

Low temperature chemical vapor deposition (CVD) is the most widely used CNT synthesis method because process variables (such as the type of protonated gas, metal catalyst, size or sharpness of the catalyzed atom, representing moiety and any additional co-catalysts, gas flow rate, CVD temperature, and CVD run time) can be conveniently tuned to stabilize diameter, length, purity, and alignment [9]. In general, carbon precursors in gaseous form are fluxed it in to a reactor vessel with another carrier gas, where a metallic catalyst is required to initiate the chemical process that leads to CNTs development [10]. The two main processes for explaining CNTs catalytic growth are tip-growth and base-growth, which are named after the location of the catalyst in relation to the substrate [11]. Detachment of the active component from the substrate and travels forward during the development of SWNTs in tip-growth mode [12]. The whole nanotube travels away from the catalyst in base-growth mode, but the catalyst remains in its original place. Under the reaction circumstances, the carbon precursor decomposes on the metal particle in both processes [13]. Carbon atoms, which are extremely versatile on metal surfaces, quickly diffuse across and through the metallic particles, generating a hexagonal tube structure. The other two major methods for creating CNTs are arc discharge and laser ablation. The first method involves a DC or AC arc discharge among two carbon electrodes (one of which is normally pure graphite) in a sealed chamber with an inert atmosphere. Substantial alterations have been done towards this approach, and more information may be found in a recent evaluation [14]. Similar to the arc-discharge approach, energy is given by a laser striking a graphite substrate holding the catalysts material. Several factors, including laser irradiation, laser power level, laser mode of operation, wavelength, target material, chamber gas, and pressure, can influence the CNTs' properties even in this circumstance [15, 16].

6.2.2 EFFECT CARBON NANOTUBES ON CANCER CELLS

The unusual resilience of cancer cells to traditional anticancer therapies (e.g., chemotherapy, radiation, and surgery), as well as undesirable reactions to these treatments, are the driving forces behind the recent rise in research interest in cancer nanomedicine. A large number of nanomaterials may be designed to operate as chemotherapeutic drug carriers, with the potential to target cancer tissues selectively owing to cutting-edge functionalization [4, 17]. Furthermore, as thoroughly discussed by, current research is increasingly concentrating on nanoparticles combination treatment, i.e., multi-drug delivery accomplished by nanoparticles capable of carrying and delivering many types of medicines at the same time. Nanoparticles' distinguishing characteristic against cancer is their capacity to infiltrate tumor tissues owing to their size, while being able to exit cancer cells due to their poor lymphatic system [18]. Enhanced permeability and retention (EPR) is a property that explains why nanoparticle dimensions should be effectively managed and improved [1]. CNTs are particularly well suited for such applications, as mentioned by Lim et al. because to their hollow interior and remarkable physical characteristics [4, 18]. Hydrophobic medicines, in particular, may be placed within CNTs via non-covalent π-π stacking. The outer surface functionalization customized for distinct cancer receptors ensures targeted medication administration. Targeted activity is necessary to prevent harm to healthy tissues, making the procedure less intrusive for the patient. CNTs, on the contrary, can do more than merely transport drugs in the battle against cancer. Engineered carbon nanotubes can be used as contrast agents (adjuvants) (CA) in a variety of imaging methods and can also improve medication cytotoxicity [19]. They may also be utilized to perform thermal ablation, detect reactive oxygen species (ROS) or particular antigens, as well as tumor indicators. Multiple functionalization, as extensively discussed in, may be used to combine all of these features to produce a multifunctional tool. There are two methods of functionalization on CNTs: covalent and non-covalent [20, 21]. The next sections focus on the synergy of all of CNTs' anticancer characteristics previously described.

6.3 CONTRAST AGENT IN MEDICAL IMAGING

6.3.1 *ULTRASONOGRAPHY*

Another new and potentially powerful application of CNTs is in diagnostic imaging [22]. Due to its cheap value per testing and intrinsic safety, ultrasonography is one of the most often used imaging modalities [23]. Ultrasound (US) is a therapeutic application of sound waves with a frequency range of 2 to 12 MHz and a spatial resolution of 0.2 to 1 mm. Functionalized MWCNTs have improved characteristics as ultrasonic contrast agents, according to Delogu et al. [24]. They functionalized MWCNTs with 1,3-dipolar azomethine ylides (ox-MWCNT-NH_3^+) and compared them to pristine MWCNTs and functionalized SWCNTs, finding that the functionalized MWCNTs exhibited a signal response equivalent to a commercial contrast agent [25]. They demonstrated the effectiveness of their procedure *in vitro* and *in vivo* on a pig. In his procedure, MWCNTs were extensively functionalized with poly-ethyleneimine (PEI) before being coupled with Fluorescein IsoThio-Cyanate (FITC) and PSCA monoclonal antibody (mAbPSCA). Several functions were combined into these nanosensors (CNT-PEI(FITC)-mAb), but the US contrast agent and the ability to target the chosen tumor marker are the most important for this evaluation. In fact, *in vivo* experiments show that the

CNT-PEI(FITC)-mAb was able to target the tumor spot properly, resulting in a clear US image [26].

6.3.2 *PHOTOACOUSTIC IMAGING*

Photoacoustic (PA) imaging is another strong and developing technology akin to ultrasonography [26]. The PA imaging signal is an acoustical wave, similar to ultrasonography, but the origin is light, which causes a tissue region being an activated acoustical source. The PA's output current is broadband [26]. Although certain tissues exhibit inherent PA behavior, many illnesses do not display PA contrast, necessitating the application of an extrinsic contrast agent [27]. PA characteristics exist in pristine CNTs, and they can be fully practice to increase the performance of pure CNTs [28–31]. The difficulty is that CNTs must be targeted to the cancer location in order to be imaged. De la Zerda et al. came up with a solution by using a double CNT functionalization. The first was using IndoCyanine Green (ICG) dye, which was used to improve PA performance by enhancing optical absorption through-stacking interactions [31]. The second was the use of cyclic arginylglycylaspartic acid–RGD peptides on the surface of PEGylated CNTs to guide CNTs to overexpressed V3 integrins in tumor vasculature. They were pitted against RAD, a non-targeted peptide that didn't bind to V3 integrins. For stomach tumor targeting, Wang's team combined the two techniques to synthesize RGD-conjugated silica-coated gold nanotubes on the surface of carbon nanotubes. The nanoprobes aggregated in the areas where stomach cancer was prevalent, and the PA signal became stronger over time as a result of this buildup [32].

6.3.3 *NEAR-INFRARED IMAGING*

In the near-infrared window, CNTs have intrinsic fluorescence and significant optical absorption (700 to 1,400 nm). Non-photobleaching fluorophores with high resolution *in vivo* imaging can make use of this feature [33]. Furthermore, the excitation wavelengths are in the near-infrared-I (NIR-I, 700–900 nm) window, whereas the emission wavelengths are in the near-infrared-II (NIR-II, 950–1,400 nm) window [34–37]. However, not all CNTs act the same way; certain CNTs chirality lacks an absorption wavelength and are hence ineffective, if not hazardous, for such applications [38]. Antaris and colleagues Just one reactive CNTs chirality was chosen and administered a very small amount (4 g) of CNTs into mice after properly combining the surfactant for biocompatibility. This technique can aid in the surgical excision of tumoral masses at an early stage, resulting in a significant improvement in post-treatment survival [39, 40].

6.3.4 MAGNETIC RESONANCE IMAGING

This technique is among the most effective diagnostic tools known today in medicine. MRI aligns the nuclear magnetization of hydrogen bond in water across the body using a high-intensity magnetic field instead of ionizing radiation, taking advantage of variances in water content within tissues to make available anatomical photographs of great quality with remarkable spatial resolution [41]. There are two types of MRI contrast agents: spin-lattice relaxation agents that have a greater impact on T1 shortening and spin-spin relaxation agents that have a greater effect on T2 shortening, where T1 and T2 are proton relaxation durations [42]. Liu et al. recently created a T2-weighted contrast agent by placing nanoparticles into the MWCN's inner cavity, super paramagnetic iron oxide (SPIO). The SPIO-MWCNT were coated with a polymer to prevent aggregation and increase vascular biocompatibility. RAFT polymerization was utilized to make di-block copolymers (PMETAC-b-PEGMA) according to the technique described in [43, 44]. Two different components make up the final polymer. The cationic charged PMETAC block has been developed. To electrostatically connect to the negatively charged oxidized CNTs, and the it was possible to develop a working PEGMA block to increase the hybrid material's water dispersion stability [44–46].

6.3.5 POSITRON EMISSION TOMOGRAPHY

Emission of positron tomography is a noninvasive nuclear imaging method that tracks cellular functions using a radioactively labeled molecular ligand (or tracer). PET, one of the nuclear imaging methods, has become a valuable tool in clinical and research settings. Two spinning detectors detect gamma (γ) rays generated by a decaying radionuclide within the patient and convert the energy into an electrical signal, which is subsequently processed into a photograph [47].

In PET imaging, radio-nuclei emit positrons that interact with electrons in the local region, resulting in the production of two extremely high-energy photons (511 keV each). The two photons with a 511-keV energy are released in opposing directions, at an angle of around 180°. Detectors in a ring detect the rays, which registers coincident rays from a single event along a particular line of response [48].

Positron-emitting radionuclides can be attached or even incorporated into carbon nanotubes for PET imaging. SWNTs that have been radiolabeled and functionalized by phospholipid bilayer carrying polyethylene-glycol (PEG) coupled with arginine-glycine-aspartic acid (RGD) peptide, Liu et al. showed tumor-targeted PET imaging for the first time. Such a combination was able to effectively target integrin-positive tumors while also providing high contrast imaging [49, 50]. Other CNTs have also been functionalized, both of them radiolabeled and tumor-targeting biomolecules, enabling multi-modality cancer theranostics. Ruggiero and colleagues created two kinds of MWCNT structures, each of which included an E4G10 antibody to target the epitope encoded in tumor angiogenic arteries [51]. The first was created to supply a potent atom producing 225Ac3+ radionuclide producer, while the second was created to transmit a positron-emitting 89Zr radionuclide for PET imaging. They achieved a five-fold increase in particular activity of PET imaging with the second construct, which enhanced the image's signal-to-noise ratio [52]. While the first build produced good results for cancer therapy. It's worth noting that a single CNT may be designed to support both imaging and therapeutic payloads on the same framework (Figure 6.2) [53].

6.3.6 MULTIMODALITY IMAGING

It should be abundantly obvious that each imaging is a valuable tool. There are benefits and drawbacks to this strategy, making it difficult for one strategy to outperform another. The next best step is to merge all of the benefits into a single technique while attempting to avoid all of the drawbacks. As a result, various research groups are working on multimodal CAs that could make use of all benefits of each approach. Because of the various sorts of functionalization that may be performed on CNTs, they are a suitable place for this task [54–56]. Cinsneros et al., developed a dual CA using CNTs. For MRI and PET systems, they loaded CNTs with Gd^{3+} and Cu^{2+}, respectively. Considering the fact that it did not assess the situation, them on actual tumors, they were able to demonstrate platform stability *in vivo* over time and confirm their accumulation, which was mostly in the lungs and liver [57]. This is one avenue in which enhanced imaging probes with changeable multimodal

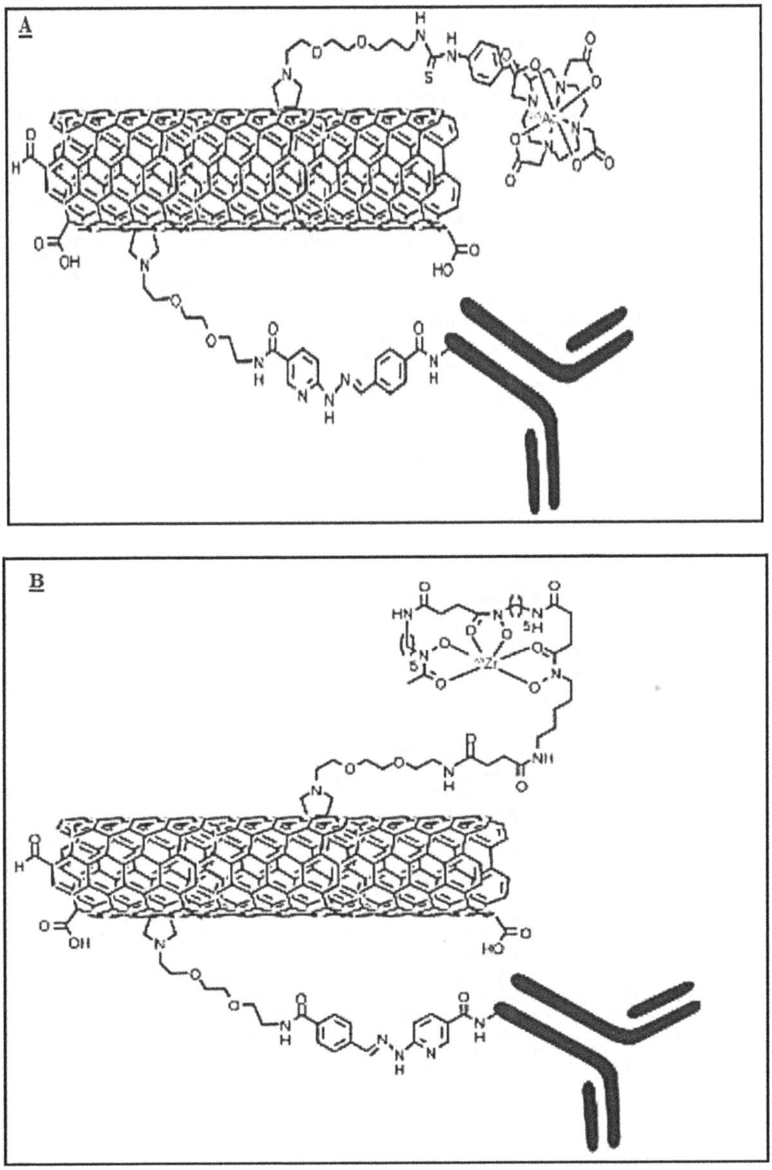

FIGURE 6.2 Covalent functionalization of water-soluble SWCNT-NH_2 with radionuclides, 1,4,7,10-tetraazacyclododecane-1,4,7,10-tetraacetic acid (DOTA), desferrioxamine B (DFO), and antibodies resulted in the addition of important moieties such as 1,4,7,10-tetraazacyclododecane-1,4,7,10-tetraacetic acid (DOT). (A) Construct I (SWCNT-([225Ac]DOTA)(E4G10)) is a radio-immunotherapeutic drug; and (B) construct II (SWCNT-([89Zr]DFO) is a radio-immunoimaging drug (E4G10).

imaging capabilities are being designed. Wang's group conceived and built a bimodal CNTs CA for SPECT and MRI in a similar fashion. The magnetic characteristics of the CNTs were provided by super-paramagnetic iron oxide nanoparticle (SPION), while the radioactivity was granted by 99 mTc. Even in this example, there was no real tumor in the test individual; instead, just the stability, dispersion, and organ aggregation were investigated. After 4 hours, distribution investigations revealed widespread aggregation in the lungs, liver, and spleen, with a steady decrease in lung uptake but no change in liver signals [58]. The hybrids' capacity as double magnetic resonance imaging and SPECT contrast agents for *in-vivo* application is demonstrated by imaging data. Zhao et al. recently developed a novel CNTs multimodal hybrid by merging SWCNT, covered with polydopamine (PDA) and PEG, with Mn^{2+} for MR imaging and 131I for nuclear imaging, and also radioisotope cancer treatment, to generate a novel multimodal hybrid made of carbon nanotubes. The scientists reported effective tumor development of SWNT@PDA-131I-PEG following systemic delivery into mice, as evidenced by MR and gamma imaging. Furthermore, they used SWCNTs great NIR absorbance to conduct NIR-triggered photothermal treatment in tandem with 131I-based radioisotope treatment to successfully eradicate cancer. These new multimodal contrast compounds will be useful for tumor imaging, also theranostic and radiation therapy [59–61].

6.4 CNTS THERAPIES IN CANCER

6.4.1 *PHOTOTHERMAL THERAPY*

Hyperthermia is a therapeutic method that raises the temperature over a biological boundary, causing cell death in a cancer-affected area of the body. Photothermal therapy is a term used to describe when a person's temperature is raised using optical light (PTT). Thermal ablation has the benefit over removal of surgical tissue in that it is less intrusive and has a lower mortality rate, also the capability to treat tumors in essential structures that cannot be removed medically [62–64]. Furthermore, when coupled along with other therapies like as chemotherapy or radiation, PTT might boost tumor cytotoxicity in a synergistic manner. Hyperthermia also improves the tumor's permeability vasculature in a preferential manner, which can improve medication transport into tumors [65]. The crucial component in the ablation of cancer cells by heat is reliably overcoming the thermal resistance of cells threshold. Because of CNTs' with the capacity to transform heat from near-infrared light A new group of hybrid has been created for cancer light therapy that is both efficient and effective [66]. Taking use of CNTs' strong NIR absorption isn't the only technique to raise their temperature. SWCNTs were coated with a polymer to prevent aggregation and injected into tumors by Gannon's team [67]. The polymer-coated CNTs were then subjected to 13.56 MHz Radio frequency field for two minutes. The tumors were entirely eliminated in all of the test samples. Tumors without CNT but under the same RF field and tumors with CNTs but no RF field, on the other side, were remained alive. These findings showed that CNTs hyperthermia therapy might allow non-invasive RF field therapies to suppress cancer cells by inflicting deadly thermal damage [68].

6.4.2 *PHOTODYNAMIC THERAPY*

As a result of aerobic metabolism, tiny quantities of reactive oxygen species (ROS) are continually produced in living. Antioxidants, which are found in living cells, help to neutralize harmful species [69]. Oxidative stress is a state that occurs when ROS levels are excessively high in comparison to antioxidants. When oxidative stress in a cell lasts too long, it can cause apoptosis, or cell death. Apoptosis and cancer are opposite processes; however, ROS have been consistently displayed to play a vital role in both. ROS are purposely produced within cancer cells to destroy them in the context of tumor therapy [70, 71]. They next adsorbed a PDT agent called Hematoporphyrin Mono-Methyl Ether (HMME) on top of HA-CNT in a second stage, as shown in Figure 6.3 [72].

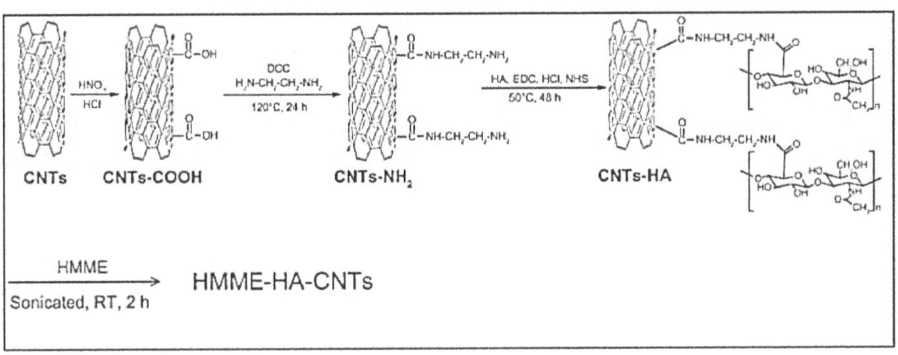

FIGURE 6.3 Photodynamic therapy.

The materials were forced to endure *in vitro* and *in vivo* experiments to determine their photodynamic and photothermal characteristics. In the case of the *in vivo* testing, comparative tests were carried out. The mice with tumors were separated into five categories and given different treatments: (i) NaCl solution; (ii) HA-CNTs treated with an 808-nm laser; (iii) HMME treated with a 532-nm laser; (iv) HMME-HA-CNTs treated both with 532- and 808-nm lasers; and (v) HMME-HA-CNTs treated with both 532- and 808-nm lasers.

6.4.3 DRUG DELIVERY SYSTEM

Chemotherapy, the most common cancer treatment, aims to supers cancer cells while causing little damage to healthy tissue. Many contemporary chemotherapeutic drugs, on another side, are far from perfect. Many of them, in fact, have a high overall toxicity [72–75]. They also have disadvantages such as low solubility and poor non-selective biodistribution. To address these issues, scientists began to employ carbon nanotubes for targeted medication delivery. CNTs, as previously noted, offer properties that may be exploited to make excellent drug nano-vectors [76]. Only a few of these qualities are improved EPR, needle-like morphology that promotes transmembrane invasion and intracellular deposition, and flexibility of molecules loading over either on the surface or within the inner core of CNTs using interactions that are both covalent and non-covalent. Ji et al. wrapped chitosan surrounding the surface of the CNTs to non-covalently functionalize SWCNTs [77]. Carbon nanotubes that are being chitosan-functionalized are more water miscible and biocompatible. Many malignancies have an overexpression of the folate receptor, Ji's team further functionalized the novel material with folic acid to target it solely to cancer cells. Finally, they added Doxorubicin, a widely recognized anti-cancer drug [78]. As a consequence, the final hybrid was evaluated *in-vitro* and *in-vivo,* and it outperformed free DOX in terms of killing tumor cells. These positive results are attributed to three main factors: more accurate tumor targeting owing to folic acid, improved capacity of CNTs to get inside cells in comparison to free DOX, and the fact that DOX release occurs in a low pH environment, which is typical of tumors [79]. Tumor targeting clearly improves effectiveness while lowering the needed therapeutic dosage. Furthermore, substantial research is being done on multifunctional CNTs, which can be utilized as imaging contrast agents while delivering medicines [80, 81].

6.4.4 INTENTIONAL CYTOTOXICITY

CNTs are now widely regarded in the scientific field as having the ability to traverse biological membranes, regardless of cell type [82]. In this light, CNTs possess two sides of the single coin: planned cytotoxicity to suppress cancer cells and unintended cytotoxicity caused by their use in other treatments, such as drug vectors, contrast agents, and so on [83]. Many research organizations are attempting to use CNTs' cytotoxicity to kill cancer cells. Garcia-group Hevia's is among the busiest in this field among them. They looked into the cytotoxicity of uncoated MWCNTs and observed that they may readily penetrate cells and intertwine to cytoskeleton protein nanofilaments, causing mitotic biomechanics to be disrupted. This activity is similar to that of other regularly prescribed anti-cancer medicines, such as paclitaxel [84, 85].

6.4.5 GENE THERAPY

Gene therapy may be characterized in the most general meaning as a means of providing genetic data to patient somatic cells in order for them to produce specific therapeutic proteins to fix or modify illness. Vectors capable of efficiently transferring genetic elements into target cells with little harm are required for successful gene therapy. Because of its high transfection effectiveness, the most widely investigated gene carriers are still viral vectors. Non-viral delivery techniques, on another side, are an appealing option due to worries about virus usage in people and other restrictions [86–88]. Non-viral vectors are especially well-suited due to their ease of use, ease of large-scale manufacture, and absence of a specific immune response. Several innovative non-viral vectors have recently been discovered that are similar to viruses in terms of transfection effectiveness. CNTs drew a lot of focus due to its potential to quickly permeate biological membranes and minimal immunogenicity. For example, in a follow-up to a prior work on tumor apoptosis, intertumoral treatment of small interfering RNA (siRNA)-functionalized MWCNTs complexes inhibited tumor development and extended life in human lung xenograft-bearing mice [89]. Guo et al. functionalized MWCNTs with appropriate siRNA, which inhibits polo-like kinase 1 (PLK1), which is thought to prevent cancer cells from reproducing (lung cancer in this case). They used intertumoral injections to compare Carbon nanotubes and liposomes as vectors [90]. They discovered that combining siPLK1 with MWCNTs made it easier for tumor cells to internalize it in a solid tumor mass *in vivo*, results in considerable PLK1 knockdown when comparing to liposomal complexes, despite the fact that the latter are normally administered systemically [91]. Similarly, Siu's group used polymer (succinate polyethyleneimine) and siRNA fragments to non-covalently functionalize CNTs and mute genes in a melanoma model [92]. In the tumors tissue, they discovered considerable absorption of administered siRNA also a functioning gene silencing effect. Over a 25-day period, this therapy [93]. As a result of the treatment, there was a drop in tumor development. These examples show the tremendous potential of gene therapy alone and in conjunction with carbon nanotubes in the battle against cancer [94, 95].

6.5 CONCLUSION

Carbon nanotubes' unusual physical qualities prompted substantial research into the structure as a nanoscale tool for a variety of cancer therapy and diagnostic applications throughout the last decade. The one-dimensional structure of CNTs and their variable length make them an excellent platform for researching shape and size effects *in vitro*, but particularly *in vivo*. CNTs, unlike conventional inorganic nanoparticles, could be functionalized in a number of ways and have intrinsic physical properties such as resonance photoluminescence, strong NIR optical absorption, and Raman scattering, which may use for static and functional imaging, passive, and active tracking, and drug and gene vectoring and targeting. The majority of these "skills" may be combined on a single CNT, making it a one-of-a-kind platform for multimodality cancer treatment and imaging. They can also be used in conjunction Using conventional cancer therapies such as chemo and radiotherapy.

Regardless of whether those multiple promising outcomes employing CNTs in tumor fighting have been reported in recent years, much more research is needed before they can be utilized in the clinic. The key problem and practical constraint to be addressed is the possible long-term toxicity. Much has been done to address this problem, particularly with polymer coating and induced biodegradation, but more effort is needed to create a hybrid that is both stable and non-toxic. With these characteristics, they have a strong chance of becoming the tumor nano-theranostic tool of the future, which combines diagnostic and therapeutic qualities in a single nanometric agent, and might open up previously unimagined possibilities for cancer detection and treatment.

KEYWORDS

- **cancer therapy**
- **carbon nanotubes**
- **carrier**
- **nanomedicine**
- **nanotechnology**

REFERENCES

1. Seeta, R. R. G., Benton, L., Pavitra, E., & Yu, J. S., (2015). Multifunctional nanoparticles: Recent progress in cancer therapeutics. *Chem. Commun., 51*, 13248–13259. doi: 10.1039/C5CC04643B.
2. Marchesan, S., Kostarelos, K., Bianco, A., & Prato, M., (2015). The winding road for carbon nanotubes in nanomedicine. *Mater. Today., 18*, 12–19. doi: 10.1016/j.mattod.2014.07.009.
3. Lacerda, L., Bianco, A., Prato, M., & Kostarelos, K., (2006). Carbon nanotubes as nanomedicines: From toxicology to pharmacology. *Adv. Drug Deliv. Rev., 58*, 1460–1470. doi: 10.1016/j.addr.2006.09.015.
4. Lim, E., Kim, T., Paik, S., Haam, S., Huh, Y. M., & Lee, K., (2015). Nanomaterials for theranostics: Recent advances and future challenges. *Chem. Rev., 115*, 327–394. doi: 10.1021/cr300213b.
5. Dresselhaus, M., Dresselhaus, G., & Saito, R., (1995). Physics of carbon nanotubes. *Carbon, 33*, 883–891. doi: 10.1016/0008-6223(95)00017-8.
6. Wilder, J. W., Venema, L. C., Rinzler, A. G., Smalley, R. E., & Dekker, C., (1998). Electronic structure of atomically resolved carbon nanotubes. *Nature, 391*, 59–62. doi: 10.1038/34139.
7. Mahar, B., Laslau, C., Yip, R., & Sun, Y., (2007). Development of carbon nanotube-based sensors–a review. *IEEE Sens. J., 7*, 266–284. doi: 10.1109/JSEN.2006.886863.
8. Siegal, M., Overmyer, D., & Provencio, P., (2002). Precise control of multiwall carbon nanotube diameters using thermal chemical vapor deposition. *Appl. Phys. Lett., 80*, 2171–2173. doi: 10.1063/1.1463204.
9. Prasek, J., Drbohlavova, J., Chomoucka, J., Hubalek, J., Jasek, O., Adam, V., & Kizek, R., (2011). Methods for carbon nanotubes synthesis—Review. *J. Mater. Chem., 21*, 15872–15884. doi: 10.1039/c1jm12254a.
10. Chen, Y., Zhang, Y., Hu, Y., Kang, L., Zhang, S., Xie, H., Liu, D., et al., (2014). State of the art of single-walled carbon nanotube synthesis on surfaces. *Adv. Mater., 26*, 5898–5922. doi: 10.1002/adma.201400431.
11. Yellampalli, S., (2011). *Carbon Nanotubes: Synthesis, Characterization, Applications.* In-Tech; Vienna, Austria.

12. Helveg, S., Lopez-Cartes, C., Sehested, J., Hansen, P. L., Clausen, B. S., Rostrup-Nielsen, J. R., Abild-Pedersen, F., & Nørskov, J. K., (2004). Atomic-Scale imaging of carbon nanofiber growth. *Nature, 427*, 426–429. doi: 10.1038/nature02278.
13. Yoshida, H., Takeda, S., Uchiyama, T., Kohno, H., & Homma, Y., (2008). Atomic-scale in-situ observation of carbon nanotube growth from solid state iron carbide nanoparticles. *Nano Lett., 8*, 2082–2086. doi: 10.1021/nl080452q.
14. Arora, N., & Sharma, N., (2014). Arc discharge synthesis of carbon nanotubes: Comprehensive review. *Diamond Relat. Mater., 50*, 135–150. doi: 10.1016/j.diamond.2014.10.001.
15. Scott, C. D., Arepalli, S., Nikolaev, P., & Smalley, R. E., (2001). Growth mechanisms for single-wall carbon nanotubes in a laser-ablation process. *Appl. Phys. A., 72*, 573–580. doi: 10.1007/s003390100761.
16. Arepalli, S., (2004). Laser ablation process for single-walled carbon nanotube production. *J. Nanosci. Nanotechnol., 4*, 317–325. doi: 10.1166/jnn.2004.072.
17. Gadde, S., (2015). Multi-Drug delivery nanocarriers for combination therapy. *Med. Chem. Commun., 6*, 1916–1929. doi: 10.1039/C5MD00365B.
18. Hernández-Rivera, M., Zaibaq, N. G., & Wilson, L. J., (2016). Toward carbon nanotube-based imaging agents for the clinic. *Biomaterials, 101*, 229–240. doi: 10.1016/j.biomaterials.2016.05.045.
19. Wong, B. S., Yoong, S. L., Jagusiak, A., Panczyk, T., Ho, H. K., Ang, W. H., & Pastorin, G., (2013). Carbon nanotubes for delivery of small molecule drugs. *Adv. Drug Deliv. Rev., 65*, 1964–2015. doi: 10.1016/j.addr.2013.08.005.
20. Singh, R., & Torti, S. V., (2013). Carbon nanotubes in hyperthermia therapy. *Adv. Drug Deliv. Rev., 65*, 2045–2060. doi: 10.1016/j.addr.2013.08.001.
21. Fard, J. K., Jafari, S., & Eghbal, M. A., (2015). A review of molecular mechanisms involved in toxicity of nanoparticles. *Adv. Pharm. Bull., 5*, 447. doi: 10.15171/apb.2015.061.
22. Zhang, L., Lv, D., Su, W., Liu, Y., Chen, Y., & Xiang, R., (2013). Detection of cancer biomarkers with nanotechnology. *Am. J. Biochem. Biotechnol., 9*, 71. doi: 10.3844/ajbbsp.2013.71.89.
23. Dinesh, B., Bianco, A., & Ménard-Moyon, C., (2016). Designing multimodal carbon nanotubes by covalent multi-functionalization. *Nanoscale, 8*, 18596–18611. doi: 10.1039/C6NR06728J.
24. Marchesan, S., Melchionna, M., & Prato, M., (2015). Wire up on carbon nanostructures! How to play a winning game. *ACS Nano, 9*, 9441–9450. doi: 10.1021/acsnano.5b04956.
25. Bilalis, P., Katsigiannopoulos, D., Avgeropoulos, A., & Sakellariou, G., (2014). Non-Covalent functionalization of carbon nanotubes with polymers. *RSC Adv., 4*, 2911–2934. doi: 10.1039/C3RA44906H.
26. Postema, M., & Gilja, O. H., (2011). Contrast-enhanced and targeted ultrasound. *World J. Gastroenterol. WJG., 17*, 28. doi: 10.3748/wjg.v17.i1.28.
27. Delogu, L. G., Vidili, G., Venturelli, E., Ménard-Moyon, C., Zoroddu, M. A., Pilo, G., Nicolussi, P., Ligios, C., Bedognetti, D., Sgarrella, F., et al., (2012). Functionalized multi-walled carbon nanotubes as ultrasound contrast agents. *Proc. Natl. Acad. Sci. USA., 109*, 16612–16617. doi: 10.1073/pnas.1208312109.
28. Wu, H., Shi, H., Zhang, H., Wang, X., Yang, Y., Yu, C., Hao, C., et al., (2014). Prostate stem cell antigen antibody-conjugated multi-walled carbon nanotubes for targeted

ultrasound imaging and drug delivery. *Biomaterials, 35*, 5369–5380. doi: 10.1016/j.biomaterials.2014.03.038.
29. Wang, L. V., & Hu, S., (2012). Photoacoustic tomography: *In vivo* imaging from organelles to organs. *Science, 335*, 1458–1462. doi: 10.1126/science.1216210.
30. Luke, G. P., Yeager, D., & Emelianov, S. Y., (2012). Biomedical applications of photoacoustic imaging with exogenous contrast agents. *Ann. Biomed. Eng., 40*, 422–437. doi: 10.1007/s10439-011-0449-4.
31. Nguyen, V. P., Oh, Y., Ha, K., Oh, J., & Kang, H. W., (2015). Enhancement of high-resolution photoacoustic imaging with indocyanine green-conjugated carbon nanotubes. *JPN. J. Appl. Phys., 54*, 07 HF04. doi: 10.7567/JJAP.54.07HF04.
32. Wu, L., Cai, X., Nelson, K., Xing, W., Xia, J., Zhang, R., Stacy, A. J., Luderer, M., Lanza, G. M., Wang, L. V., et al., (2013). A green synthesis of carbon nanoparticles from honey and their use in real-time photoacoustic imaging. *Nano Res., 6*, 312–325. doi: 10.1007/s12274-013-0308-8.
33. Zanganeh, S., Li, H., Kumavor, P. D., Alqasemi, U., Aguirre, A., Mohammad, I., Stanford, C., et al., (2013). Photoacoustic imaging enhanced by indocyanine green-conjugated single-wall carbon nanotubes. *J. Biomed. Opt., 18*, 096006. doi: 10.1117/1.JBO.18.9.096006.
34. De La Zerda, A., Zavaleta, C., Keren, S., Vaithilingam, S., Bodapati, S., Liu, Z., Levi, J., Smith, B. R., Ma, T. J., Oralkan, O., et al., (2008). Carbon nanotubes as photoacoustic molecular imaging agents in living mice. *Nat. Nanotechnol., 3*, 557–562. doi: 10.1038/nnano.2008.231.
35. De La Zerda, A., Liu, Z., Bodapati, S., Teed, R., Vaithilingam, S., Khuri-Yakub, B. T., Chen, X., et al., (2010). Ultrahigh sensitivity carbon nanotube agents for photoacoustic molecular imaging in living mice. *Nano Lett., 10*, 2168–2172. doi: 10.1021/nl100890d.
36. De La Zerda, A., Bodapati, S., Teed, R., May, S. Y., Tabakman, S. M., Liu, Z., Khuri-Yakub, B. T., et al., (2012). Family of enhanced photoacoustic imaging agents for high-sensitivity and multiplexing studies in living mice. *ACS Nano, 6*, 4694–4701. doi: 10.1021/nn204352r.
37. Kim, J. W., Galanzha, E. I., Shashkov, E. V., Moon, H. M., & Zharov, V. P., (2009). Golden carbon nanotubes as multimodal photoacoustic and photothermal high-contrast molecular agents. *Nat. Nanotechnol., 4*, 688–694. doi: 10.1038/nnano.2009.231.
38. Wang, C., Bao, C., Liang, S., Fu, H., Wang, K., Deng, M., Liao, Q., & Cui, D., (2014). RGD-Conjugated silica-coated gold nanorods on the surface of carbon nanotubes for targeted photoacoustic imaging of gastric cancer. *Nanoscale Res. Lett., 9*, 1–10. doi: 10.1186/1556-276X-9-264.
39. Antaris, A. L., Robinson, J. T., Yaghi, O. K., Hong, G., Diao, S., Luong, R., & Dai, H., (2013). Ultra-low doses of chirality sorted (6, 5) carbon nanotubes for simultaneous tumor imaging and photothermal therapy. *ACS Nano, 7*, 3644–3652. doi: 10.1021/nn4006472.
40. Ghosh, D., Bagley, A. F., Na, Y. J., Birrer, M. J., Bhatia, S. N., & Belcher, A. M., (2014). Deep, noninvasive imaging and surgical guidance of submillimeter tumors using targeted M13-stabilized single-walled carbon nanotubes. *Proc. Natl. Acad. Sci. USA, 111*, 13948–13953. doi: 10.1073/pnas.1400821111. [.
41. Hu, Z., Yang, W., Liu, H., Wang, K., Bao, C., Song, T., Wang, J., & Tian, J., (2014). From PET/CT to PET/MRI: Advances in instrumentation and clinical applications. *Mol. Pharm., 11*, 3798–3809. doi: 10.1021/mp500321h.

42. Brown, M. A., & Semelka, R. C., (2011). *MRI: Basic Principles and Applications.* John Wiley & Sons; London, UK.
43. Liu, Y., Hughes, T. C., Muir, B. W., Waddington, L. J., Gengenbach, T. R., Easton, C. D., Hinton, T. M., et al., (2014). Water-Dispersible magnetic carbon nanotubes as T 2-weighted MRI contrast agents. *Biomaterials, 35*, 378–386. doi: 10.1016/j.biomaterials.2013.09.079.
44. Maciejewska, B. M., Warowicka, A., Baranowska-Korczyc, A., Załęski, K., Zalewski, T., Kozioł, K. K., & Jurga, S., (2015). Magnetic and hydrophilic MWCNT/Fe composites as potential T 2-weighted MRI contrast agents. *Carbon, 94*, 1012–1020. doi: 10.1016/j.carbon.2015.07.091.
45. Al Faraj, A., (2016). SWCNTs as novel theranostic nanocarriers for cancer diagnosis and therapy: Towards safe translation to the clinics. *Nanomedicine, 11*, 1431–1445. doi: 10.2217/nnm-2016–0065.
46. Al Faraj, A., Shaik, A. S., & Al Sayed, B., (2015). Preferential magnetic targeting of carbon nanotubes to cancer sites: Noninvasive tracking using MRI in a murine breast cancer model. *Nanomedicine, 10*, 931–948. doi: 10.2217/nnm.14.145.
47. Al Faraj, A., Shaik, A. P., & Shaik, A. S., (2015). Magnetic single-walled carbon nanotubes as efficient drug delivery nanocarriers in breast cancer murine model: Noninvasive monitoring using diffusion-weighted magnetic resonance imaging as sensitive imaging biomarker. *Int. J. Nanomed., 10*, 157. doi: 10.2147/IJN.S75074.
48. Liu, Y., Hao, X., Waddington, L. J., Qiu, J., & Hughes, T. C., (2014). Surface modification of multi-walled carbon nanotubes with engineered self-assembled RAFT diblock coatings. *Aust. J. Chem., 67*, 151–158. doi: 10.1071/CH13401.
49. Liu, Y., Muir, B. W., Waddington, L. J., Hinton, T. M., Moffat, B. A., Hao, X., Qiu, J., & Hughes, T. C., (2015). Colloidally stabilized magnetic carbon nanotubes providing MRI contrast in mouse liver tumors. *Biomacromolecules, 16*, 790–797. doi: 10.1021/bm501706x.
50. Caravan, P., Ellison, J. J., McMurry, T. J., & Lauffer, R. B., (1999). Gadolinium (III) chelates as MRI contrast agents: Structure, dynamics, and applications. *Chem. Rev., 99*, 2293–2352. doi: 10.1021/cr980440x.
51. Richard, C., Doan, B. T., Beloeil, J. C., Bessodes, M., Tóth, É., & Scherman, D., (2008). Noncovalent functionalization of carbon nanotubes with amphiphilic Gd^{3+} chelates: Toward powerful T1 and T2 MRI contrast agents. *Nano Lett., 8*, 232–236. doi: 10.1021/nl072509z.
52. Louie, A., (2010). Multimodality imaging probes: Design and challenges. *Chem. Rev., 110*, 3146–3195. doi: 10.1021/cr9003538.
53. Al Faraj, A., Shaik, A. S., Al Sayed, B., Halwani, R., & Al Jammaz, I., (2016). Specific targeting and noninvasive imaging of breast cancer stem cells using single-walled carbon nanotubes as novel multimodality nanoprobes. *Nanomedicine, 11*, 31–46. doi: 10.2217/nnm.15.182.
54. Wang, J. T. W., Cabana, L., Bourgognon, M., Kafa, H., Protti, A., Venner, K., Shah, A. M., Sosabowski, J. K., Mather, S. J., Roig, A., et al., (2014). Magnetically decorated multi-walled carbon nanotubes as dual MRI and SPECT contrast agents. *Adv. Funct. Mater., 24*, 1880–1894. doi: 10.1002/adfm.201302892.
55. Zhao, H., Chao, Y., Liu, J., Huang, J., Pan, J., Guo, W., Wu, J., Sheng, M., Yang, K., Wang, J., et al., (2016). Polydopamine coated single-walled carbon nanotubes as a

versatile platform with radionuclide labeling for multimodal tumor imaging and therapy. *Theranostics, 6*, 1833. doi: 10.7150/thno.16047.
56. Hong, G., Diao, S., Antaris, A. L., & Dai, H., (2015). Carbon nanomaterials for biological imaging and nanomedicinal therapy. *Chem. Rev., 2015.* doi: 10.1021/acs.chemrev.5b00008.
57. Li, Q., Ruan, H., & Li, H., (2014). Nanocarbon materials for photodynamic therapy and photothermal therapy. *Pharm. Nanotechnol., 2*, 58–64. doi: 10.2174/2211738502666140929211831.
58. Beik, J., Abed, Z., Ghoreishi, F. S., Hosseini-Nami, S., Mehrzadi, S., Shakeri-Zadeh, A., & Kamrava, S. K., (2016). Nanotechnology in hyperthermia cancer therapy: From fundamental principles to advanced applications. *J. Controll. Release, 235*, 205–221. doi: 10.1016/j.jconrel.2016.05.062.
59. Hahn, G. M., (2012). *Hyperthermia and Cancer.* Springer Science & Business Media; New York, NY, USA.
60. Falk, M., & Issels, R., (2001). Hyperthermia in oncology. *Int. J. Hyperth., 17*, 1–18. doi: 10.1080/02656730150201552.
61. Schaaf, L., Schwab, M., Ulmer, C., Heine, S., Mürdter, T. E., Schmid, J. O., Sauer, G., et al., (2016). Hyperthermia synergizes with chemotherapy by inhibiting PARP1-dependent DNA replication arrest. *Cancer Res., 76*, 2868–2875. doi: 10.1158/0008-5472.CAN-15-2908.
62. Hainfeld, J. F., Lin, L., Slatkin, D. N., Dilmanian, F. A., Vadas, T. M., & Smilowitz, H. M., (2014). Gold nanoparticle hyperthermia reduces radiotherapy dose. *Nanomed.: Nanotechnol. Biol. Med., 10*, 1609–1617. doi: 10.1016/j.nano.2014.05.006.
63. Li, L., Ten, H. T. L., Haeri, A., Soullie, T., Scholten, C., Seynhaeve, A. L., Eggermont, A. M., & Koning, G. A., (2014). A novel two-step mild hyperthermia for advanced liposomal chemotherapy. *J. Controll. Release., 174*, 202–208. doi: 10.1016/j.jconrel.2013.11.012.
64. Gong, F., Hongyan, Z., Papavassiliou, D. V., Bui, K., Lim, C., & Duong, H. M., (2014). Mesoscopic modeling of cancer photothermal therapy using single-walled carbon nanotubes and near infrared radiation: Insights through an off-lattice Monte Carlo approach. *Nanotechnology, 25*, 205101. doi: 10.1088/0957-4484/25/20/205101.
65. Liang, C., Diao, S., Wang, C., Gong, H., Liu, T., Hong, G., Shi, X., et al., (2014). Tumor metastasis inhibition by imaging-guided photothermal therapy with single-walled carbon nanotubes. *Adv. Mater., 26*, 5646–5652. doi: 10.1002/adma.201401825.
66. Zhang, B., Wang, H., Shen, S., She, X., Shi, W., Chen, J., Zhang, Q., et al., (2016). Fibrin-Targeting peptide CREKA-conjugated multi-walled carbon nanotubes for self-amplified photothermal therapy of tumor. *Biomaterials, 79*, 46–55. doi: 10.1016/j.biomaterials.2015.11.061.
67. Khan, S. A., Kanchanapally, R., Fan, Z., Beqa, L., Singh, A. K., Senapati, D., & Ray, P. C., (2012). A gold nanocage–CNT hybrid for targeted imaging and photothermal destruction of cancer cells. *Chem. Commun., 48*, 6711–6713. doi: 10.1039/c2cc32313c.
68. Iancu, C., & Mocan, L., (2011). Advances in cancer therapy through the use of carbon nanotube-mediated targeted hyperthermia. *Int. J. Nanomed., 6*, 1675–1684. doi: 10.2147/IJN.S23588.
69. Murali, V. S., Mikoryak, C., Wang, R., & Draper, R. K., (2014). Effect of carbon nanotube amount and subcellular location on the near infrared (NIR) photothermal ablation of cells. *Cancer Res., 74*, 5374. doi: 10.1158/1538-7445.AM2014-5374.

70. Hashida, Y., Tanaka, H., Zhou, S., Kawakami, S., Yamashita, F., Murakami, T., Umeyama, T., et al., (2014). Photothermal ablation of tumor cells using a single-walled carbon nanotube–peptide composite. *J. Controll. Release, 173*, 59–66. doi: 10.1016/j.jconrel.2013.10.039.
71. Gao, F., Xie, S. X., Sitharaman, B., Booske, J. H., & Hagness, S. C., (2014). Functionalized carbon nanotube theranostic agents for microwave diagnostic imaging and thermal therapy of tumors. *Proceedings of the 8th European Conference on Antennas and Propagation (EuCAP 2014)* (pp. 691–693). The Hague, The Netherlands.
72. Truong, N. P., Whittaker, M. R., Mak, C. W., & Davis, T. P., (2015). The importance of nanoparticle shape in cancer drug delivery. *Expert Opin. Drug Deliv., 12*, 129–142. doi: 10.1517/17425247.2014.950564.
73. Kostarelos, K., Lacerda, L., Pastorin, G., Wu, W., Wieckowski, S., Luangsivilay, J., Godefroy, S., Pantarotto, D., Briand, J. P., Muller, S., et al., (2007). Cellular uptake of functionalized carbon nanotubes is independent of functional group and cell type. *Nat. Nanotechnol., 2*, 108–113. doi: 10.1038/nnano.2006.209.
74. Wang, J. T. W., & Al-Jamal, K. T., (2015). Functionalized carbon nanotubes: Revolution in brain delivery. *Nanomedicine, 10*, 2639–2642. doi: 10.2217/nnm.15.114.
75. Martincic, M., & Tobias, G., (2015). Filled carbon nanotubes in biomedical imaging and drug delivery. *Expert Opin. Drug Deliv., 12*, 563–581. doi: 10.1517/17425247.2015.971751.
76. Marega, R., & Bonifazi, D., (2014). Filling carbon nanotubes for nanobiotechnological applications. *New J. Chem., 38*, 22–27. doi: 10.1039/C3NJ01008B.
77. Shao, W., Paul, A., Zhao, B., Lee, C., Rodes, L., & Prakash, S., (2013). Carbon nanotube lipid drug approach for targeted delivery of a chemotherapy drug in a human breast cancer xenograft animal model. *Biomaterials, 34*, 10109–10119. doi: 10.1016/j.biomaterials.2013.09.007.
78. Ji, Z., Lin, G., Lu, Q., Meng, L., Shen, X., Dong, L., Fu, C., & Zhang, X., (2012). Targeted therapy of SMMC-7721 liver cancer *in vitro* and *in vivo* with carbon nanotubes-based drug delivery system. *J. Colloid Interface Sci., 365*, 143–149. doi: 10.1016/j.jcis.2011.09.013.
79. Lee, Y. K., Choi, J., Wang, W., Lee, S., Nam, T. H., Choi, W. S., Kim, C. J., Lee, J. K., Kim, S. H., Kang, S. S., et al., (2013). Nullifying tumor efflux by prolonged endolysosome vesicles: Development of low dose anticancer-carbon nanotube drug. *ACS Nano, 7*, 8484–8497. doi: 10.1021/nn4041206.
80. Singh, R. K., Patel, K. D., Kim, J. J., Kim, T. H., Kim, J. H., Shin, U. S., Lee, E. J., et al., (2014). Multifunctional hybrid nanocarrier: Magnetic CNTs ensheathed with mesoporous silica for drug delivery and imaging system. *ACS Appl. Mater. Interfaces, 6*, 2201–2208. doi: 10.1021/am4056936.
81. Jeyamohan, P., Hasumura, T., Nagaoka, Y., Yoshida, Y., Maekawa, T., & Kumar, D. S., (2013). Accelerated killing of cancer cells using a multifunctional single-walled carbon nanotube-based system for targeted drug delivery in combination with photothermal therapy. *Int. J. Nanomed., 8*, 2653–2667.
82. Liu, J., Wang, C., Wang, X., Wang, X., Cheng, L., Li, Y., & Liu, Z., (2015). Mesoporous silica coated single-walled carbon nanotubes as a multifunctional light-responsive platform for cancer combination therapy. *Adv. Funct. Mater., 25*, 384–392. doi: 10.1002/adfm.201403079.

83. Zhang, Y., Lai, J. C., & Bhushan, A., (2013). Biomedical and pharmaceutical sciences department, college of pharmacy, division of health sciences differential effects of functionalized and non-functionalized short multi-wall carbon nanotubes on survival and cell signaling in pancreatic cancer cells. *Cancer Res., 73*, 4414. doi: 10.1158/1538-7445.AM2013-4414.
84. García-Hevia, L., Villegas, J. C., Fernández, F., Casafont, Í., González, J., Valiente, R., & Fanarraga, M. L., (2016). Multiwalled carbon nanotubes inhibit tumor progression in a mouse model. *Adv. Healthc. Mater., 2016.* doi: 10.1002/adhm.201500753.
85. Mady, M. M., (2011). Cationic liposomes as gene delivery system. *Afr. J. Pharm. Pharmacol., 5*, 2007–2012.
86. Boulaiz, H., Marchal, J. A., Prados, J., Melguizo, C., & Aranega, A., (2004). Non-Viral and viral vectors for gene therapy. *Cell. Mol. Biol. (Noisy-le-Grand, France), 51*, 3–22.
87. El-Aneed, A., (2004). An overview of current delivery systems in cancer gene therapy. *J. Controll. Release., 94*, 1–14. doi: 10.1016/j.jconrel.2003.09.013.
88. Sun, N., Liu, Z., Huang, W., Tian, A., & Hu, S., (2014). The research of nanoparticles as gene vector for tumor gene therapy. *Crit. Rev. Oncol. Hematol., 89*, 352–357. doi: 10.1016/j.critrevonc.2013.10.006.
89. Ibraheem, D., Elaissari, A., & Fessi, H., (2014). Gene therapy and DNA delivery systems. *Int. J. Pharm., 459*, 70–83. doi: 10.1016/j.ijpharm.2013.11.041.
90. Bates, K., & Kostarelos, K., (2013). Carbon nanotubes as vectors for gene therapy: Past achievements, present challenges and future goals. *Adv. Drug Deliv. Rev., 65*, 2023–2033. doi: 10.1016/j.addr.2013.10.003.
91. Chakrabarti, M., Kiseleva, R., Vertegel, A., & Ray, S. K., (2015). Carbon nanomaterials for drug delivery and cancer therapy. *J. Nanosci. Nanotechnol., 15*, 5501–5511. doi: 10.1166/jnn.2015.10614.
92. Klumpp, C., Kostarelos, K., Prato, M., & Bianco, A., (2006). Functionalized carbon nanotubes as emerging nanovectors for the delivery of therapeutics. *Biochim. Biophys. Acta (BBA)-Biomembr., 1758*, 404–412. doi: 10.1016/j.bbamem.2005.10.008.
93. Podesta, J. E., Al-Jamal, K. T., Herrero, M. A., Tian, B., Ali-Boucetta, H., Hegde, V., Bianco, A., et al., (2009). Antitumor activity and prolonged survival by carbon-nanotube-mediated therapeutic siRNA silencing in a human lung xenograft model. *Small, 5*, 1176–1185. doi: 10.1002/smll.200801572.
94. Guo, C., Al-Jamal, W. T., Toma, F. M., Bianco, A., Prato, M., Al-Jamal, K. T., & Kostarelos, K., (2015). Design of cationic multi-walled carbon nanotubes as efficient siRNA vectors for lung cancer xenograft eradication. *Bioconjugate Chem., 26*, 1370–1379. doi: 10.1021/acs.bioconjchem.5b00249.
95. Siu, K. S., Chen, D., Zheng, X., Zhang, X., Johnston, N., Liu, Y., Yuan, K., et al., (2014). Non-covalently functionalized single-walled carbon nanotube for topical siRNA delivery into melanoma. *Biomaterials, 35*, 3435–3442. doi: 10.1016/j.biomaterials.2013.12.079.

CHAPTER 7

Carbon Nanotubes: A Novel Approach in Management of Fatal Disease Cancer

UMESH LADDHA,[1] EKNATH AHIRE,[1] KHEMCHAND SURANA,[2] SWATI TALELE,[3] GOKUL TALELE,[4] SANJAY KSHIRSAGAR,[1] and NILIMA THOMBRE[1]

[1]*Department of Pharmaceutics, MET's Institute of Pharmacy, Affiliated to Savitribai Phule Pune University, BKC, Adgaon, Nashik, Maharashtra, India*

[2]*Department of Pharmaceutical Chemistry, Shreeshakti Shaikshanik Sanstha, Divine College of Pharmacy, Satana, Nashik, Maharashtra, India*

[3]*Department of Pharmaceutical Chemistry, Sandip Institute of Pharmacy, Nashik, Maharashtra, India*

[4]*Department of Pharmaceutical Chemistry, Matoshri College of Pharmacy, Eklahare, Nashik, Maharashtra, India*

ABSTRACT

Cancer is a generic term associated with abnormal and uncontrolled cell proliferation, which results in the development of tumor. Till date more than 200 types of cancers have been identified, of which lung, stomach, liver, colon, and breast cancer are the most recurrent types as per World Health Organization. Currently, it is treated by chemotherapy, radiotherapy, surgical resection or a blend of these three approaches. Conventional cancer treatment is associated with several limitations like systemic toxicity, bystander effects, nephrotoxicity, infertility, hair loss, myocardial infarction and many more. There is an imperative need to develop some novel treatment to target

Carbon Nanotubes for Biomedical Applications and Healthcare.
Chin Hua Chia, Swati Gokul Talele, Ann Rose Abraham, and A. K. Haghi, (Eds.)

cancer cells. Researchers have concluded two major requisite for cancer management as designing the treatment in such a way that it targets to only cancer cell with less harm to normal cells and to target high dose to cancer cells to improve drug efficacy. In the last few years, (CNTs) have increased attention of many biomedical researchers owing to their inimitable features. Carbon nanotubes are essentially cylindrical molecules of carbon atoms having a diameter of around 1 nm. It possesses disguised properties like size in nano-range, high surface area, high aspect ratio and possibility of surface fictionalization. CNTs are thrashing the biomedical field as the most promising and dynamic drug carrier in cancer. It has proved its ability to deliver drugs, peptides, proteins, Plasmid DNA and interfering RNA. It has the potential to use as imaging tool as well as the drug transporter. Various researchers have already unveiled the use of carbon nanotubes in animal model. CNTs in combination with light energy (photo-thermal therapy) showed destructive effect on cancer cell without affecting normal tissues. Moreover, injection of PEGylated-CNTs in mice not show any toxicity even after several months. Henceforth; in this chapter we seek to provide insight to biomedical applications of CNTs in context with cancer.

7.1 INTRODUCTION

Abnormal and uncontrolled cell proliferation results in development of one of the most life threatening disease known as the cancer which simultaneously damages the normal tissues as well as organs [1–3]. Cancerous cells get modified in terms of resistance to the signals and process that causes cell apoptosis and also acquire the power to multiply with high number in comparison to normal cell [4]. One of the cruelest characteristics of cancer is to rapidly create abnormal cell having the power to invade bordering cells, tissues, and spread to all other parts. This process is known as the metastases.

Cancer is the second most leading cause of death which contributes 13% in total global death of which 70% deaths are from low to middle income countries [5]. Addiction of tobacco and alcohol, low intake of fruits and vegetables, high weight and less physical activity further worsen the brutality of cancer. So far 200 different types of cancers have been identified. According to the World Health organization, based on the number of new cases in the year 2020, the most common type of cancer includes breast, lungs, colon, prostate, and skin and stomach cancer (Figure 7.1).

On another hand, lung, colon, liver, stomach, and breast cancer are the most common type of cancer that ends with the death of patients (Figure 7.2) [6–8]. At present, cancer is treated with chemotherapy, radiotherapy, surgical removal of tumor part or blend of it. One of the crucial aim of cancer treatment is to prevent metastasis [9]. Researchers have set two strategies to improve efficacy of cancer treatment viz. destruction of cancer cells with lowest impact on normal cells and to deliver high dose of anti-tumor moiety to cancer cells [10, 11]. Current treatment of cancer results in severe type of complications which limits its application in terms of patient compliance (Figure 7.3).

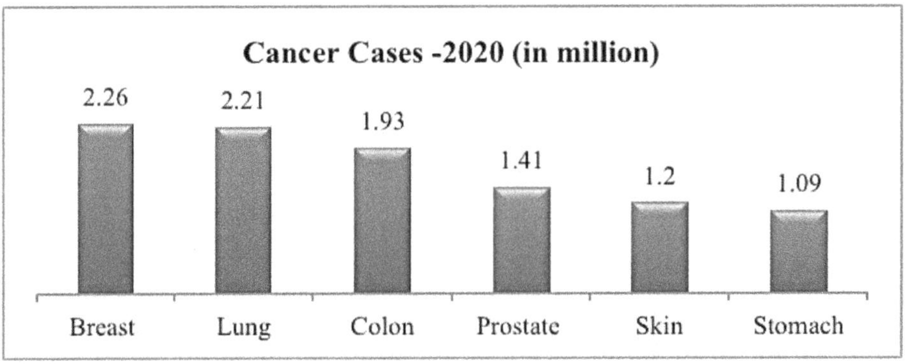

FIGURE 7.1 Reported cancer cases in year 2020.

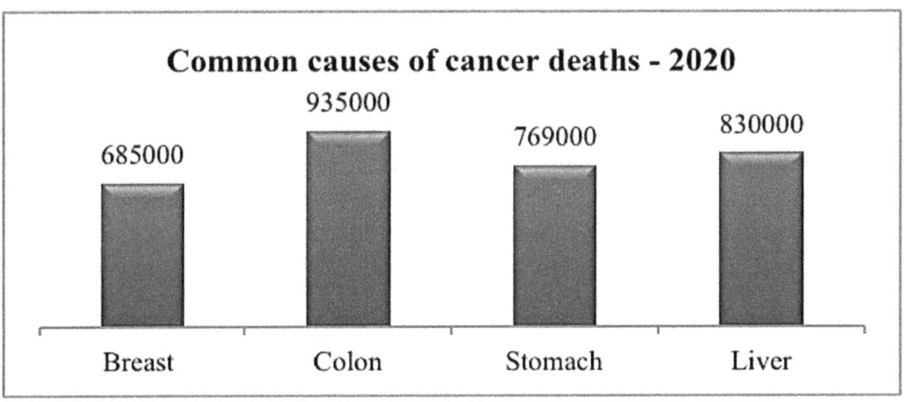

FIGURE 7.2 Common causes of cancer deaths.

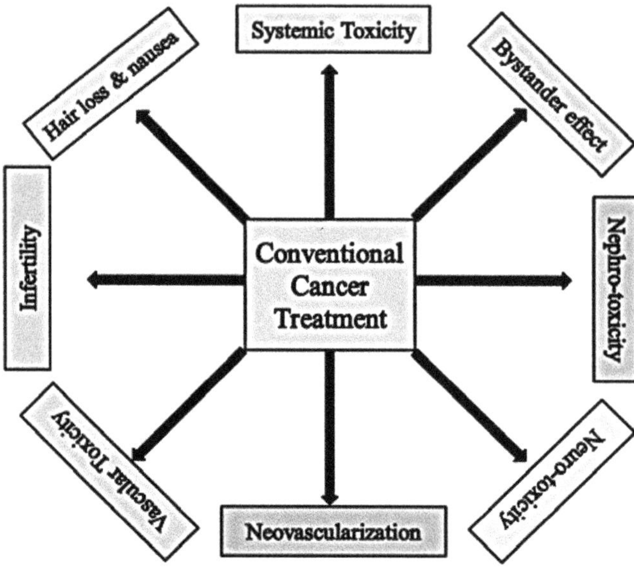

FIGURE 7.3 Limitations conventional cancer.

There is urgent need to develop novel approach to target cancer cells in order to increases survival of patient. In last couple of decades, biological nano-materials has attracted attention of many researchers to treat life threatening diseases like cancer. It includes use of polymeric nanoparticles, silver, and gold nanoparticles, quantum dots, carbon nanotubes (CNT) and liposomes [12]. Comparatively, CNT have proved its more dynamic role in cancer treatment than others because of their unique properties [13].

CNTs are essentially graphene sheets converted into open ended or capped seamless cylinder with high aspect ratio. It is made up of carbon atoms with a diameter of 1 nm and variable length. Basically CNTs are of two types viz. single walled nanotubes (SWNT) and multi-walled nanotubes (MWNT). SWNT consist of single graphene sheet, while number of graphene sheet together forms MWNT (Figure 7.4) [14]. With appropriate functionalization, one can use CNTs for transfer of anticancer drug, genes, and proteins. CNTs can also play a vital role as mediator in few anticancer therapies such as PTT (photothermal therapy) and PDT (photodynamic therapy) to destroy cancer cells (Figure 7.5) [15].

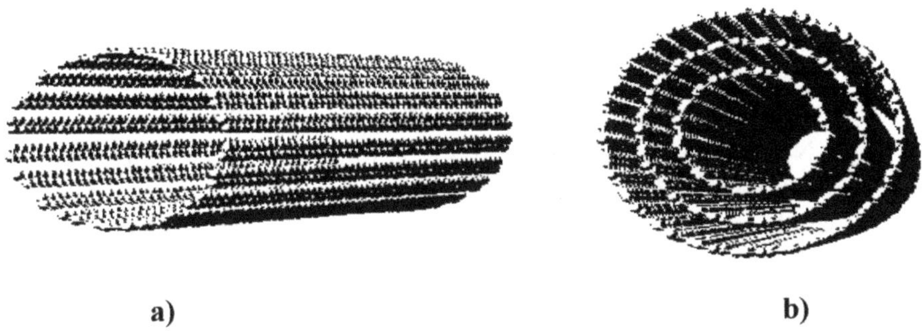

FIGURE 7.4 (a) Single walled nanotubes (SWNT); and (b) multi-walled nanotubes (MWNT).

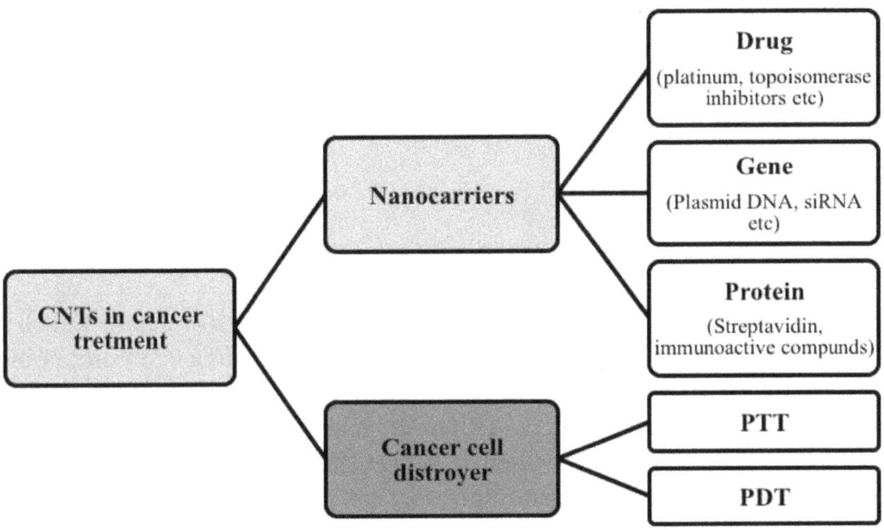

FIGURE 7.5 Involvement of CNTs in cancer treatment.

7.1.1 ADVANTAGES OF CNTS IN MANAGEMENT OF CANCER

- CNTs can serve for dual role as cancer cell imaging as well as drug carrier.
- Possesses unique physical, biological, and chemical properties.
- Ability to maintain desired functional group on surface as per need of therapy.

- Needle like shape allows CNTs to enter the cell by different mechanisms such as passive diffusion and endocytosis.
- Due to hollow monolithic structure act as more prominent carriers for a wide range of anticancer molecules.
- CNTs can be functionalized by reactions with strong acid or coated with polyethylene glycol to make them more water soluble and stable in serum which ultimately helps to improve biocompatibility [15–21].

7.2 CNT-BASED CANCER TREATMENT

Conventional cancer was treated by means of radiation and surgery. Later on several anti-cancer drugs have been developed but they are also associated with solemn limitations like narrow therapeutic window and non-specificity of drug delivery which also harms to the normal cells and tissues. CNTs have shown promising results as drug carrier as well as mediators in cancer cell destruction methods. The major advantage of CNTs is it can direct target to cancer cells only [22, 23].

7.2.1 CNTS AS ANTICANCER MOLECULE CARRIERS

Anticancer drugs can be packed in hollow parts of CNTs or can be attached to the surface of CNTs by covalent or non-covalent bonding by hydrophobic, electrostatic, and π-π stacking. Covalent bonding is more feasible and stable in comparison to non-covalent. However; sometimes it leads to chemical changes in anticancer drug which in terns affects the efficacy of the drug. Non-covalent bonding comparatively does not causes chemical changes, but the drug may get detached from CNTs before it reaches to target cell [24–27].

Cancer cells are associated with over-expression of folic acid receptors. It has also been reported by many researchers that lymph nodes retained non-spherical structure for long time period than spherical structure. By taking the above facts into consideration, researchers have developed CNTs functionalized with folic acid to target lymph node cancer [28, 29]. Magnetic nanoparticles of cisplatin were loaded in folic acid engineered MWNT's found to be more effective in specific lymph node cancer treatment. Yang et al. investigated gemcitabine as magnetic MWNT's in mice for lymph node cancer and reported high activity against metastasis for a long duration of time [30]. Sahoo et al. prepared polyvinyl alcohol functionalized MWNT's of poorly water soluble camptothecin and found significant effect in the management of breast and skin cancer [31].

Topoisomerase inhibitors are the chemotherapeutic agents with the potential to inhibit the activity of topoisomerase which helps to slow down cancerous cell growth. These agents are classified into two types, viz. Topoisomerase I inhibitors (e.g., irinotecan, topotecan, camptothecin, etc.) and Topoisomerase II inhibitors (e.g., etoposide, teniposide, doxorubicin, epirubicin, etc.). Tian et al. developed camptothecin loaded MWNT's functionalized with Pluronic P123 to make it more hydrophilic [32]. Cell line study showed significantly improved antitumor activity than un-complexed drug. More promising results were also reported by Wu et al. and Tripisciano et al. for camptothecin analogs 10-hydroxycamptothecin and irinotecan, respectively [33, 34]. In another study, Liu et al. developed doxorubicin loaded SWNT which was further functionalized by using polyethylene glycol (PEG) [35]. Engineering of SWNT by PEG showed increased loading efficiency (400%) with improved stability in buffers, serum, and acidic environment. Cytotoxicity study on cell lines MCF-7 and U87MG showed enhanced results in comparison to pure doxorubicin. Similar results were also observed by work carried out by Ali-Boucetta et al. by forming doxorubicin loaded MWNTsv [36]. Furthermore; biding of doxorubicin with folic acid, antibody or estradiol helps to make it more target specific [37, 38].

Paclitaxel is a less water soluble anticancer drug available in the market as Taxol. Major issues with taxol included less circulation time and use of Cremophor EL to increase solubility which is more toxic in nature. Liu et al. developed SWNTs conjugated with paclitaxel through PEG and further investigated its impact in 4T1 breast cancer animal model [39]. They found deeply improved cellular uptake by cancer cells with long circulation time. Similar findings were also reported with MWNT of Paclitaxel by using cancer cell line studies by many of researchers. Just like folic acid receptors, biotin receptors have been reported in many of cancers cells, which need to be explored more by conjugation between anticancer molecule and CNTs functionalized with biotin [39].

7.2.2 CNTS AS PLATINUM (PT)-BASED DRUG DELIVERY

Platinum based drug compounds are well known in management of cancer which works by chelating DNA and leads to death of cancer cells. Many of researchers have investigated CNTs for platinum based drug delivery [40]. Inert Pt(IV) prodrug and combination Pt(II) drugs and carriers are widely studied class.

Pt(IV) conjugated with CNTs developed for transportation of cisplatin (cis-dicholro-diammine-platinum, i.e., CDDP). A 'longboat delivery system' for CDDP with SWNT functionalized by amine was developed by Dhar et al. which showed entry in cancer cells by endocytocis [41]. Tripisciano et al. prepared CDDP loaded SWNTs and checked the anticancer effect on PC-3 and DU145 prostate cancer cells. Additionally, magnetic engineered CNTs with Pt-based anticancer drug were also found to be more effective against specific target. Yang et al. investigated magnetic CNTs with anticancer drugs such as cisplatin which was functionalized with PEG and FA to target lymph node [42]. *In vivo* investigation showed delivery of magnetic CNTs specifically to lymph node with drug release for several days, which leads to selective killing of cancer cells. Carboplatin which is the Pt-anticancer molecule was loaded into MWNTs by Hampel et al. and evaluated its effect on urinary bladder cancer cells [43]. *In vitro* study showed inhibiting effect on the growth of cancer cells in comparison to placebo CNTs and free drug.

7.2.3 INVOLVEMENT OF CNTS IN DELIVERY OF GENETIC MATERIAL, PROTEINS, AND IMMUNOACTIVE COMPOUNDS

Gene therapy is the method by means of which genetic materials are transferred to targeted cells or tissues that will clear the root cause of disease. However; entry of genetic material is restricted due to their large size as well as hydrophilicity. Henceforth; there is need to use of viral or non-viral vectors to deliver gene to target site and further internalization. Even though non-viral vectors like CNTs are short lived and less effective, but they are safer than viral vectors and hence preferred by many of researchers [44, 45]. It has also been suggested to perform functionalization of CNTs to enhance uptake of it by the mechanism of endocytosis [46].

Pantarotto and coworkers prepared SWNT-DNA and found better expression inside to cell. Kam et al. proved the efficiency of CNTs are vector for macromolecules like protein and DNA by using confocal microscopy and flow cytometry. In previous work, Kam et al. also found internalization of DNA linked with SWNT significantly than plain DNA at 37°C. While at 4°C, he found no internalization which might be because of possible mechanism of gene transport follows the energy dependent mechanism.

Recent advancement in gene-therapy coined the term 'gene silencing' which involves use of siRNA found to be effective in treatment of cancer. In cancer, because of SOCS1, i.e., suppressors of cytokine signaling-1, our own antitumor activity is inhibited. Loading or surface attachment of siRNA with SWNTs which are further functionalized by phospholipids confirmed efficient gene silencing and subsequent target cell death [47]. Podesta et al. developed the siRNA-MWNTs and investigated effect in lung cancer in animal model [48]. They found tumor suppressant effect with long animal survival.

Protein like streptavidin is known for its anticancer effect. However, because of high molecular weight it fails to penetrate in cell to produce a noticeable effect. Kam et al. form the complex of streptavidin and biotin-SWNTs and investigates on cancer cell line. In comparison to plain streptavidin, complexed form showed significantly increased cell accumulation by adsorption mediated endocytosis. Extension in the progress of CNTs combination with genetic material and protein, researchers have also tested CNTs with immunotherapy. Meng et al. conjugated the tumor lysate protein as an antigen to MWNTs and found a significant increase in anticancer immune response. Similarly, Ruggiero et al. attached the E4G10 (angiogenesis targeting antibodies) to SWNTs and found long survival of cancer induced animal along with reduction in tumor size.

7.2.4 CNTS IN PHOTOTHERMAL CANCER THERAPY

Photothermal therapy (PTT) and photodynamic therapy (PDT) can be used for non-invasive cancer treatment with fewer side effects in comparison to existing radiotherapy [37]. CNTs have been identified as ideal material in PTT and PDT which satisfy the two major requirements as efficacy and safety.

In PTT method, CNT absorbs the NIR light and absorbed NIR light transmits heat to the nanotubes. Henceforth; when the optical coupling effect of light and CNT is applied, external heat energy can be transmitted inside to the body. This property can be used to kill cancer cells (Figure 7.6). Investigation of CNTs in PTT method is summarized in Table 7.1.

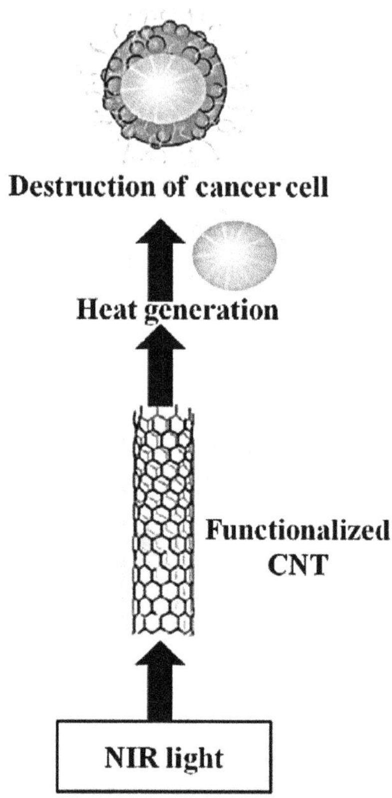

FIGURE 7.6 Mechanism of action of photothermal therapy (PTT).

TABLE 7.1 Investigation of CNTs in PTT

CNT System	Type of Study	Model/Cell Line	Significant Outcome	References
SWNT	*In vivo*	Rabbits bearing hepatic VX2 tumors.	SWNT-treated tumors showed complete necrosis in comparison to Kentera alone.	[49]
SWNT	*In vitro*	EMT6	SWNT showed significant control in breast cancer.	[50]
SWNT	*In vivo*	Mice	PTT showed complete destruction of the tumor with no occurrence during 6 months.	[51]
MWNT	*In vitro*	Kidney cancer cells.	Wavelengths 700–1,100 nm is desirable to kill the tumor.	[52]
MWNT	*In vitro*	EAC	Within 1.5 minutes of NIR irradiation 95% cell were died.	[53]

In application of PDT, it involves the use of light source, photosensitizer, and molecular oxygen in CNT (CNT acts as a carrier). CNT enters in to cancer cell, photosensitizer is activated by light which in terns transfer energy to oxygen molecules. Oxygen gets changed in to excited state which is cytotoxic in nature. Ultimately, cytotoxic oxygen starts to damage the cancer cells (Figure 7.7). Investigation of CNTs in the PDT method is summarized in Table 7.2.

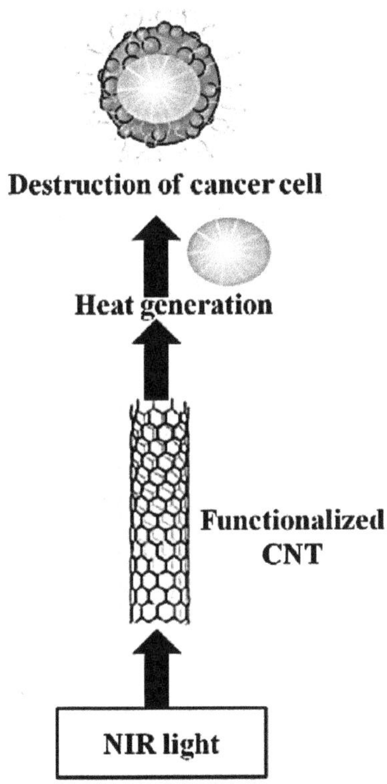

FIGURE 7.7 Mechanism of action of photodynamic therapy (PDT).

TABLE 7.2 Investigation of CNTs in PDT

CNT System	Type of Study	Model/Cell Line	Significant Outcome	References
SWNT	*In vitro*	MCF-7	95% decrease in cell viability.	[54]
SWNT	*In vitro*	HeLa	SWNT showed significant toxicity in HeLa cells.	[55]
MWNT	*In vitro*	MGC 803	At 632 nm MWNT with PDT treatment showed cell destruction.	[56]

7.3 CONCLUSION

Carbon nanotubes (CNTs) are one of the reliable carrier systems for both micro- as well as macromolecules. Their unique characteristics make them more promising systems in the management of cancer either as drug carriers or mediators in tumor destruction methodologies such as photothermal therapy and photodynamic therapy with minimal side effects. Furthermore, CNTs can be made more cancer cells specific by functionalization with suitable agent like folic acid, biotin, etc., to avoid harmful effects of anticancer drug molecules on normal cells and tissues. CNTs have exclusive property of cell uptake by both diffusion as well as endocytosis mechanisms. However; involvement of CNTs in cancer management is introduced in recent years and hence, extensive research is expected in upcoming years to further confirm safety and efficacy of CNTs.

ACKNOWLEDGMENT

We thank MET's, Institute of Pharmacy, BKC, affiliated under Savitribai Phule Pune University, Nashik, Divine College of Pharmacy Satana and Sandip Institute of Pharmaceutical Science for their constant support and providing all facilities to complete this work. We are also thankful to the Ministry of Tribal Affairs Government of India for providing financial assistance in the form of fellowship (Award No.: 202021-NFST-MAH-01235).

KEYWORDS

- **cancer**
- **carbon nanotube**
- **disease management**
- **fatal disease**

REFERENCES

1. Kuk, H. S., Jeong, H. H., & Jin, W. L., (2016). Carbon nanotubes as cancer therapeutic carriers and mediators. *International Journal of Nanomedicine*, 5163–5185.

2. Bandyopadhyay, A., Das, T., & Yeasmin, S., (2015). *Nanoparticles in Lung Cancer Therapy: Recent Trends* (pp. 1–15). Berlin, Germany: Springer International Publishing.
3. Seyed, Y. M., Naghmeh, N., Oshani, D., Aaron, T., & Alexander, M., S., (2011). A new era of cancer treatment: Carbon nanotubes as drug delivery tools. *International Journal of Nanomedicine*, 2963–2979.
4. Luo, J., Solimini, N. L., & Elledge, S. J., (2009). Principles of cancer therapy: Oncogene and nononcogene addiction. *Cell, 136*(5), 823–837.
5. Rajpal, S., Kumar, A., & Joe, W., (2018). Economic burden of cancer in India: Evidence from cross-sectional nationally representative household survey, 2014. *PloS One, 13*(2), e0193320. https://doi.org/10.1371/journal.pone.0193320.
6. https://www.who.int/news-room/fact-sheets/detail/cancer (accessed on 27 February 2023).
7. Utreja, P., Jain, S., & Tiwary, A. K., (2010). Novel drug delivery systems for sustained and targeted delivery of anti-cancer drugs: Current status and future prospects. *Curr. Drug Deliv., 7*, 152–161.
8. Zhuang, L., Kai, C., Corrine, D., et al., (2008). Drug delivery with carbon nanotubes for *in vivo* cancer treatment. *Cancer Res., 68*, 6652–6660.
9. Dhar, S., Liu, Z., Thomale, J., Dai, H., & Lippard, S. J., (2008). Targeted single-wall carbon nanotube-mediated Pt (IV) prodrug delivery using folate as a homing device. *J. Am. Chem. Soc., 130,* 11467–11476.
10. Chang, T. M., & Prakash, S., (2001). Procedures for microencapsulation of enzymes, cells and genetically engineered microorganisms. *Mol. Biotechnol., 17*, 249–260.
11. Sahoo, N. G., Bao, H., Pan, Y., et al., (2011). Functionalized carbon nanomaterials as nanocarriers for loading and delivery of a poorly water-soluble anticancer drug: A comparative study. *Chem. Commun. (Camb)., 47*, 5235–5237.
12. Ahire, E. D., Swati, G. T., & Heena, S. S., (2020). Nanoparticles as a promising technology in microbial pharmaceutics. *Applied Pharmaceutical Science and Microbiology* (pp. 133–158). Apple Academic Press.
13. Lamprecht, C., Liashkovich, I., Neves, V., et al., (2009). AFM imaging of functionalized carbon nanotubes on biological membranes. *Nanotechnology, 20*, 43400.
14. Beg, S., Rizwan, M., Sheikh, A. M., Hasnain, M. S., Anwer, K., & Kohli, K., (2011). Advancement in carbon nanotubes: Basics, biomedical applications and toxicity. *J. Pharm. Pharmacol., 63,* 141–163.
15. Bianco, A., Kostarelos, K., & Prato, M., (2005). Applications of carbon nanotubes in drug delivery. *Curr. Opin. Chem. Biol., 9*, 674–679.
16. Shi, K. N. W., Jessop, T. C., Wender, P. A., & Dai, H., (2004). Nanotube molecular transporters: Internalization of carbon nanotube-protein conjugates into mammalian cells. *J. Am. Chem. Soc., 126*, 6850–6851.
17. Kam, N. W., & Dai, H., (2005). Carbon nanotubes as intracellular protein transporters: Generality and biological functionality. *J. Am. Chem. Soc., 127*, 6021–6026.
18. Dayana Alonso, David Hernández-Castillo, Luis Almagro, Roy González-Alemán, Dolores Molero, M. Ángeles Herranz, Erick Medina-Páez, Julieta Coro, Roberto Martínez-Álvarez, Margarita Suárez, & Nazario Martín. (2020). Diastereoselective Synthesis of Steroid–[60]Fullerene Hybrids and Theoretical Underpinning. *The Journal of Organic Chemistry, 85*(4) , 2426–2437. https://doi.org/10.1021/acs.joc.9b03121.

19. Hampel, S., Kunze, D., Haase, D., et al., (2008). Carbon nanotubes filled with a chemotherapeutic agent: A nanocarrier mediates inhibition of tumor cell growth. *Nanomedicine, 3*(2), 175–182.
20. Wu, W., Li, R., Bian, X., et al., (2009). Covalently combining carbon nanotubes with anticancer agent: Preparation and antitumor activity. *ACS Nano, 3*(9), 2740–2750.
21. Li, Y., Cousins, B. G., Ulijn, R. V., & Kinloch, I. A., (2009). A study of the dynamic interaction of surfactants with graphite and carbon nanotubes using Fmoc-amino acids as a model system. *Langmuir, 25*, 11760–11767.
22. Liu, Z., Fan, A. C., Rakhra, K., et al., (2009). Supramolecular stacking of doxorubicin on carbon nanotubes for *in vivo* cancer therapy. *Angew Chem. Int. Ed. Eng., 48*, 7668–7672.
23. Gottesman, M. M., Fojo, T., & Bates, S. E., (2002). Multidrug resistance in cancer: Role of ATP-dependent transporters. *Nat. Rev. Cancer, 2*, 48–58.
24. Reddy, S. T., Rehor, A., Schmoekel, H. G., Hubbell, J. A., & Swartz, M. A., (2006). *In vivo* targeting of dendritic cells in lymph nodes with poly(propylene sulfide) nanoparticles. *Journal of Controlled Release, 112*(1), 26–34.
25. Yang, F., Fu, D. L., Long, J., & Ni, Q. X., (2008). Magnetic lymphatic targeting drug delivery system using carbon nanotubes. *Medical Hypotheses, 70*(4), 765–767.
26. Yang, F., Hu, J., Yang, D., et al., (2009). Pilot study of targeting magnetic carbon nanotubes to lymph nodes. *Nanomedicine, 4*(3), 317–330.
27. Sahoo, N. G., Bao, H., Pan, Y., et al., (2011). Functionalized carbon nanomaterials as nanocarriers for loading and delivery of a poorly water-soluble anticancer drug: A comparative study. *Chemical Communications, 47*(18), 5235–5237.
28. Tian, Z., Yin, M., Ma, H., Zhu, L., Shen, H., & Jia, N., (2011). Supramolecular assembly and antitumor activity of multiwalled carbon nanotube–camptothecin complexes. *J. Nanosci. Nanotechnol., 11*(2), 953–958.
29. Wu, W., Li, R., Bian, X., et al., (2009). Covalently combining carbon nanotubes with anticancer agent: Preparation and antitumor activity. *ACS Nano, 3*(9), 2740–2750.
30. Tripisciano, C., Rummeli, M. H., Chen, X. C., & Borowiak-Palen, E., (2010). Multiwall carbon nanotubes-a vehicle for targeted irinotecan drug delivery. *Physica Status Solidi B., 247*, 2673–2677.
31. Liu, Z., Sun, X., Nakayama-Ratchford, N., & Dai, H., (2007). Supramolecular chemistry on water-soluble carbon nanotubes for drug loading and delivery. *ACS Nano, 1*(1), 50–56.
32. Ali-Boucetta, H., Al-Jamal, K. T., McCarthy, D., Prato, M., Bianco, A., & Kostarelos, K., (2008). Multiwalled carbon nanotube–doxorubicin supramolecular complexes for cancer therapeutics. *Chem. Commun., 4*, 459–461.
33. Heister, E., Neves, V., Tilmaciu, C., et al., (2009). Triple functionalization of single-walled carbon nanotubes with doxorubicin, a monoclonal antibody, and a fluorescent marker for targeted cancer therapy. *Carbon N Y., 47*, 2152–2160.
34. Lodhi, N., Mehra, N. K., & Jain, N. K., (2013). Development and characterization of dexamethasone mesylate anchored on multi walled carbon nanotubes. *J. Drug Target, 21*(1), 67–76.
35. Liu, Z., Chen, K., Davis, C., et al., (2008). Drug delivery with carbon nanotubes for *in vivo* cancer treatment. *Cancer Research, 68*(16), 6652–6660.
36. Wang, D., & Lippard, S. J., (2005). Cellular processing of platinum anticancer drugs. *Nat. Rev. Drug Discov., 4*(4), 307–320.

37. Dhar, S., Liu, Z., Thomale, J., Dai, H. J., & Lippard, S. J., (2008). Targeted single-wall carbon nanotube-mediated Pt(IV) prodrug delivery using folate as a homing device. *J. Am. Chem. Soc., 130*(34), 11467–11476.
38. Yang, F., Fu De, L., Long, J., & Ni, Q. X., (2008). Magnetic lymphatic targeting drug delivery system using carbon nanotubes. *Med. Hypotheses, 70*(4), 765–767.
39. Hampel, S., Kunze, D., Haase, D., et al., (2008). Carbon nanotubes filled with a chemotherapeutic agent: A nano-carrier mediates inhibition of tumor cell growth. *Nanomedicine (Lond), 3*(2), 175–182.
40. Elhissi, A. M., Ahmed, W., Hassan, I. U., Dhanak, V. R., & D'Emanuele, A., (2012). Carbon nanotubes in cancer therapy and drug delivery. *J. Drug Deliv., 2012*, 837327.
41. Rochat, T., & Morris, M. A., (2002). Gene therapy for cystic fibrosis by means of aerosol. *Journal of Aerosol Medicine, 15*(2), 229–235.
42. Kam, N. W. S., Liu, Z., & Dai, H., (2005). Carbon nanotubes as intracellular transporters for proteins and DNA: An investigation of the uptake mechanism and pathway. *Angewandte Chemie, 44*, 1–6.
43. Pantarotto, D., Singh, R., McCarthy, D., et al., (2004). Functionalized carbon nanotubes for plasmid DNA gene delivery. *Angewandte Chemie International Edition, 43*(39), 5242–5246.
44. Kam, N. W. S., Jessop, T. C., Wender, P. A., & Dai, H., (2004). Nanotube molecular transporters: Internalization of carbon nanotube-protein conjugates into mammalian cells. *Journal of the American Chemical Society, 126*(22), 6850–6851.
45. Kam, N. W. S., Liu, Z., & Dai, H., (2005). Functionalization of carbon nanotubes via cleavable disulfide bonds for efficient intracellular delivery of siRNA and potent gene silencing. *Journal of the American Chemical Society, 127*(36), 12492–12493.
46. Podesta, J. E., Al-Jamal, K. T., Herrero, M. A., et al., (2009). Antitumor activity and prolonged survival by carbon-nanotube-mediated therapeutic siRNA silencing in a human lung xenograft model. *Small, 5*(10), 1176–1185.
47. Meng, J., Duan, J., Kong, H., et al., (2008). Carbon nanotubes conjugated to tumor lysate protein enhance the efficacy of an antitumor immunotherapy. *Small, 4*(9), 1364–1370.
48. Ruggiero, Villa, H. C., Holland, J. P., et al., (2010). Imaging and treating tumor vasculature with targeted radiolabeled carbon nanotubes. *International Journal of Nanomedicine, 5*(1), 783–802.
49. Li, Q., Ruan, H., & Li, H., (2014). Nanocarbon materials for photodynamic therapy and photothermal therapy. *Pharmaceutical Nanotechnol., 2*(2), 58–64.
50. Gannon, C. J., Cherukuri, P., Yakobson, B. I., et al., (2007). Carbon nanotube enhanced thermal destruction of cancer cells in a noninvasive radiofrequency field. *Cancer, 110*(12), 2654–2665.
51. Zhou, F., Wu, S., Wu, B., Chen, W. R., & Xing, D., (2011). Mitochondria-targeting single-walled carbon nanotubes for cancer photothermal therapy. *Small, 7*(19), 2727–2735.
52. Moon, H. K., Lee, S. H., & Choi, H. C., (2009). *In vivo* near-infrared mediated tumor destruction by photothermal effect of carbon nanotubes. *ACS Nano, 3*(11), 3707–3713.
53. Torti, S. V., Byrne, F., Whelan, O., et al., (2007). Thermal ablation therapeutics based on CNx multi-walled nanotubes. *Int. J. Nanomed., 2*, 707–714.
54. Burlaka, A., Lukin, S., Prylutska, S., et al., (2010). Hyperthermic effect of multiwalled carbon nanotubes stimulated with near infrared irradiation for anticancer therapy: *In vitro* studies. *Exp. Oncol., 32*(1), 48–50.

55. Ogbodu, R. O., Limson, J. L., Prinsloo, E., & Nyokong, T., (2015). Photophysical properties and photodynamic therapy effect of zinc phthalocyanine spermine-single walled carbon nanotube conjugate on MCF-7 breast cancer cell line. *Synthetic Met., 204*, 122–132.
56. Xiao, H. R., Zhu, B. S., Wang, D. L., et al., (2012). Photodynamic effects of chlorin e6 attached to single wall carbon nanotubes through noncovalent interactions. *Carbon N Y., 50*, 1681–1689.

CHAPTER 8

Carbon Nanotubes: Application in Management of Alzheimer's Disease

UTKARSHA P. PATIL, HARSHADA U. BAGUL, AKASH M. BHOITE, SWATI G. TALELE, and ANIL G. JADHAV

Department of Pharmaceutics, Sandip Institute of Pharmaceutical Sciences, Nashik, Maharashtra, India

ABSTRACT

Carbon nanotubes (CNTs) are a promising innovation in nanomedicine that has great potential to treat neurological disorders like Alzheimer's. A CNTs is a graphitic allotrope of carbon made up of a cylindrical tube with a diameter measured typically in nanometers and a length of several millimeters. The CNTs often refer to single-wall carbon nanotubes (SWCNTs) and multi-wall carbon nanotubes (MWCNTs). Known medically as Alzheimer's disease, Alzheimer's causes brain cells to die and the brain to shrink over time. This disease is associated with abnormal self-assembly of amyloid-β peptides into toxic β-rich aggregates. It is the most prevalent type of dementia and can be defined as a Degenerative disease of the nervous system, marked by neurotic plaques, amyloid-β peptides accumulation and discrepancy of acetylcholine concentration, and other neurotransmitters imbalance. For proper and improved treatment of Alzheimer's disease in the last few years, CNTs have increased attention of many biomedical researchers. CNTs has its ability to proper delivery of drugs at the specific site of action, also they inhibit the formation of β-sheet rich oligomers of Alzheimer's amyloid-β peptide and to deliver the acetylcholine. The behavior of degradation and excretion of CNTs can be carefully tailored based on the intended *in vivo* application.

Carbon Nanotubes for Biomedical Applications and Healthcare.
Chin Hua Chia, Swati Gokul Talele, Ann Rose Abraham, and A. K. Haghi, (Eds.)

8.1. INTRODUCTION

Scientists have been focusing on the characteristics of novel delivery materials since 1991 when carbon nanotubes were revolutionized. Nanotechnology is a big Research field and modern manufacturing technology that is growing rapidly. Nanomaterials have a size not larger than 100 nanometers, including drugs and possess magnetic, electronic, mechanical, or optical properties. This broad class of materials offers the possibility of many new applications. In terms of nanomaterials, nanotubes are the most promising among them. Iijima which was the Japanese scientist first observed carbon nanotubes using a TEM (Transmission Electron Microscopy), and this led to the discovery of the field of carbon nanotubes.

Carbon nanotubes are made of rolled up sheets of graphite which have diameter in micrometer while diameter of around 100 nm. The carbon atoms in CNTs are arranged in a condensed benzene ring sequence and rolled into a tubular structure. Nanotubes are a family of carbon allotropes, in which multiple carbon atoms bind collectively to form a cylindrical structure. The CNTs possess a variety of distinctive properties that may result in their utilization as a drug delivery system. Graphite and diamond are naturally occurring nanomaterials that are sp^3 (cubic) and sp^2 (planar) forms of carbon, respectively. This novel artificial nanomaterial is part of the fullerene family, the Carbon with a third allotrope. Nanotube diameters in relation to each other is $>10^6$ in the nanorange; length is upto several mm containing high surface area. CNTs have Near-high absorbance at infrared region (NIR). The high surface area, excellent chemical stability, complex electronic structure, and rich polyaromatic properties of CNTs make them ideal as adsorbents and conjugates for a broad range of therapeutic molecules (including proteins, drugs, antibodies, enzymes, DNA, etc.). Because of their capability to penetrate directly into the cells and maintain the drug without transformation during transport in the body, they have proven to be excellent vehicles for drug delivery. In the treatment and diagnosis of various diseases, carbon nanotubes are used for various applications, such as antioxidants, in the therapy of cancer, as biosensors, in gene therapy by DNA delivery, in infection therapy, in neurological disorders, etc.

Alzheimer's disease (AD) is a brain disorder characterized by the degeneration of brain cells, slowly destroys thinking skills and memory and leads to behavioral problems also, the loss of reasoning capabilities and a lack of performance daily activities independently, which is a chief cause of dementia. There are three stages of its symptoms, mild, moderate, and severe, which can be seen in an X-ray image. Often, the condition as time goes on, it gets worse. A number of conjectures have been preferred for the cause of AD, the two main hypotheses being cholinergic and amyloid. AD can be treated only by two classes of drugs, including inhibitors of the cholinesterase enzyme and NMDA antagonists, which neither cure nor prevent AD, but treat its symptoms. Alzheimer's symptoms can currently be treated, and researchers are still searching for new ways to prevent Alzheimer's symptoms by lowering the deterioration of memory, enhancing quality of life tasks and improving quality of daily life (Figure 8.1).

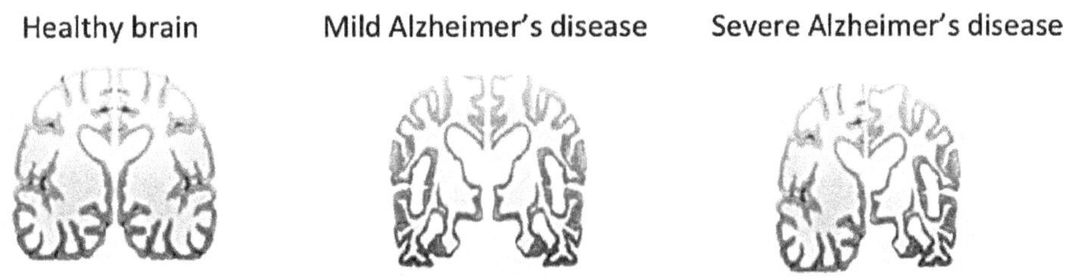

FIGURE 8.1 Diagram showing brain's conditions in Alzheimer's disease.

Source: https://www.vecteezy.com/free-vector/diagram

Since CNTs are a promising biomedical material, they have been utilized in neuroscience. Their tiny dimensions and external modifications allow them to penetrate the blood-brain barrier by multiple processes in order to act as effective delivery carriers for target molecules in the brain. A study by Yang et al. has demonstrated that it was successful to deliver acetylcholine using SWCNTs to mice affected by Alzheimer's disease while exhibiting a wide safety range. In general, these studies indicate that CNT conjugates with therapeutic molecules promote neuronal growth more efficiently than the drugs alone [1–11, 21, 23].

8.2 CLASSIFICATION OF CARBON NANOTUBES

Nanotubes are structures made up of a thin layer of carbon atoms joined by a hexagonal mesh. This one-atom thick layer called graphene, and carbon nanotubes are formed when carbon nanosheets are wrapped around each other as cylinders. The outer walls of nanotubes can consist of only one wall or of more than one wall. They are generally divided into two categories:

(i) single-walled carbon nanotubes; and
(ii) multi-walled carbon nanotubes.

8.2.1 *SINGLE-WALLED CARBON NANOTUBES*

Single-walled carbon nanotubes are made up of a single graphene cylinder whose diameter varies between 0.4 and 2 nm, and most commonly exist in hexagonal bundles. As SWCNTs exhibit a large number of electronic properties, they can be put to use to replace micro-electromechanical systems as the basis for miniaturizing electronics.

Nanotubes with single walls It's possible to make it in three distinct ways: armchair, chiral, and zigzag. Each shape is determined by the manner in which graphene is wrapped around a cylinder (Figure 8.2).

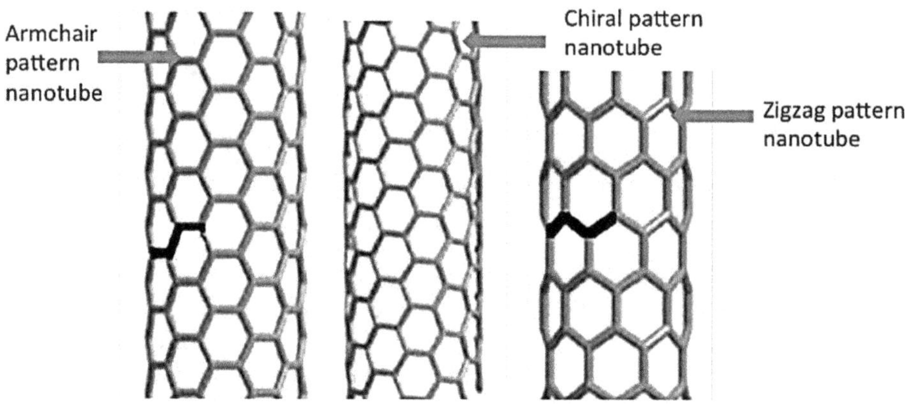

FIGURE 8.2 Carbon nanotubes with single wall.

8.2.2 *MULTI-WALLED CARBON NANOTUBES*

In multiwalled carbon nanotubes, the outer walls protect the inner carbon nanotubes from chemical interactions with outside materials, although the properties are similar to those of single-walled nanotubes. The tensile strength of multiwalled nanotubes is also higher than its single-walled counterpart.

Multiwalled carbon nanotubes can be structured in two ways:

1. **Russian Doll Model:** Carbon nanotubes are enclosed within another nanotube in the Russian doll model. The circumference of the inner nanotube is smaller than the circumference of the outer nanotube.
2. **Parchment Model:** Graphene sheets are rolled up like scrolls of paper in the parchment model, where a single sheet is rolled up multiple times (Figure 8.3).

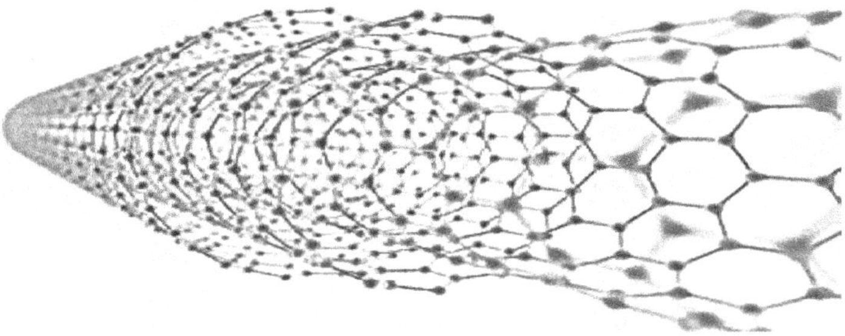

FIGURE 8.3 Carbon nanotubes with multiple walls.

8.3 SYNTHESIS OF CARBON NANOTUBES [18–23]

Depending on a CNT's need, SWCNTs and MWCNTs can be synthesized. They may include small-scale requirements, for example, CNTs used in laboratory studies. Such a type of CNTs generated by utilizing the local method, but the problem that arises is they do not possess purity and also contain some flaws and other inadequacies. CNTs required for industrial operations, especially in the electrical, mechanical, and thermal fields. For that purification, perfection, and freedom from deformation are needed. As a result, highly precise methods are required to manufacture them. For example, the factor which determines the properties of MWCNTs is investigated using the plasma-enhanced chemical vapor decomposition method. CNTs can be grown using various techniques, like the common chemical vapor decomposition method, electric arc method, and laser ablation method. Alternatively, CNTs also produced locally at room temperature by using a mixed solution of acids in that graphite powder placed in sulfuric acid and nitric acid with potassium chromate. Iijima discovered MWCNTs in 1991 using the electric arc method, a technique that had long been employed in the synthesis of carbon fibers and fullerenes. Afterward, the laser ablation method was used to produce SWCNTs, and in later years, Yacaman et al., discovered how to grow CNTs by catalytic means using a CVD method. Both types of CNTs can be produced via three distinct methods, as in Figure 8.4.

8.3.1 ELECTRIC ARC DISCHARGE METHOD

With a power supply of 10–20 A, an inert gas, such as helium, is present in the presence of two graphite electrodes that create a hot plasma discharge, resulting in the creation of carbon nanotubes. A certain amount of helium

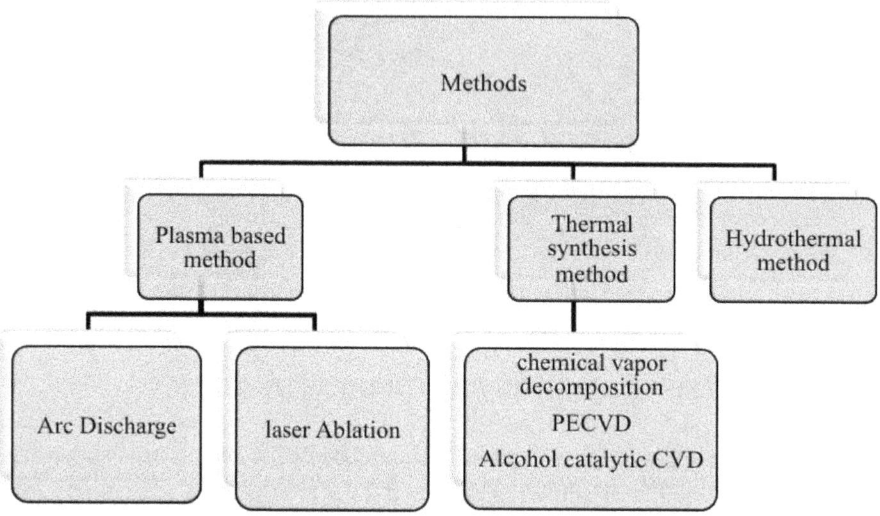

FIGURE 8.4 Methods for the production of carbon nanotubes.

pressure created into the chamber can increase the yield of carbon nanotubes, but beyond that value, it decreases. Lowering the supply current can improve the quality of the carbon nanotubes. The use of CF4 and nitrogen instead of helium was also employed (Figure 8.5).

8.3.2 LASER ABLATION METHOD

It involves passing a high beam of laser on a target, and then the carbons in the tube will evaporate into nanotubes. After passing through the copper collector, the argon will sweep the atoms of carbon from high-temperature zone into the low-temperature zone, where they condense into nanotubes having of 10–100 nm in size and 90–100 m long. Factors such as wavelength dependence, pulse width and repetition rate dependence, density, and power dependencies, single-laser, and multiple sequences, etc., all affect the laser ablation process. The method is very expensive since it requires high power supplies (Figure 8.6).

8.3.3 CHEMICAL VAPOR DECOMPOSITION METHOD

The decomposition of volatile carbon compounds such as methane and ethylene present in the chamber onto metal substrates, which act as catalysts and nucleation sites that allow carbon nanotubes to grow in temperatures

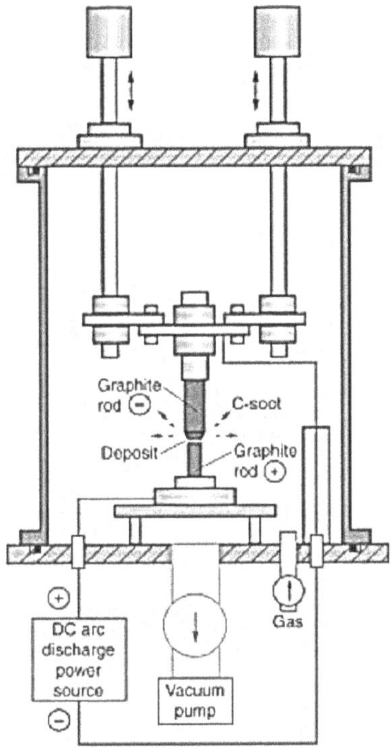

Electric arc discharge assembly

FIGURE 8.5 Assembly for electric arc discharge.

Source: Venkataraman et al. (2019). http://creativecommons.org/licenses/by/4.0/ [49]

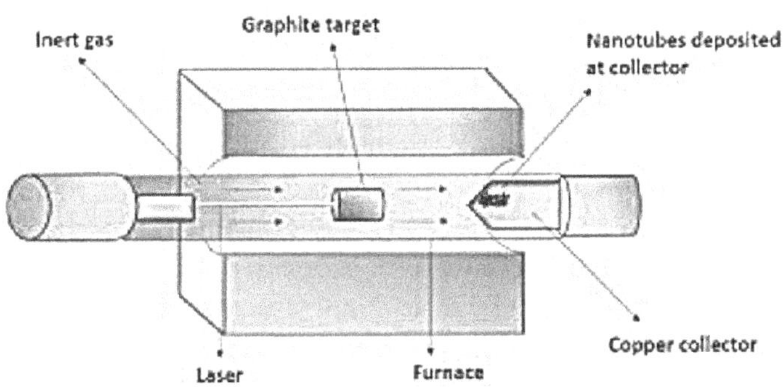

Laser ablation assembly

FIGURE 8.6 Assembly showing laser ablation.

Source: Yahya et al. (2020) [18]

between 500 and 1,000°C and at atmospheric pressure. A key factor in the formation of carbon nanotubes is the selection of the catalyst and substrate. Fe, Co, and Ni are considered fine catalysts, and porous silicon is thought to be a substrate (Figure 8.7).

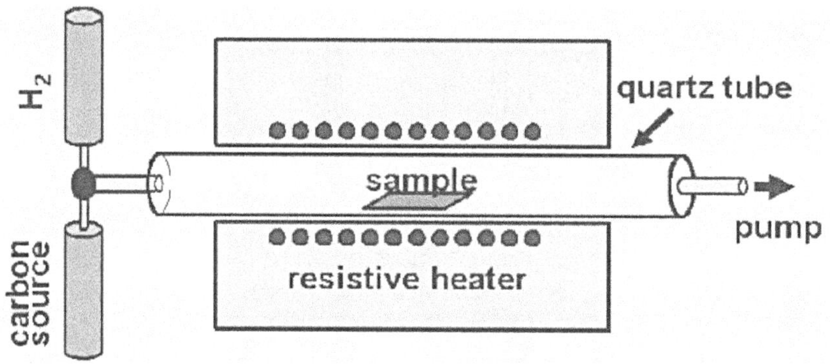

Chemical vapor decomposition assembly

FIGURE 8.7 Assembly for chemical vapor decomposition.

Source: Yahya et al. (2020) [18]

8.4 UTILIZATION OF CARBON NANOTUBES IN DELIVERY OF DRUGS IN ALZHEIMER'S DISEASE [24–48]

The brain is protected by the BBB which has a low permeability endothelium which is joined by tight junctions which avert the passage of most drugs from the bloodstream to the brain. Yet, CNTs are the nanoparticles capable of transferring drugs into the central nervous system (CNS) at the point of action. Therefore, CNTs are a good means of transferring the medication to treat Alzheimer's disease. Anti-Alzheimer's drugs can be very effectively delivered with carbon nanotubes.

Alzheimer, a disease characterized by memory loss, can be treated with tacrine (TAC). In order to increase TAC's effectiveness, several efforts have been created to characterize its features. Nanostructures are also used to deliver TAC and this work investigated the features of loading TAC at CNT using *in silico* computer simulation. TAC is loaded non-covalently on the surface of a model structure that is indicative of CNT. For the purpose of loading TAC onto CNT, a nanostructure-based model is chosen. The main achievements of this work with respect to the goal of loading TAC onto CNT for drug delivery purposes. A molecular scale study was performed to demonstrate clearly how such complex formation affects the properties of its counterpart, especially for the TAC counterpart. As part of targeted drug delivery systems, appropriate carriers for drugs are chosen so that the drugs reach the target in a safe manner. However, this goal couldn't be achieved through conventional methods. Initially, this research optimizes 3-D molecular models of the TAC molecule and a representative CNT for minimum energy structure. Molecular distribution patterns of HOMO (highest occupied molecular orbital) and LUMO (lowest unoccupied molecular orbital) which are molecular orbitals energy levels located at both ends of the molecule. By further optimizing the interacting molecular system, ESP (electrostatic potential) surfaces can depict the localization of charge at the investigated molecules. Such single molecule analyses are used to study the complex formation of TAC@CNT. Intriguingly, the HOMO and LUMO distributions are located exclusively in the CNT counterpart, not in the TAC counterpart of the TAC@CNT complex. This shows that CNT plays a key role in carrying the loaded TAC drug. HOMO and LUMO distributions are placed only at CNT when the drug is loaded at the CNT, which leads to a loss of reactivity. The continuous ESP representation of TAC@CNT is found to indicate in agreement with the complex formation. Besides serving as a carrier to deliver the loaded drug, CNTs could also act as a biosensor in this case. In conclusion, TAC@CNT complex formation could aid in targeted drug delivery by emphasizing the role of CNT in achieving the target (Figure 8.8).

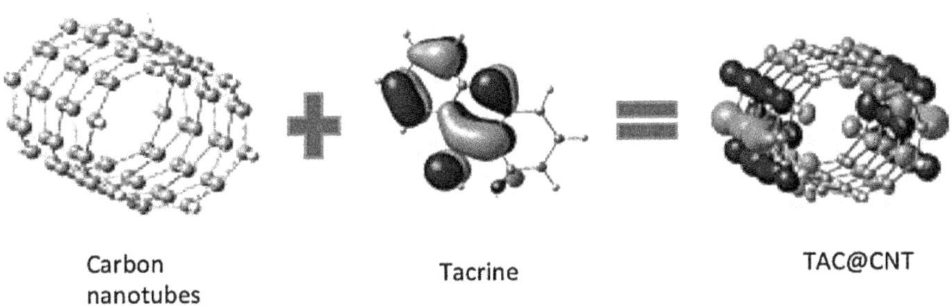

FIGURE 8.8 Formation of TAC@CNT complex.

Also, another way of treating Alzheimer's disease with the use of CNTs is through the development of berberine-loaded multiwalled carbon nanotubes. The current study is concerned with the synthesis of berberine (BRB) and polysodium and phospholipid-coated multiwalled carbon nanotubes (MWCNTs) for the treatment of Alzheimer's Disease (AD). Comparatively to other groups, phospholipid-, and polysorbate-coated MWCNTs were remarkably effective in recovering memory function from 18th to 20th days. It has been proven that these coated MWCNTs reduce β-amyloid-induced AD symptoms by preserving normal biochemical levels in brain tissue. Polysorbate/phospholipid coated MWCNTs of BRB have significant potential in treating AD holistically, based on the results of the studies.

An important neurotransmitter of the neuromuscular junction and the autonomic ganglia, acetylcholine (ACh) is a fast-acting, point-to-point neurotransmitter. Despite being the primary excitatory neurotransmitter in peripheral areas, ACh appears to have neuromodulatory effects in the brain. Yang et al. demonstrated that small-sized carbon nanotubes (SWCNTs) with diameters of 0.8 to 1.6 nm and varying lengths of 5 to 300 nm are successfully delivered into the brain, targeting lysosomes and not mitochondria. ACh drug effectiveness can be increased by using the SWCNT because of its lack in brain areas. The lack of ACh can be overcome by using SWCNT as a carrier with high bio-safety. Because ACh cannot be delivered direct to the brain at low doses because of its poor lipophilicity. The lack of ACh can be overcome by using highly biocompatible nanomaterials (SWCNT). This can be achieved due to ACh's poor lipophilicity, making it hard to deliver to the brain at low doses. Therapeutic effects can be achieved with SWCNTs without undesirable side effects by delivering ACh into targeted lysosomes.

Amyloid-β (Aβ) peptides, which are produced by the body, are abnormally self-assembled into toxic amyloid-β-rich aggregates in Alzheimer's disease. By inhibiting Aβ nucleation, hydrophobic nanoparticles retard fibrillation. However, their effect on Aβ oligomeric structures remains elusive. Independent of their surface physicochemical properties, carbon nanotubes inhibit/promote amyloid formation by increasing or decreasing nucleation lag times, which suggest a surface-modulated nucleation mechanism. By performing extensive all-atom replica exchange molecular dynamics simulations in explicit solvent, investigating the conformations of Aβ (16–22) octamers in the presence and absence of a single-walled carbon nanotube (SWCNT). The addition of SWCNT into an Aβ (16–22) solution prevents the formation of β-sheets when simulations starting with eight random chains. Simulations of Aβ (16–22) solutions starting from random chains show that SWCNT destabilizes the β-sheet structure. Simulations of Aβ (16–22) solutions starting from a prefibrillar β-sheet octamer show that SWCNT prevents β-sheet formation. SWCNTs are hydrophobic tubes, they are able to penetrate easily into the cytoplasm and nucleus through the lipid bilayer and SWCNT have no long term or short-term side effects. The computational study suggests that SWCNT inhibits full-length Aβ fibrillation and Aβ (16–22).

8.5 CONCLUSION

(CNTs) have recently been utilized in a wide variety of areas in the pharmacy and medical field, as outlined in this chapter. Since bionanotechnology has enabled us to carry drugs, genes, biomolecules, vaccines, and so on deeply into cells or organs that were previously unobtainable, the discovery of CNTs has opened up new alternatives to the ancient drug delivery methods. It is also possible to use collagen carbon nanotubes as scaffolds for tissue regeneration and artificial implants since CNTs resist biodegradation and are more feasible to use for tissue regeneration and artificial implants than other existing materials. As well, CNTs have been used as excellent diagnostic or therapeutic tools by combining them with biosensors or other materials in various areas, such as for drug analysis. As a health maintenance tool, functionalized CNTs can be developed for their free radical scavenger properties. These nanotechnologies could revolutionize the treatment of many incurable diseases in the near future, bringing hope for the treatment of some of the most difficult to treat ailments.

In this chapter, the use of CNTs for delivery of some drugs like tacrine, berberine, and acetylcholine for the management of Alzheimer's disease was conducted at the molecular level to establish the properties of materials without external interference. Analyzing quantitative and qualitative results, it was found that CNTs-mediated attraction to TAC drug was observed in both singular and complex models. As a conclusion of the present study, the complex of TAC@CNT could be utilized for targeted drug delivery systems due to CNT's advantage of carrying the drugs. Before CNTs could be used in clinical studies and then marketed worldwide, further toxicological studies are highly recommended from intact CNTs to functionalized CNTs and their conjugates.

KEYWORDS

- **Alzheimer's disease**
- **biomedical**
- **carbon nanotubes**
- **neurodegenerative disease**
- **neurological disorders**

REFERENCES

1. Hua, H., Pham-Huy, L., Pierre, D., Deli, X., Pengli, Z., & Pham-Huy, C., (2013). *Carbon Nanotubes: Applications in Pharmacy and Medicine*, 1–12.
2. Iijima, S., (1991). Helical microtubules of graphitic carbon. *Nature, 354*(6348), 56–58.
3. Dresselhaus, M. S., Dresselhaus, G., & Eklund, P. C., (1996). *Science of Fullerenes and Carbon Nanotubes.* Academic Press, San Diego, CA.
4. Hirlekar, R., Yamagar, M., Garse, H., Vij, M., & Kadam, V., (2009). Carbon nanotubes and its applications: A review. *Asian Journal of Pharmaceutical and Clinical Research, 2*(4), 17–27.
5. Singh, B. G. P., Baburao, C., & Pispatietal, V., (2012). Carbon nanotubes. A novel drug delivery system. *International Journal of Research in Pharmacy and Chemistry, 2*(2), 523–532.
6. Usui, Y., Haniu, H., Tsuruoka, S., & Saito, N., (2012). Carbon nanotubes innovate on medical technology. *Medicinal Chemistry, 2*(1), 1–6.
7. Zhang, Y., Bai, Y., & Yan, B., (2010). Functionalized carbon nanotubes for potential medicinal applications. *Drug Discovery Today, 15*(11, 12), 428–435.
8. Marta, R., & Dimitrios, G. F., (2013). Biomedical applications of carbon nanotubes. *Annual Reports Section C (Physical Chemistry)*, 10–35.
9. Dresselhaus, M., Dresselhaus, G., & Saito, R., (1995). Physics of carbon nanotubes. *Carbon, 33*, 883–891.
10. Surabhi, & Singh, B. K., (2019). Alzheimer's disease: A comprehensive review. International *Journal of Pharmaceutical Sciences and Research, 10*(3), 993–1000.
11. Lamberti, M., Pedata, P., Sannolo, N., Porto, S., Rosa, A. De., & Caraglia, M., (2015). Carbon nanotubes: Properties, biomedical application, advantages and risks in patients and occupationally-exposed workers. *International Journal of Immunopathology and Pharmacology, 28*(1), 4–13.
12. Yang, Z., Zhang, Y., Yang, Y., et al., (2010). Pharmacological and toxicological target organelles and safe use of single-walled carbon nanotubes as drug carriers in treating Alzheimer's disease. *Nanomedicine, 6*(3), 427–441.
13. Wang, J., (2005). Carbon-nanotube based electrochemical biosensors: Are view. *Electroanalysis, 17*(1), 7–14.
14. Kateb, B., Yamamoto, V., Alizadeh, D., et al., (2010). Multi-walled carbon nanotube (MWCNT) synthesis, preparation, labeling, and functionalization. *Methods in Molecular Biology, 651*, 307–317.
15. Casey, A., Herzog, E., Lyng, F. M., Byrne, H. J., Chambers, G., & Davoren, M., (2008). Single walled carbon nanotubes induce indirect cytotoxicity by medium depletion in A549 lung cells. *Toxicology Letters, 179*(2), 78–84.
16. Yang, D., Yang, F., Hu, J., Long, J., Wang, C., Fu, D., & Ni, Q., (2009). Hydrophilic multi-walled carbon nanotubes decorated with magnetite nanoparticles as lymphatic targeted drug delivery vehicles. *Chemical Communications*, 4447–4449.
17. Rajwant, K., Pooja, V., & Mandeep, K., (2018). Carbon nanotubes: A review article. *International Journal for Research in Applied Science & Engineering Technology, 6*(IV), 5075–5079.
18. Yahya, S. I., Chifu, E. N., & Tasia, A., (2020). Carbon nanotubes: A review of synthesis and characterization methods/techniques. *The International Journal of Science & Technology, 8*, 43–50.

19. Siegal, M., Overmyer, D., & Provencio, P., (2002). Precise control of multiwall carbon nanotube diameters using thermal chemical vapor deposition. *Appl. Phys. Lett., 80*, 2171–2173.
20. Prasek, J., Drbohlavova, J., Chomoucka, J., Hubalek, J., Jasek, O., Adam, V., & Kizek, R., (2011). Methods for carbon nanotubes synthesis—Review. *J. Mater. Chem., 21*, 15872–15884.
21. Rajesh, J. H. N., Sankaranarayanan, R., Kathiresan, M., Senthamaraikannan, P., Anish, K., Abdullah, M. A., & Imran, K., (2019). Synthesis, properties, and characterization of carbon nanotube-reinforced metal matrix composites. *Woodhead Publishing Series in Composites Science and Engineering*, 805–830.
22. Chen, Y., Zhang, Y., Hu, Y., Kang, L., Zhang, S., Xie, H., Liu, D., et al., (2014). State of the art of single-walled carbon nanotube synthesis on surfaces. *Adv. Mater., 26*, 5898–5922.
23. Yellampalli, S., (2011). *Carbon Nanotubes: Synthesis, Characterization, Applications.* Intech; Vienna, Austria.
24. Mirali, M., Jafariazar, Z., & Mahmoud, M., (2021). Loading tacrine Alzheimer's drug at the carbon nanotube: DFT approach. *Lab-in-Silico, 30*(3–8).
25. Mirzaei, M., (2010). The NMR parameters of the SiC-doped BN nanotubes: A DFT study. *Physica E., 42*, 1954–1957.
26. Mirzaei, M., Hadipour, N. L., Seif, A., & Giahi, M., (2008). Density functional study of zigzag BN nanotubes with equivalent ends. *Physica E., 40*, 3060–3063.
27. Mirzaei, M., & Mirzaei, M., (2010). A computational study of oxygen-termination of a (6, 0) boron nitride nanotube. *Monatshefte für Chemie., 141*, 491–494.
28. Mirzaei, M., & Mirzaei, M., (2010). Electronic structure of sulfur terminated zigzag boron nitride nanotube: A computational study. *Solid State Sciences, 12*, 1337–1340.
29. Wilson, B., Samanta, M. K., Santhi, K., Kumar, K. S., Ramasamy, M., & Suresh, B., (2010). Chitosan nanoparticles as a new delivery system for the anti-Alzheimer drug tacrine. *Nanomedicine: Nanotechnology, Biology and Medicine, 6*, 144–152.
30. Tahmasebi, E., & Shakerzadeh, E., (2020). Potential application of B40 fullerene as an innovative anode material for Ca-ion batteries: In silico investigation. *Lab-in-Silico, 1*, 16–20.
31. Eagger, S. A., Levy, R., & Sahakian, B. J., (1991). Tacrine in Alzheimer's disease. *The Lancet, 337*, 989–992.
32. Sameem, B., Saeedi, M., Mahdavi, M., & Shafiee, A., (2017). A review on tacrine-based scaffolds as multi-target drugs (MTDLs) for Alzheimer's disease. *European Journal of Medicinal Chemistry,* 128, 332–345.
33. Lohan, S., Raza, K., Mehta, S. K., Bhatti, G. K., Saini, S., & Singh, B., (2017). Anti-Alzheimer's potential of berberine using surface decorated multi-walled carbon nanotubes: A preclinical evidence. *International Journal of Pharmaceutics*, 263–278.
34. Asai, M., Iwata, N., Yoshikawa, A., Aizaki, Y., Ishiura, S., Saido, T. C., & Maruyama, K., (2007). Berberine alters the processing of Alzheimer's amyloid precursor protein to decrease abeta secretion. *Biochemical and Biophysical Research Communications, 352*, 498–502.
35. Cai, Z., Wang, C., & Yang, W., (2016). Role of berberine in Alzheimer's disease. *Neuropsychiatric Disease and Treatment, 12*, 2509–2520.

36. Kafa, H., Wang, J. T., Rubio, N., Venner, K., Anderson, G., Pach, E., Ballesteros, B., et al., (2015). The interaction of carbon nanotubes with an *in vitro* blood-brain barrier model and mouse brain *in vivo. Biomaterials, 53*, 437–452.
37. Kulkarni, S. K., & Dhir, A., (2010). Berberine: A plant alkaloid with therapeutic potential for central nervous system disorders. *Phytotherapy Research: PTR, 24*, 317–324.
38. Hakim, A. G., (2018). Modeling of the usefulness of carbon nanotubes as antiviral compounds for treating Alzheimer disease. *Advances in Alzheimer's Disease, 7*, 79–92.
39. Huiyu, L., Yin, L., Philippe, D., & Guanghong, W., (2011). Carbon nanotube inhibits the formation of β-sheet-rich oligomers of the Alzheimer's amyloid-β (16-22) peptide. *Biophysical Journal*, 2267–2276.
40. Pitschke, M., Prior, R., & Riesner, D., (1998). Detection of single amyloid β-protein aggregates in the cerebrospinal fluid of Alzheimer's patients by fluorescence correlation spectroscopy. *Nature Medicine*, 832–834.
41. Jeong, E. K., & Minyung, L., (2003). Fullerene inhibits β-amyloid peptide aggregation. *Biochemical and Biophysical Research Communication*, 576–579.
42. Ma, B., & Nussinov, (2002). *Stabilities and Conformations of Alzheimer's Beta–Amyloid Peptideoligomers (Abeta 16-22, Abeta 16-35, and Abeta 10-35): Sequence Effects*, 14126–14131.
43. Ren, H. X., Chen, X., & Huang, X. J., (2010). Toxicity of single-walled carbon nanotube: How we were wrong. *Mater. Today, 13*, 6–8.
44. Kaiser, J. P., Roesslein, M., & Wick, P., (2011). Carbon nanotubes—Curse or blessing. *Ciurr. Med. Chem., 18*, 2115–2128.
45. Balbach, J. J., Ishii, Y., & Tycko, R., (2000). Amyloid fibril formation by A *β* 16-22, a seven-residue fragment of the Alzheimer's *β*-amyloid peptide, and structural characterization by solid state NMR. *Biochemistry, 39*, 13748–13759.
46. Shi, K. N. W., Jessop, T. C., & Dai, H., (2004). Nanotube molecular transporters: Internalization of carbon nanotube-protein conjugates into mammalian cells. *J. Am. Chem. Soc., 126*, 6850, 6851.
47. Porter, A. E., Gass, M., & Welland, M., (2007). Direct imaging of single-walled carbon nanotubes in cells. *Nat. Nanotechnol., 2*, 713–717.
48. Röhrig, U. F., Laio, A., & Petronzio, R., (2006). Stability and structure of oligomers of the Alzheimer peptide A*β*16-22: From the dimer to the 32-mer. *Biophys. J., 91*, 3217–3229.
49. Venkataraman, A., Amadi, E.V., Chen, Y. et al. Carbon Nanotube Assembly and Integration for Applications. Nanoscale Res Lett 14, 220 (2019).

PART III

New Horizons in Sensing Technologies, Biomedical Imaging, and Health Care

CHAPTER 9

Recent Advances in Carbon Nanotube-Based Electrochemical and Optical Biosensors

GREESHMA SARA JOHN,[1,2] ATHIRA MARIA JOHNSON,[1,2] P. ARJUN SURESH,[1,2] N. V. UNNIKRISHNAN,[3] and K. V. ARUN KUMAR[1,2]

[1]*Department of Physics, CMS College (Autonomous), Kottayam, Kerala, India*

[2]*Nanotechnology and Advanced Materials Research Center, CMS College (Autonomous), Kottayam, Kerala, India*

[3]*School of Pure and Applied Physics, Mahatma Gandhi University, Kottayam, Kerala, India*

ABSTRACT

Carbon nanomaterials are one of the fascinating research fields due to their significant optical, chemical, electronic, mechanical, and thermal properties. In the past few decade's researchers looking to exploit carbon-based materials in developing advanced technology for sensing applications. The function of nanomaterials inside sensors has opened a pathway for the detection of analytes or target molecules. Large surface area to volume ratio and superior signal-to-noise ratio, biocompatibility, high-quality sensitivity, and selectivity than other structures are some of the added advantages of carbon nanomaterials in sensing applications. A wide range of detection of chemical to biological molecules is another advantage of carbon nanomaterials. Here we discussed the recent development of carbon-based nanomaterials in the application of virus detection, biosensor, electrochemical biosensors, cancer detection, etc.

Carbon Nanotubes for Biomedical Applications and Healthcare.
Chin Hua Chia, Swati Gokul Talele, Ann Rose Abraham, and A. K. Haghi, (Eds.)

9.1 INTRODUCTION

A large number of microorganisms are harmful to human life, many of them cause diseases which is leading to a large number of demises per annum. Many of communicable diseases significantly affect a lot of individuals and continuously cause major health issues. For the past century huge number of people affected by communicable diseases like COVID-19, dengue, hepatitis virus, Ebola virus, influenza virus (H5N1 and H1N1), Zika virus, human immunodeficiency virus (HIV), etc., and caused death in a large percentage. In the traditional way detection and culture of pathogens is often tedious and time-consuming work, moreover, this method needs trained personnel and cannot be afforded by all laboratories as it is still expensive. The limitations of these drawbacks can be overcome with the advance of micro-and nano-electronics which brought about the development of new kinds of biosensor designs for the identification of pathogenic microorganisms [1–4, 8]. In the healthcare field, the detection of pathogens, biological molecules, and other disease biosensors have a great role in the future. The biosensors are chemical sensors that utilize the recognition properties of the biomolecules in their sensitive layer. Three important parts of a normal biosensor are: (i) a recognition molecule that can be a protein, enzyme, antibody, or DNA, etc.; (ii) a transducer that records the interactivity of the analyte or target with the recognition molecule and produces a signal; (iii) a signal processor [1–8]. For the detection of microorganisms, different biosensor formats have been used like optical biosensors such as integrating waveguide biosensors, photodiode-based detection, or electrochemical detection systems, with a very good limit of detection. In the case of virus detection, electrochemical impedance spectroscopy or surface plasmon resonance assays have proven successful for the detection of bacteriophages. Due to the recognition properties of biomolecules to hold the target molecules on the surface of the electrode, an electrochemical biosensor is attached to these molecules. As a result of this process, a reaction signal is converted into an electrical signal like the voltage, current, impedance, etc., which can be easily detected. The majority of the biosensors that have been developed are electrochemical. The electrochemical biosensors have been used to study the quantitative as well as the qualitative aspects of the detected molecule. The electrochemical biosensors are highly sensitive to ensure detection, highly selective to avoid the interference of other species, cost-effective, small in size, and easy to use. Amongst the nanomaterials utilized for fabricating nano-sensors, carbon-based nanomaterials are a more promising candidate among sensors, as they can respond better to signals and can be used in various sensing applications. In addition to their high surface area, carbon-based nanomaterials are biocompatible materials and are advantageous in terms of simplicity, rapidity, and sensitivity, rendering them a high position to be considered in up-to-date technologies for viral recognition [6–10]. Carbon nanomaterial-based biosensors for viral recognition at the level of the virus type. Dengue virus, influenza virus (H5N1 and H1N1), Ebola virus, human immunodeficiency virus (HIV), Hepatitis virus, Zika virus, and Adenovirus. Due to its abundance in nature, carbon is widely applied in scientific and technological areas. A variety of carbon allotropes can be synthesized by changing the combinations of sp, sp^2, and sp^3 hybridization and an array of carbon structures and nanostructures have been presented up to the present time. The specifications of carbon nanomaterials are exclusive, due to their chemical stability, good electrical conductivity, and also it shows broad functional surface area. This section discusses the diagnostic applications of carbon nanomaterials. We discussed here the advanced level of application of carbon nanotube in electrochemical and optical biosensors [11–18].

9.2 BIOSENSORS

Biosensors are diagnostic techniques used in the medical field to detect various viral or bacterial diseases. Biosensors are mainly classified into electrochemical biosensors and optical biosensors. Compared to optical biosensors, electrochemical biosensors suffer from poor durability and poor selectivity. The average size of COVID-19 virus is found using a transmission electron microscope (TEM) and it's in the range 60–140 nm. That is the size of the virus lies in the nanoscale. Thus, by using nanomaterial as biosensors will give accurate results. Carbon nanotube (CNT) is one of the best materials that can be used in optical and electrochemical biosensors. Due to its conductivity, chemical stability, and tensile stress, it can be considered a suitable candidate for the same [19].

9.3 OPTICAL BIOSENSORS

Optical biosensors are the most popular biosensors used for diagnosing diseases. Its work is based on detecting the biological element by analyzing the interaction with change in its fluorescence, phosphorescence, refraction, surface plasmon resonance (SPR), etc. The optical biosensors can be classified mainly into direct and indirect biosensors. In indirect biosensors labeling such as fluorophores, chromophores are used for finding the analyte. In direct biosensors, the sensing is done by analyzing the optical properties like change in refractive index (RI) [20, 21]. Direct, real-time, and label-free detection is possible for optical biosensors compared to others [22].

An Optical biosensor is a device consisting of a biorecognition element that is connected to an optical transducer system. The biosensor is capable of generating signals that are proportional to the concentration of the analyte and can give real-time data. SPR (surface plasmon resonance) based biosensors, LSPR (localized surface plasmon resonance) based biosensor, SWIR (shortwave-infrared-red) based biosensors, SERS (surface-enhanced Raman spectroscopy) based sensors, SEF (Surface-enhanced fluorescence) based biosensor are the most popular optical biosensors. Among these biosensors, the sensor which is based on LSPR is suitable for detecting various types of analytes. For enhancing fluorophore excitation rate via local enhancement of the electric field, the metal nanoparticles are placed near fluorophores. This could change the radiative decay rate of an excited fluorophore [23].

9.4 SURFACE-ENHANCED RAMAN SPECTROSCOPY (SERS) BIOSENSOR

SERS biosensors are the most studied diagnostic tool against the COVID-19 virus. It is based on vibrational spectroscopy technique, and it can provide much more information compared to an electronic spectroscopy technique [24]. It has numerous advantages compared to other optical sensors which include its photostability, high sensitivity, and fast detection of molecules. Figure 9.1 shows the schematic diagram of the SERS-based biosensor. An enhanced electric field is developed due to the surface plasmon resonance on the metal surface when it is irradiated with laser. Due to the enhanced electric field, the molecules placed in the field become more polarized and hence the Raman signal is enhanced. When the electromagnetic field is increased in the plasmonic mode of the nanoparticles there will be enhanced Raman emission in the SERS mode. The adsorption peak corresponds to the stage at which the frequency of the incident light to metal nanoparticles is equal to the frequency of the surface plasmon.

It is found that using plasmonic materials like Ag, Au as active substrate, will enhance the Raman signal intensity to a great extent. SERS biosensors have the ability to detect biomolecules like cancer cells, viruses, bacteria, etc. In the early stages of infection of COVID-19, the presence of viruses in the sample will be significantly low. It is very hard to detect the presence using the conventional method of diagnosing. By using plasmonic particles the Raman scattering of the particles can be enhanced and hence it is easy to find its presence in the sample [25]. By using the Raman spectroscopy analysis tool, researchers identify the COVID-19 virus from an infected person's saliva. It shows a sensitivity of about 92.5% and an accuracy of about 91.6%. Thus, by using the plasmonic particle, we can even detect the presence of the virus without staining or labeling [26].

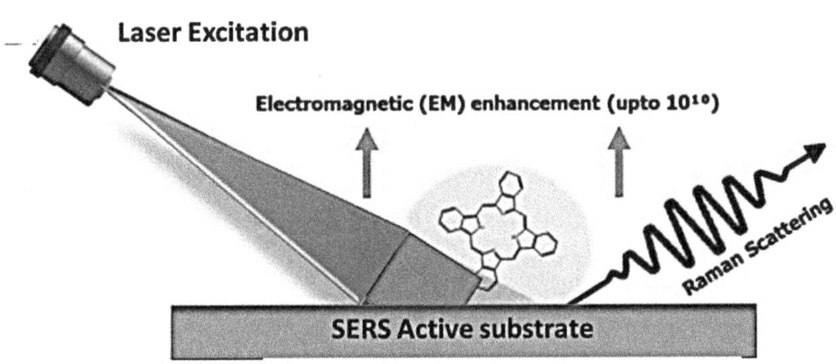

FIGURE 9.1 SERS based biosensor.

A carbon nanotube is a worthy candidate for making SERS biosensors. It is found that Silver coated CNT shows an excitation wavelength from visible to near infrared (NIR). The CNT can be classified into single-walled carbon nanotube (SWCNT) and multi-walled CNT (MWCNT). Among these two structures, SWCNT shows strong resonance Raman scattering. Thus, by introducing the plasmonic effect into the biosensor will increase the sensitivity. One of the drawbacks of SERS is its slow imaging speed compared to other optical biosensors.

9.5 ELECTROCHEMICAL BIOSENSORS

Carbon nanotube and its derivatives exhibit numerous properties due to its large surface area, conductivity, etc. [27]. Due to its properties, it can be used for biosensing purposes. Carbon derivatives are already used in electrochemical biosensors for finding different viruses. Electrochemical biosensors are not a recent invention, it is already established, and it is used for finding different viruses (Figure 9.2).

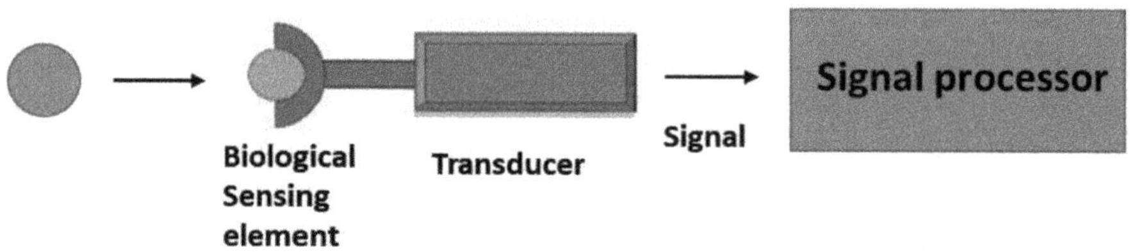

FIGURE 9.2 Schematic diagram of a biosensor.

The biosensor consists of a combination of a biological sensing element and a transducer which converts the data from the biological process into electrical signals. It is then given to the signal processing unit which consists of an amplifier and filter. The amplifier amplifies the electrical signal, and it is filtered through a low pass filter. Finally, it is passed through a microcontroller and get analyzed [28, 29].

In recent years Chandra et al. formulated a smartphone-assisted diagnostic test of the COVID-19 virus. It is based on Electrochemical impedance spectroscopy (EIS) and the electrode used in the device are carbon-based derivatives – carbon nanotube, graphene oxide, etc. He also designed an electrochemical Geno sensor, and its aim was to detect the genetic material of the COVID-19 virus [30]. The sensor contains a trans-impedance enhancer, a detector, and a primary converter. The surface of the sensor is covered with silica-coated nanoparticles which are used to increase the hydrophobicity. Single-walled carbon nanotubes are also used to enhance the sensitivity of electrodes and to amplify the signal. This sensor can be used not only to identify the COVID-19 virus but also for identifying various respiratory diseases [31]. Electrochemical biosensors work based on studying the changes caused in the conductometric, potentiometric, capacitive, amperometric, or piezoelectric properties of the species [32].

9.6 CARBON NANOTUBE AS ELECTRODE-ELECTROCHEMICAL BIOSENSOR

The electrode is an important candidate in the working of electrochemical biosensors. The material that is used as an electrode must have certain peculiarities. It must be inert when the electrochemical reaction takes place, also it must be conductive. Generally, gold, silver, platinum is used as electrodes [33].

Recently carbon derivatives have also been used. Even though carbon derivatives are not much conductive as gold or silver, it has a huge surface area and also it is chemically inert with electroactive species. For an electrochemical biosensor generally, three electrodes are used: they are reference electrode, auxiliary electrode, working electrode. In these three electrodes, the reference electrode shows a constant potential, generally, Ag or AgCl is used as reference electrode, auxiliary electrode supplies the current to the working electrode by connecting through the electrolyte, and the working electrode acts as a transducer. The auxiliary electrode and working electrode must be chemically stable and conductive. Gold, silver, platinum, or carbon compounds are generally used as an electrode [34, 35].

Moreover, the diameter of the SARS-CoV-2 virus is in the range of 50–200 nm and it is very close to the longitudinal dimension of CNT. The high surface-to-volume ratio of nanomaterials will increase the signal-to-noise ratio and that will increase efficiency [36]. Carbon nanotube electrodes are already used for certain types of biosensors due to their mechanical properties, high surface area, high electrolytic activity, high chemical stability [37].

9.7 CARBON NANOTUBE IN FET-BASED BIOSENSOR

Field effect transistors biosensors are gaining more popularity today. The FET biosensor was first generated by Bergveld in 1970. Even though conventional diagnosing techniques give an accurate result, FET can reduce the diagnosing time to a great extent, and also it is much cheaper [38].

FET is a device that can control the electroconductivity between source and drain terminals by third gate electrode through an insulator. When the analyte binds to the bio-receptor the electrostatic surface potential of the semiconductor changes and this potential acts as a gate voltage in a MOSFET. The analyte can be detected by measuring the change in the current [39]. Nanomaterials are also used to increase the sensitivity of FET. Exposing the target analytes to a biosensor, the transducer converts the chemical changes to a measurable signal [40]. Carbon derivatives like Carbon nanotube and graphene are the most common materials used for making nano-transducers (Figure 9.3) [41].

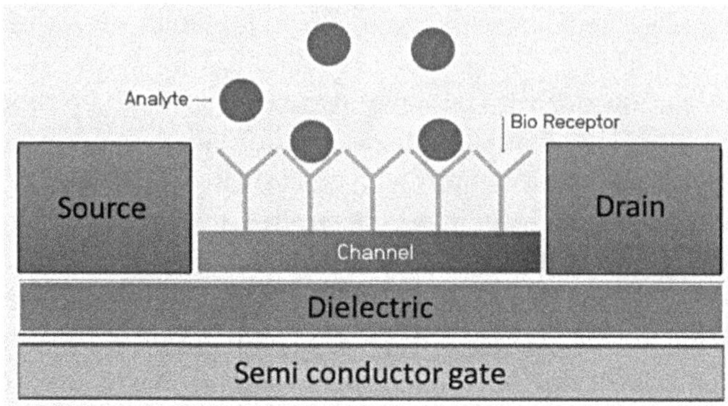

FIGURE 9.3 Schematic diagram of FET biosensor.

Research is going on to find an effective and fast method for diagnosing COVID-19, CNT-based FET is in the development stage. CNT-based FETs are prepared on a polymer substrate and the sensor is made by immobilizing the RdRp gene sequence of the COVID-19 virus on the CNT channel. It has shown a limit of detection of about ~ 10 fM [42]. SWCNT (Single-walled carbon nanotube) based FET is also drawing attention in the field of biosensors. SWCNT-based FET decorated with the binding antibodies of COVID-19 spike protein are under development. It has a LOD of about ~0.55 fg./ml [43].

9.8 APPLICATIONS OF CARBON-BASED MATERIALS FOR VIRUS DETECTION

9.8.1 CARBON NANOTUBES IN HUMAN VIRUS DETECTION

Human pathogenic viruses are one of the major causes of serious illness and deaths around the world. The incidence of such infectious diseases affecting the human life has risen tremendously. Speedy primary diagnostics is crucial for proper and timely treatments. Effectual therapies require rapid, specific, and sensitive diagnostic tests [1].

Biosensors, which consist of biochemical recognition element and a physical transducer [44] are attractive alternative methods to the conventional diagnostic tests. Particular focus has been laid on miniaturization of biosensors by making use of nanomaterials for their nano-size and exclusive electronic, optical, mechanical, and magnetic properties; to obtain sensors of extreme sensitivity and minimal invasivity [1].

Carbon nanomaterials are favorable materials for improved sensing and recognition functionality [1]. The extraordinaire mechanical and electronic properties and large specific area of CNTs made them attractive candidates for biosensing applications, especially electrochemical biosensing [12]. CNTs are novel detection components of biosensors for rapid diagnosis and more cost-effective, stable, and selective biosensing technologies. Biocompatibility and simplicity also make them advantageous in the viral detection technologies [1].

Electrochemical biosensors use CNTs as electrodes to sense the analyte by detecting the electric response that results from the electrochemical reaction that happens between the analyte and the electrode surface of the sensor. In optical biosensors, which measures the variation in light emanation during target detection, CNTs can be fluorescent quenching agents [1]. CNT electrodes in electrochemical biosensor have improved electron transport rate as an advantage of its high aspect ratio, and large surface area. Exclusive optical properties that CNTs have, its high luminous intensity, make them perfect for optical biosensors [1].

The recognition of virus can be done by detecting the antibodies that result from the infection, detecting nucleic acid from the virus, or by detecting the entire virus [1].

Biosensors, with great application in the medical field, were found to be prominent since the 1950s [45]. The electrochemical biosensor was the first to get described which then paved the way to optical as well as other biosensors. The invention of biosensors started with the electrochemical oxygen biosensor followed by advancements in those with the introduction of enzyme electrodes and enzyme transducer to catalyze an electrochemical reaction [45]. After that, a number of biosensors were developed which could be used for both *in vivo* and *in vitro* applications. The large classification of biosensors includes immune-biosensors, thermal biosensors, microbial biosensors, etc. [45]. The recent advancement is the addition of nanobiosensors [45].

9.8.2 ROLE OF CARBON NANOTUBES IN BIOSENSORS

The most versatile physicochemical properties of nanomaterials were responsible for the introduction of nanotechnologies and nanomaterials into the world of biosensors thus owing to the invention of nanobiosensors [45]. This class of biosensors employs nanotubes as well as nanoparticles [45]. It is a small size and large surface to volume of the nanomaterials that helps in the functionality of the nanobiosensors [45]. The small size of the nanomaterials could be employed in the increased performance by enhancing the sensitivity and lower detection limits [45]. They could also act as transducers.

CNTs with its unique structural, mechanical, electronic, and optical properties could be used to assemble many probes that could be used in medical as well as other applications [45]. They have the ability to multifunctionalize and thus to multiplex which is opposed by mono-conjugated biosensor species [45]. They could also be used for signal transduction, conduct electricity, and also could account for higher thermal conductivity. The CNTs act as a promising candidate in medical applications due to their ability to overcome biological membranes thus could account for *in vivo* applications. CNTs-based biosensors could be classified into electronic transducers, electrochemical CNTs biosensors, immunosensors, and optical CNTs-based biosensors which have different target recognition and transduction [45]. These CNTs-based biosensors are potential probe for detecting cancer by using cancer biomarkers [45].

Biosensors based on CNTs comprise a large variety of which the electrochemical and optical biosensors are the area of our interest. Thus, detailing the above-mentioned class of biosensors and the method of employing them for cancer detection and treatment.

9.8.3 ROLE OF ELECTROCHEMICAL AND ELECTRONIC CNT-BASED BIOSENSORS

Electrochemical biosensors with the advantages of small size, fast response time, ease of use, and low cost is the larger part of biosensors discovered to date [45]. The basis biosensor comprises of a reference electrode, a working electrode, and a counter electrode. Target is recognized by the enzyme placed on the working electrode [45]. Enzymes possess the advantage of high catalytic activity.

CNTs is employed in electrochemical biosensors due to their good and efficient capability to transfer electrons, high conductivity, large surface area, small size, sensitivity, and high chemical stability [45]. These biosensors could be used to develop protein biomarkers and detect metabolites.

9.8.4 CNTs-BASED ELECTROCHEMICAL BIOSENSORS FOR CANCER DETECTION AND TREATMENT

Biosensors are developed for the detection of cancer cells. Studies done to date shows the increasing response in the detection of cancer cells by the modification of bipolar electrode (BPE) with multi-walled nanotubes (MWCNT). They were specifically used to detect drugs useful for breast cancer [45]. Another class of biosensors tricosane (C23H48)-functionalized SWCNTs biosensor was employed for the detection of lung cancer [45]. Biosensors modified with SWCNT or MWCNT could show greater advancement in the detection of gastric cancer cells and many other cancer cells [45]. Research have confirmed that the properties of both SWCNTs and MWCNTs could be employed in the early stage detection of prostate cancer [45].

9.8.5 ROLE OF OPTICAL CNT-BASED BIOSENSORS

This class of biosensors depends on the changes in the emission of light to detect the target. Optical biosensors are categorized based on the method employed to detect the target either surface plasmon resonance, absorbance, reflectance, fluorescence, phosphorescence, luminescence, wavelength intensity, lifetime, anisotropy, quenching, and fluorescence energy transfer [45]. There exist colorimetric biosensors that depend on the changes in light absorption and photometric light intensity biosensors that depend on the difference in fluorescence [45].

CNT is a potential nanomaterial for biosensors for biomarker detection. SWNT with photoluminescence between 650 and 1,400 nm has the ability to penetrate through biological tissues. The stability they offer to photobleaching makes it suitable for biomedical imaging applications [45].

9.8.6 DIAGNOSIS OF COVID-19

The world is now facing a serious disease caused due to coronavirus. The coronavirus was first reported in Wuhan, and it is further spread into other parts of the globe. Coronavirus has the ability to spread through the air, and the spreading of the virus can be limited to some extent by using masks, sanitizers, etc. It is caused by the SARS-CoV-2 virus, and it causes respiratory illness. The SARS-CoV-2 virus enters the body first binds with entry receptors present on the surface of the cell, such as ACE2 (angiotensin-converting enzyme 2). ACE2 is commonly present in the human body, mainly in the lungs and small intestine. Then the COVID-19 virus replicates the genomic RNA inside the cell and creates full-length copies [46]. Even though vaccines against coronavirus were invented, they are successful only up to some extent. It is found that the effectiveness of the COVID-19 vaccine is slightly lower in delta variants compared to others. The easy way to reduce its spreading is by fast and economically diagnosing its presence. Fast diagnosing the disease and isolating the infected persons can reduce the spreading to a great extent [47–49].

The diagnosis of COVID-19 is usually based on: (i) virus detection; (ii) antibody detection; and (iii) antigen protein detection. The samples required for the study are collected either from blood or from saliva. Various diagnostic techniques are used for analyzing its presence. PCR (Polymerase chain reaction) and RT-qPCR (Reverse transcriptase-quantitative chain reaction) techniques are the most commonly used methods. But they are time-consuming and expensive, also they have a higher false-negative rate. Thus, researchers are working hard to find an alternate method for diagnosing the disease [50–52].

9.8.6.1 NAKED EYE DIAGNOSTIC TEST OF COVID-19 VIRUS

Fast diagnosing of the coronavirus is essential for decreasing the spreading of the virus. Availability of testing kits, equipment, limited test centers is the factor that decreases the rate of testing. In such a situation finding an alternative way of testing SARS-CoV-2 is important. Moitra et al. suggest a diagnostic technique for diagnosing the COVID-19 virus by using the naked eye. It doesn't require any advanced types of equipment for diagnosing. The author suggests the usage of nanotechnology-based colorimetric bioassays which don't require any complex instruments or trained staff. In the field of colorimetric-based biosensors, gold nanoparticles (AuNPs) have gained more attention in recent days. Due to their good optical properties, inherent photo-stability, and localized surface plasmon resonance, they are used for optical biosensors. In this diagnostic test, the author utilizes the intrinsic properties of plasmonic AuNP and also uses the targeting ability of Antisense oligonucleotides (ASOs). The researchers discovered three SARS-related viral genomes. They are RNA-dependent RNA polymerase gene (RdRP), Envelope protein gene (E gene), and Nucleocapsid phosphoprotein gene (N gene). Thus, the author finds a way of finding the N gene sequence of the COVID-19 virus and uses gold nanoparticles as the most important anisotropic plasmonic nanostructures which can diagnose the COVID-19 virus [53].

9.8.7 DIAGNOSIS OF DENGUE VIRUS

Dias et al. developed an immunosensor based on CNTs-screen printed electrodes (CNTs-SPEs) by dispersing carboxylated CNTs in carbon ink for detecting NS1 protein, a non-structural protein of dengue virus. Dengue virus attack is identified by detecting the NS1 protein [1, 2]. CNT-SPE is the working electrode on which anit-NS1 antibodies were immobilized through deposited ethylenediamine (EDA) film on the electrode [2].

A 190% increase in the electroactive surface area was observed. Constant redox peaks from voltammograms showed that electrodes with CNTs are more stable than that without CNTs. The limit of detection (LOD) was much lower when compared to the LOD of microbalance immunosensor using quartz crystal. The immunosensor showcased excellent reproducibility and good repeatability. The repeatability was tested by measuring 10 replicated using the same CNT-SPE [2].

A label free chemiresistive immunosensor was offered by Wasik et al. for the detection of the dengue NS1 protein by functionalizing a network of SWCNTs with anti-dengue monoclonal antibodies. Contaminated synthetic human saliva within concentration ranges of clinical standard was tested for the virus. Selective and sensitive detection of the NS1 protein was possible [1].

Palomar et al. have given a picture of impedimetric biosensor for dengue virus antibody detection by functionalizing CNTs by immobilizing dengue virus 2 NS1 glycoprotein on them via electrogenerated polypyrrole-NHS by covalent amide joining. This offers required selectivity towards the NS1 antibody [1].

9.8.8 DIAGNOSIS OF INFLUENZA VIRUS

Tam et al. developed a DNA sensor using dual interdigitated electrodes that works on multi-walled carbon nanotubes (MWCNTs) for label-free and for directly detecting influenza virus (type A). The functionalized MWCNTs work as linkers for the immobilization of the DNA strands probe onto the sensor. The sensors have potential application for controlling this disease apart from the advantages like high selectivity, cost effectiveness, and rapid diagnosis. The MWCNTs used were synthesized by chemical vapor deposition (CVD) [11].

The LOD of this sensor (0.5 nM concentration of the virus sample) was lesser when compared with the electrochemical transducer which aids fluorescence and square wave voltammetry done by Li et al. The response time was less than 4 minutes. The alteration in conductance forming the metal-CNT's contact was the sensing process used [11].

Lee et al. worked on plasmon-assisted fluoroimmunoassay (PAFI). Plasmonic resonance energy transfer (PRET) phenomenon is the thrust of PAFI by which a photoluminescence (PL) strengthening happens as a result of the synergism between the semiconducting nanoparticles and the plasmonic nanoparticles. In this type of biosensors, interactions of an antibody with its antigen are detected. In this particular work, gold nanoparticles (Au NPs) which exhibit surface plasmon resonance, decorated CNTs and CdTe quantum dots (QDs) are used. CdTe QDs are fluorescent nanoparticles. Apart from the surface plasmon resonance exhibited by the Au NPs, other advantage of the biosensors is the exhibition of electrical conductivity and the accommodation of many π electrons on their surfaces. AuCNTs were utilized as influenza virus detection platforms [8].

Influenza virus/New Caledonia/20/99IvR116 (H1N1), Influenza virus A/Beijing/262/95 (H1N1) and the clinically isolated Influenza virus A/Yokohama/110/2009 (H3N2) were the three viruses tested. The PL intensities as a function of concentration of the influenza virus were measured for the virus detection. The combined effect between the fluorescent nanoparticles and the plasmonic nanoparticles led to the PL enhancement. The MWCNTs mediates the plasmon-coupling interaction between adjacent Au NPs which could enhance the optical property of the hybrid structure. A non-symmetric and broadened plasmonic band was obtained for the Au NPs. Surface enhanced Raman scattering (SERS) and enhanced electrical conductivity were achieved. The LOD improved by about 10 times when compared to other PAFI systems. A 100-fold higher selectivity was attained for this sensing system in comparison with commercial diagnostic kit [8].

CNTs can be used to produce fluorescent labels because of their near-infrared photoluminescence. A high signal-to-noise ratio could be achieved. A stable fluorescence measurement was possible as the CNTs do not exhibit fluorescent photobleaching. The lower quantum yield of CNTs is a limiting factor for the fluorescent label performance. Ashiba et al. evaluated the performance of CNTs fluorescent label for influenza virus detection using surface plasmon resonance-assisted fluoroimmunoassay (SPRF) in a V-trench biosensor. The study concentrated on (8,3) CNTs. The system was excited at 670 nm and gave an emission at 970 nm which is detectable by making use of visible charge-coupled device (CCD) [9].

The result was obtained that CNTs labels were tolerant against quenching. CNTs-labeled anti-body binding to the target analyte offered enhanced sensitivity than unlabeled antibody binding to the target analyte. Modifying CNTs by the introduction of defects by covalent or oxidation functionalization greatly enhanced CNTs luminous intensity which can further improve the CNTs label performance. Work has to be done to overcome the low labeling efficiency of CNTs, poor reactivity [9].

9.8.9 DIAGNOSIS OF HUMAN IMMUNODEFICIENCY VIRUS (HIV)

Fang et al. developed an electrochemical immunosensor with enhanced sensitivity for detecting human immunodeficiency virus p24 (HIV-p24). A multi-enzyme amplification strategy is followed by encapsulation of enzymes in CNTs-silica matrix. Graphene oxide (GO) acts as a nanocarrier. The LOD was for this biosensor was found to be lower than the traditional electrochemical sensor for HIV-p24. The sensor has shown favorable reproducibility and stability. The sensor was proved to be simple and cost effective. MWCNTs were used which improved the electron transfer kinetics and and electrochemical stability [3].

Ma et al. developed molecularly imprinted polymers (MIPs) electrochemical biosensor on MWCNTs. Differential pulse voltammetry (DPV) transducer was used. The sensor exhibited high specificity for the HIV-p24 virus, good stability, sensitivity, reproducibility, and repeatability. The virus detection test was done in real human serum samples, which gave acceptable results, increasing the importance of the sensor. ELISA test was also done to come the reliability and accuracy of the sensor [4].

9.8.10 DIAGNOSIS OF IN CANCER DETECTION

SWNTs when conjugated with different cyclic groups such as Indocyanine Green (ICG) were observed to act on tumor-bearing mice [45]. The optical biosensors were developed to detect cyclin A, which was overexpressed in certain human cancer. Thus, it could be used as a probe to detect cancer at the very early stages [45].

Thus, CNTs based biosensors could be used to detect different types of deadly cancer disease like lung cancer, ovarian cancer, and pancreatic cancer.

9.8.10.1 DETECTION OF LUNG CANCER

Lung cancer is one of the deadliest cancers with a very high mortality rate. Thus, there is a necessity for the early detection of lung cancer and for this purpose biosensors were developed which could sense the exhaled gas of lung cancer patients [54]. The sensor technology works on the basis of the difference between the exhaled gas of a healthy person and a cancer patient. The major advantage of this type of sensory detection is the painless nature [54]. CNTs was incorporated into the sensing devices due to the advantages of low cost, high sensitivity, quick response and environment friendly nature [54]. CNTs added with transition metal was found to increase its adsorption ability and thus increasing the sensory action towards gases [54]. Studies confirms the presence of benzene is potential lung cancer patients which was detected by Rh doped CNTs based biosensor [54]. The amount of carbon dioxide also varies for a lung cancer patient as their lungs got weak by the cancer cells [54]. The Rh-CNTs shows appreciable sensitivity towards benzene and aniline, two typical gases exhaled from a lung cancer patient thus a promising candidate for early diagnosis of lung cancer. The major advantage of this novel Rh-CNTs based biosensor used for the prognosis of lung cancer is the simple technology employed and the ease to use either one needs no expertise to use this biosensor [54]. This bioisensor is proposed on the basis of DFT and could be made by experimentalist in the near future.

9.8.10.2 DETECTION OF OVARIAN CANCER

Ovarian cancer is the most widespread cancer found in women with a very high mortality rate. Although they have a very high survival rate at stage 1, they are mostly diagnosed in stage 3 and stage 4 which results in high mortality rates [55]. The biomarker for ovarian cancer is CA-125 suffers a low sensitivity at early stages and it shoots up at the later stages, making it a top biomarker for ovarian cancer [55]. The sensing devices existed were of high cost and low sensitivity thus there arises a need for a potential biosensor for ovarian cancer. CNTs were used as a significant candidate due to their exceptional electrochemical and electrical properties and also their ultra-high specific surface area [55]. They could also detect biological species at very low concentration because of their high surface to volume ratio [55]. With the additional advantage of higher stability, longer durability and better electron transfer they could be employed in biosensing devices [55]. A functional carboxylic CNTs based biosensor was developed with interdigitated electrodes which could increase the sensitivity of the CA-125 antigens [55].

9.8.10.3 DETECTION OF PANCREATIC CANCER

The biosensors were used for the detection of pancreatic cancer, one with a very low survival rate, due to their high sensitivity and selectivity. The biosensor used was fabricated using interdigitated gold electrodes and CNTs in a layer fashion [56]. The biomarker employed is CA19-9. CNTs with its unique properties could attribute to enhance the sensitivity of the biosensor [56]. Biosensor for detecting pancreatic cancer was developed using MWCNTs they possess a number of binding sites for antibodies due to their hollow shell structure [56]. The purpose of this biosensor was to detect the biomarker CA19-9, antigen for the pancreatic cancer. The method of detection was based on the impedance spectroscopy [56].

Thus, biosensors could considerably contribute to the early detection of the highly dangerous cancer cell. We could conclude by emphasizing on the importance of nanomaterials specifically CNTs for the development of biosensors in detecting cancer.

KEYWORDS

- **biosensor**
- **carbon nanotube**
- **COVID**
- **electrochemical sensor**
- **optical sensor**
- **surface plasmon resonance**

REFERENCES

1. Hamide, E. (2020). *Journal of Science: Advanced Materials and Devices.* doi.org/10.1016/j.jsamd.2020.09.005.
2. Ana, C. M. S. D., Gomes-Filho, S. L. R., Mı´zia, M. S. S., & Rosa, F. D., (2013). *Biosensors and Bioelectronics, 44*, 216–221.
3. Yi-Shan, F., Xin-Jian, H., Li-Shi, W., & Ju-Fang, W., (2015). *Biosensors and Bioelectronics, 64*, 324–332.
4. Ya, M., Xiao-Lei, S., Qiang, Z., Hai-Shui, W., & Li-Shi, W., (2017). *Talanta, 164*, 121–127.
5. García-Aljaro, C., Lakshmi, N. C., Dhamanand, J. S., Miso, P., Francisco, J. M., Marylynn, V. Y., & Ashok, M., (2010). *Biosensors and Bioelectronics, 26*, 1437–1441.
6. Ravinder, K., Sandeep, A., Sheng-Joue, Y., Vinay, G., Pankaj, B., & Ajit, K., (2020). *Journal of the Electrochemical Society*, 167037555.
7. Sebastian, K., Andrew, J. H., Jingqing, Z., Nigel, F. R., Bin, M., & Michael, S. S. (2013). doi.org/10.1016/j.addr.2013.07.015.

8. Jaewook, L., Syed, R. A., Sangjin, O., Jeonghyo, K., Tetsuro, S., Kaushik, P., Simon, S. P., et al., (2015). *Biosensors and Bioelectronics, 64*, 311–317.
9. Hiroki, A., Yoko, I., Toshiya, O., Xiaomin, W., & Makoto, F., (2017). *Sensors, 17*, 2569.
10. Jin-Ha, C., Jin-Ho, L., Joohyung, S., & Jeong-Woo, C., (2020). *Sensors, 20*, 1003.
11. Phuong, D. T., Nguyen, V. H., Nguyen, D. C., Anh-Tuan, L., & Mai, A. T., (2009). *Journal of Immunological Methods, 350*, 118–124.
12. Minghui, Y., Yordan, K., & Avraham, R., (2008). *International Journal of Food Microbiology, 127*, 78–83.
13. Bakr, A. T., Yousif, A. M., Nur, N. B., Ahmad, A., Mohd, H. H. M., Mohd, S. D. B. Z., & Norhana, A., (2021). *Diagnostics, 11*, 1119.
14. Thanihaichelvana, M., Surendran, S. N., Kumanan, T., Sutharsini, U., Ravirajan, P., Valluvan, R., & Tharsika, T. (2022). *Materials Today: Proceedings*. doi.org/10.1016/j.matpr.2021.05.011.
15. Wei, Y. L., Boon, L. L., & Narayanan, R., (2021). *Biosensors, 11*, 434.
16. Tahriri, M., Del, M. M., Moghanian, A., Tavakkoli, Y. M., Torres, R., Yadegari, A., & Tayebi, L., (2019). *Mater. Sci. Eng. C, 102*.
17. Hamide, E., Zeinab, B., & Yaghoubi-Avini, M., (2019). *Environ. Nanotechn. Monitor. Manag., 12,* 100274.
18. Hamide, E., Zeinab, B., Farzaneh, E., & Mohammad, M. A., (2018). *J. Mol. Liq., 265*, 565e571.
19. Shahabi, D., & Tavakol, H., (2017). DFT, NBO and molecular docking studies of the adsorption of fluoxetine into and on the surface of simple and sulfur-doped carbon nanotubes. *Applied Surface Science, 420*, 267–275.
20. Frías, I. A., Avelino, K. Y., Silva, R. R., Andrade, C. A., & Oliveira, M. D., (2015). Trends in biosensors for HPV: Identification and diagnosis. *Journal of Sensors, 2015*.
21. Wang, R., & Li, Y., (2016). Biosensors for rapid detection of avian influenza. *Steps Forwards in Diagnosing and Controlling Influenza, 61*.
22. Dey, D., & Goswami, T., (2011). Optical biosensors: A revolution towards quantum nanoscale electronics device fabrication. *Journal of Biomedicine and Biotechnology, 2011*.
23. Shrivastav, A. M., Cvelbar, U., & Abdulhalim, I., (2021). A comprehensive review on plasmonic-based biosensors used in viral diagnostics. *Communications Biology, 4*(1), 1–12.
24. McCreery, R. L., (2005). *Raman Spectroscopy for Chemical Analysis* (Vol. 225). John Wiley & Sons.
25. Moore, T. J., Moody, A. S., Payne, T. D., Sarabia, G. M., Daniel, A. R., & Sharma, B., (2018). *In vitro* and *in vivo* SERS biosensing for disease diagnosis. *Biosensors, 8*(2), 46.
26. Taha, B. A., Al Mashhadany, Y., Bachok, N. N., Bakar, A. A., Hafiz, M. M. H., Dzulkefly, B. Z. M. S., & Arsad, N., (2021). Detection of COVID-19 virus on surfaces using photonics: Challenges and perspectives. *Diagnostics, 11*(6), 1119.
27. Jiang, Z., Feng, B., Xu, J., Qing, T., Zhang, P., & Qing, Z., (2020). Graphene biosensors for bacterial and viral pathogens. *Biosensors and Bioelectronics*, 112471.
28. Purohit, B., Vernekar, P. R., Shetti, N. P., & Chandra, P., (2020). Biosensor nanoengineering: Design, operation, and implementation for biomolecular analysis. *Sensors International*, 100040.

29. Khan, M. Z. H., Hasan, M. R., Hossain, S. I., Ahommed, M. S., & Daizy, M., (2020). Ultrasensitive detection of pathogenic viruses with electrochemical biosensor: State of the art. *Biosensors and Bioelectronics*, 112431.
30. Tripathy, S., & Singh, S. G., (2020). Label-free electrochemical detection of DNA hybridization: A method for COVID-19 diagnosis. *Transactions of the Indian National Academy of Engineering, 5*, 205–209.
31. Cesewski, E., & Johnson, B. N., (2020). Electrochemical biosensors for pathogen detection. *Biosensors and Bioelectronics, 159*, 112214.
32. Kumar, N., Hu, Y., Singh, S., & Mizaikoff, B., (2018). Emerging biosensor platforms for the assessment of water-borne pathogens. *Analyst, 143*(2), 359–373.
33. Grabowska, I., Malecka, K., Jarocka, U., Radecki, J., & Radecka, H., (2014). Electrochemical biosensors for detection of avian influenza virus--current status and future trends. *Acta Biochimica Polonica, 61*(3).
34. Ali, M. B., Korpan, Y., Gonchar, M., El'Skaya, A., Maaref, M. A., Jaffrezic-Renault, N., & Martelet, C., (2006). Formaldehyde assay by capacitance versus voltage and impedance measurements using bi-layer bio-recognition membrane. *Biosensors and Bioelectronics, 22*(5), 575–581.
35. Thévenot, D. R., Toth, K., Durst, R. A., & Wilson, G. S., (2001). Electrochemical biosensors: Recommended definitions and classification. *Biosensors and Bioelectronics, 16*(1, 2), 121–131.
36. Carpenter, A. C., Paulsen, I. T., & Williams, T. C., (2018). Blueprints for biosensors: Design, limitations, and applications. *Genes, 9*(8), 375.
37. Zhou, M., Shang, L., Li, B., Huang, L., & Dong, S., (2008). Highly ordered mesoporous carbons as electrode material for the construction of electrochemical dehydrogenase-and oxidase-based biosensors. *Biosensors and Bioelectronics, 24*(3), 442–447.
38. Syedmoradi, L., Ahmadi, A., Norton, M. L., & Omidfar, K., (2019). A review on nanomaterial-based field effect transistor technology for biomarker detection. *Microchimica Acta, 186*(11), 1–23.
39. Matsumoto, A., & Miyahara, Y., (2013). Current and emerging challenges of field effect transistor-based bio-sensing. *Nanoscale, 5*(22), 10702–10718.
40. Lee, C. S., Kim, S. K., & Kim, M., (2009). Ion-sensitive field-effect transistor for biological sensing. *Sensors, 9*(9), 7111–7131.
41. Rajan, N. K., Duan, X., & Reed, M. A., (2013). Performance limitations for nanowire/nanoribbon biosensors. Wiley interdisciplinary reviews: *Nanomedicine and Nanobiotechnology, 5*(6), 629–645.
42. Thanihaichelvan, M., Surendran, S. N., Kumanan, T., Sutharsini, U., Ravirajan, P., Valluvan, R., & Tharsika, T., (2021). Selective and electronic detection of COVID-19 (Coronavirus) using carbon nanotube field effect transistor-based biosensor: A proof-of-concept study. *Materials Today: Proceedings.*
43. Shao, W., Shurin, M. R., Wheeler, S. E., He, X., & Star, A., (2021). Rapid detection of SARS-CoV-2 antigens using high-purity semiconducting single-walled carbon nanotube-based field-effect transistors. *ACS Applied Materials & Interfaces, 13*(8), 10321–10327.
44. Yang, M., Sapsford, K. E., Sergeev, N., Sun, S., & Rasooly, A., (2009). Meeting current public health needs: Optical biosensors for pathogen detection and analysis. In: Frontiers in *Pathogen Detection: From Nanosensors to Systems* (Vol. 7167, p. 716702). International Society for Optics and Photonics.

45. Tîlmaciu, C. M., & Morris, M. C., (2015). Carbon nanotube biosensors. *Frontiers in Chemistry, 3,* 59.
46. Hamming, I., Timens, W., Bulthuis, M. L. C., Lely, A. T., Navis, G. V., & Van, G. H., (2004). Tissue distribution of ACE2 protein, the functional receptor for SARS coronavirus. A first step in understanding SARS pathogenesis. *The Journal of Pathology: A Journal of the Pathological Society of Great Britain and Ireland, 203*(2), 631–637.
47. Lopez, B. J., Andrews, N., Gower, C., Gallagher, E., Simmons, R., Thelwall, S., & Ramsay, M., (2021). Effectiveness of COVID-19 vaccines against the B. 1.617. 2 (delta) variants. *N. Engl. J. Med.*, 585–594.
48. Chan, J. F. W., Kok, K. H., Zhu, Z., Chu, H., To, K. K. W., Yuan, S., & Yuen, K. Y., (2020). Genomic characterization of the 2019 novel human-pathogenic coronavirus isolated from a patient with atypical pneumonia after visiting Wuhan. *Emerging Microbes & Infections, 9*(1), 221–236.
49. Novir, S. B., & Aram, M. R., (2020). Quantum mechanical simulation of chloroquine drug interaction with C60 fullerene for treatment of COVID-19. *Chemical Physics Letters, 757*, 137869.
50. Singh, P., (2017). Surface plasmon resonance: A boon for viral diagnostics. *Reference Module in Life Sciences.*
51. Boeckh, M., & Boivin, G., (1998). Quantitation of cytomegalovirus: Methodologic aspects and clinical applications. *Clinical Microbiology Reviews, 11*(3), 533–554.
52. Lim, W. Y., Lan, B. L., & Ramakrishnan, N., (2021). Emerging biosensors to detect severe acute respiratory syndrome coronavirus 2 (SARS-CoV-2): A review. *Biosensors, 11*(11), 434.
53. Azzi, L., Carcano, G., Gianfagna, F., Grossi, P., Dalla, G. D., Genoni, A., & Baj, A., (2020). Saliva is a reliable tool to detect SARS-CoV-2. *Journal of Infection, 81*(1), e45–e50.
54. Wan, Q., Xu, Y., Chen, X., & Xiao, H., (2018). Exhaled gas detection by a novel Rh-doped CNT biosensor for prediagnosis of lung cancer: A DFT study. *Molecular Physics, 116*(17), 2205–2212.
55. Mandal, D., Nunna, B. B., Zhuang, S., Rakshit, S., & Lee, E. S., (2018). Carbon nanotubes-based biosensor for detection of cancer antigens (CA-125) under shear flow condition. *Nanostructures & Nano-Objects, 15,* 180–185.
56. Thapa, A., Soares, A. C., Soares, J. C., Awan, I. T., Volpati, D., Melendez, M. E., & Oliveira, Jr. O. N., (2017). Carbon nanotube matrix for highly sensitive biosensors to detect pancreatic cancer biomarker CA19-9. *ACS Applied Materials & Interfaces, 9*(31), 25878–25886.

CHAPTER 10

Role of Carbon Nanotube in Biosensor Developments

KHEMCHAND SURANA,[1] EKNATH AHIRE,[2] PANKAJ AHER,[3] UMESH LADDHA,[2] SWATI TALELE,[4] SUNIL MAHAJAN,[5] SANJAY KSHIRSAGAR,[2] and SHILPA GAJBHIYE[2]

[1]Department of Pharmaceutical Chemistry, Shreeshakti Shaikshanik Sanstha, Divine College of Pharmacy, Satana, Nashik, Maharashtra, India

[2]Department of Pharmaceutics, MET's Institute of Pharmacy, Affiliated to Savitribai Phule Pune University, BKC, Adgaon, Nashik, Maharashtra, India

[3]Department of Pharmaceutical Chemistry, Loknete Dr. J. D. Pawar College of Pharmacy, Manur, Kalwan, India

[4]Department of Pharmaceutical Chemistry, Sandip Institute of Pharmacy, Nashik, Maharashtra, India

[5]Department of Pharmaceutical Chemistry, MGV's Pharmacy College, Panchavati, Nashik, Maharashtra, India

ABSTRACT

Nanomaterials own particular features which cause them to mainly appealing for biosensing applications. Carbon nanotube (CNTs) based completely biosensors are diagnosed to be a next generation constructing block for ultrasensitive and ultra-fast biosensing systems. Especially, carbon nanotubes (CNTs) can withstand characteristic scaffolds for immobilization of biomolecules at their surface. Moreover, it holds various excellent, chemical, optical characteristics, electrical, and also the physical properties which make them one of the most magnificent, relevant materials for the transduction of signs related with the recognition that of metabolites and more important is

Carbon Nanotubes for Biomedical Applications and Healthcare.
Chin Hua Chia, Swati Gokul Talele, Ann Rose Abraham, and A. K. Haghi, (Eds.)

disease biomarkers. Many evaluations pertaining to life threatening diseases are generally used for the detection of organic marketers usually in battles or some terrorist attacks. Now biosensors have become a captious of modern life. A new variety of branded biosensors are available with carbon nanotubes as a sensing element. As of now, many identical nanomaterial graphemes emerge as unrolled nanotube. With this, evidence we can foresee the enormous use of biosensors containing carbon nanomaterials. It is delightfully arranged to appraise by virtue of what trend is beneficially contributing to this new era and modern applications of biosensors.

10.1 INTRODUCTION

As the atomic number of a chemical element like carbon is 6, having 6 electrons that occupy $1s^2$, $2s^2$, and $2p^2$ atomic orbital rings. It follows hybridization sp, sp^2, or sp^3. With the discoveries of sp^2 carbon bonded substances that are very constant nanometer size along with many other sp^2 carbon bonds like graphene, carbon nanotubes, and fullerenes have validated making inquiries in this field. Graphene is generally used to estimate the physical properties of carbon nanotubes. Graphene contains carbon atom which are profoundly prepared in an ordinary sp^2-bonded atomic-scale. It appears as honeycomb namely hexagonal pattern, and this sample is a fundamental structure for different sp^2 carbon bonded substances (allotropes) along with fullerenes and carbon nanotubes. CNTs consist of theoretically well-defined cylinder which is fabricated of rolled up grapheme sheet. This graphene can be divided into single nicely or more than one well. Nanotubes with single nicely are defined as single-wall carbon nanotubes (SWCNTs) and had been first stated in 1993, even as those with multiple nicely are multiwall carbon nanotubes (MWCNTs) and had been first observed in 1991 by Iijima [1].

10.2 STRUCTURAL ASSEMBLY AND PROPERTIES OF CARBON NANOTUBES

Carbon can bond in distinctive approaches to assemble systems with absolutely distinct properties. The sp^2 hybridization of carbon construct a layer production with susceptible out-of-plane bonding of the van der Waals form and sturdy in plane bounds. Few little tens with concentric cylinders having regular periodic interlayer spacing were noticed for spherical regular applicable hole and made MWCNTs. The real space assessment of multiwall nanotube images has demonstrated numerous interlayers Spacing in a range of 0.34 to 0.39 nm. The internal diameter of MWCNTs primarily diverge from 0 that usually depends from forms of layers. Four nm up to three nanometers and outer diameter varies regularly from 2 nm up to a range of 20 nm to 30 nm. As both the tips of MWCNTs normally been closed and their ends are capped through dome fashioned having pentagonal defects, half-fullerene molecules. The axial duration differs from 1 µm up to 3 cm. The function of the pentagonal ring defect of half-fullerene molecule is to serve in the ultimate of the tube at the two ends. On different hand, SWCNT diameters ranges from 0.4 to between 2 and 3 nm and usually their length is in micrometer range. SWCNTs commonly can come collectively and shape bundles (ropes). In a package structure, SWCNTs are hexagonally prepared to shape a crystal-like production [2].

Depending on their wide variety of walls, CNTs are particularly single-walled (SWCNTs) or may be multi-walled (MWCNTs). SWNTs having diameter in nanometer or less can be easily grown up to 20 cm its length having a cylinder shape. Hexagonal lattice of carbon atoms are generally used to fabricate the side walls of these tubes. Alike to the grapheme atomic planes that are capped at every end with the beneficial resource that uses one half of the fullerene-like molecule. SWNTs morphology represents as a single rolled up graphene sheet. Depending upon the tube axis orientation to that of hexagonal lattice, the shape of a nanotube can be definitely defined through its chiral vector, as the useful resource of the utilization of the chiral indices (n, m). By using geometric arrangement of the carbon atoms SWCNTs are categorized on the bases of the seam of the cylinders. While maximum SWCNTs are chiral ($m = n$), a number of the SWCNTs are present in different configurations, i.e., armchair configuration which is $m = n$ and zigzag configuration that is $m = 0$ [3].

In the maximum popular case, a CNTs consists of a concentric arrangement of numerous cylinders. Such MWCNTs can attain diameters of as much as a 100 nm and the space among partitions may be very near the space among graphene layers in graphite (~3.5 Å). But in double-walled carbon nanotubes (DWNTs), a unique case of MWCNTs, composed of simply concentric cylinders. Properties of each form of CNTs can be cumulated by forming DWNTs bridge among distance between SWNTs and MWNTs. Altogether DWNTs resembles SWNTs that is associated to their small diameter, capacity as well as length to form bundles, however their mechanical stability is a good deal extra than that of the SWNTs, mainly while covalently functionalized. As that of MWNTs, the outer wall of DWMTs are functionalized that works without affecting the mechanical and electrochemical houses of the internal tube [4].

Besides, CNTs have a huge specific surface area (SSA), which permits immobilization of a huge wide variety of purposeful devices on the carbon nanotube surface, which have biosensing applications with help of receptor moieties. In reality the growth withinside the wide variety of walls, results in a decrease in CNTs SSA. In fact the insignificant properties of CNTs can also additionally fluctuate extensively among MWNTs and SWNTs. SWNTs are precise nanostructures with uncommon electronic properties, due to the quantum effect that is one-dimensional. CNTs can be both semi-carrying out and semi-metal, which depends on their diameter and chirality. For example, the armchair shape behaves as a metallic material, even as the zigzag shape has semi-conductor or quasi-metallic houses. In the last instance, as there is an increase of CNT diameter, it results in a decrease of the width of the band hole of the semi-conductor.

Two properties are liable for the excessive electric conductivity of metal CNTs: As they have few defects to scatter electrons and that they present an excellent stability at excessive temperatures that may be 300°C in air and 1,500°C in vacuum. Hence, an excellent ballistic conduction is likewise detected. In addition with excellent mechanical properties and combining immoderate energy with excessive stiffness. Though the SWNTs tensile strength of is ready 20 instances that of metal and the metal fibers are very tiny as compared to the Young's modulus of CNTs. CNTs can also present a excellent or bad magneto resistance, as a feature of the applied magnetic field as well as temperature. For example, in a prone magnetic field, nanotubes show off massive diamagnetic and paramagnetic responses, counting on the Fermi energy, size of the nanotubes, helicity, and sphere direction [5].

10.3 HISTORY BEHIND BIOSENSOR DEVELOPMENT

For detection of analytes, the first biosensors seemed with developed electrochemical devices withinside the 1950s. The first and maximum well-known of those is the electrochemical oxygen biosensor defined with the aid of using Leland Clark Jr. in 1956, together with a platinum cathode with respect to oxygen is decreased and having a silver/silver chloride reference electrode. Clark and Lyons later blended this electrode with glucose oxidase included in a dialysis membrane to that of degree the concentration of glucose in solution. For few years later stated by Updike and Hicks in 1967, the primary "enzyme electrode" changed into defined with the aid of using quantify glucose in a solution and also in tissues *in vitro*, that was engineered via immobilization of glucose oxidase with in a membrane of polymerized gelatin that covered a polarographic oxygen electrode, that will serve as enzyme transducer for catalyzing an electrochemical reaction upon reputation of glucose [6].

In 1969 the primary potentiometric enzyme electrode changed into evolved with the aid of using the urea sensor called Guilbault and Montalvo, primarily based totally urease that immobilizes onto electrode having ammonium-selective liquid membrane. Ever because of the reality that a large kind of biosensors have been used having advanced *in vitro* and *in vivo* applications, also used in study of polypeptide, enzymatic, nucleic acids based, nucleic acids based, antibody and also aptamers. Similarly the biosensors has evolved with mechanism of transduction in generation available and used from electrochemical and virtual biosensors to thermic biosensors.

The change in temperature is mainly associated with the amount of heat that is generated during enzyme-catalyzed reaction. Microbial biosensors having physical transducer integrate microorganisms, including an electrochemical device, to show specific analytes or biomarkers normally via modifications in respiratory pastime or manufacturing of electroactive metabolites; immunobiosensors primarily based totally on popularity of goal species via way of means of various techniques like antibody fragments, recombinant antibodies. Generally optical biosensors primarily based totally on variations in optical diffraction, modifications withinside the emission of mild indicators upon popularity in their goal; and greater these days nanobiosensors primarily based totally on nanomaterials which started to seem on the flip of the 20th century (Figure 10.1) [7].

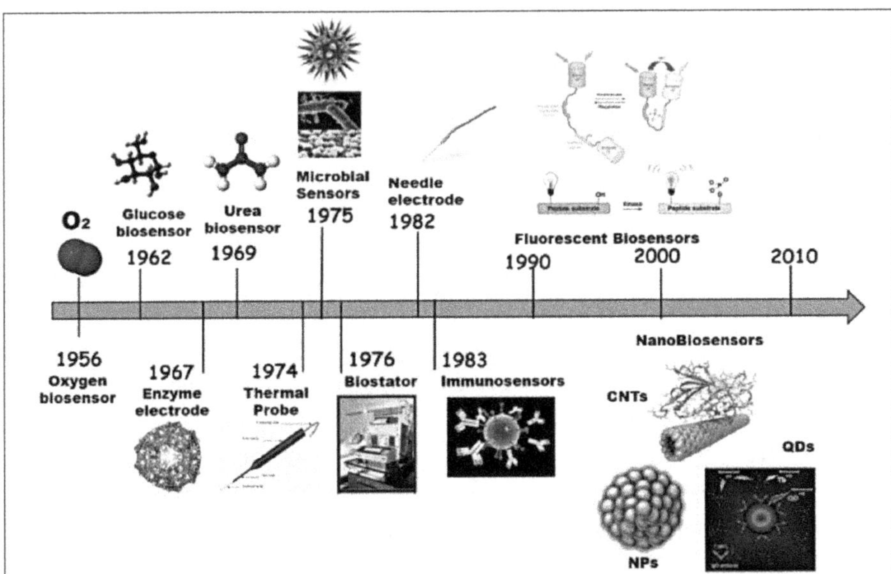

FIGURE 10.1 Timeline for biosensor development.

10.4 APPLICATIONS OF CARBON NANOTUBES FOR BIOSENSING

With the advancement in nanotechnologies and the emerging trends of nanomaterials with specific physicochemical properties, a brand new elegance of biosensors called nanobiosensors, which are developed using benefits of nanomaterials with incorporation of nanoparticles and nanotubes, appreciably their small size and big surface/volume ratio, with the capability of "macro"-biosensors. Nanomaterials provide appealing possibilities for biosensing applications, to boom sensitivity and decrease detection limits. This greater overall performance is related to the small length of nanomaterials, which endows them with a big surface/quantity ratio. This excessive precise region permits immobilization of bioreceptor units with extra concentrations relative to biosensor surface/quantity. Moreover, many biomaterials behave like transducers due to their inherent physicochemical [8].

CNTs provide numerous properties for detection purposes. With the help of distinctive feature in their unparalleled structural properties. Also the mechanical, electronic, and optical properties of CNTs provide numerous functions of interest to engineer new era probes. First, they represent scaffolds/structures which can be functionalized via conjugation of numerous entities, thereby probably improving reputation and signal transduction processes, instead of mono-conjugated biosensor species, however additionally imparting way to multifunctionalize and consequently to multiplex. Through their capacity to conduct electricity (about a 100 instances extra than copper wires), CNTs are properly suitable for transduction of electrical alerts generated upon reputation of a goal and their thermal properties are much better than diamond. Their power is about a 100 instances extra than steel. Last however now no longer least, the capacity of CNTs to move organic membranes simply makes them relevant *in vivo* with minimum invasiveness, and they'll in addition be hired for photoacoustic imaging [9].

An ever-developing variety of CNTs-conjugates were evolved for detection purpose used in various fields like cell-surface sugars, enzymes, DNA biomarkers as well as protein receptors. Depending on their mechanism of goal reputation and transduction, those biosensors are extensively categories depending upon their use some like electrochemical CNTs-biosensors, electronic transducers, immunosensors, and more important is optical CNTs-primarily based totally biosensors [10].

Different types of CNTs biosensors had been evolved to probe a huge type of cancers. Biomarkers can be processed by conjugation or complexation using DNA or aptamers, various antibodies and a number of peptides, different types of proteins, or enzymes. Thus advancement in the incorporation of CNTs into biosensing devices has enabled the improvement of rather touchy electrochemical biosensors for early-level detection of biomarkers with various sicknesses, including most of the cancers.

CNTs-primarily based totally immunosensors are nonetheless withinside the nascent level, and there are numerous demanding situations to triumph over for the successful commercialization of the concepts. Latest trends have caused utility of CNTs biosensors as imaging probes, mainly for photo acoustic imaging [11–15].

10.5 ELECTROCHEMICAL AND ELECTRONIC CNT BIOSENSORS

The huge part of biosensors advanced to this point is electrochemical. They are famous due to their low-cost, easy to use and handle due to small size and as a substitute rapid reaction times. The enzymatic catalysis of a reaction that produces electro-active species mostly depends upon enzyme-coupled electrochemical biosensors where they generate a measurable electric powered signal.

The biosensor typically consists of a working electrode, reference electrode and a counter electrode. Using enzymes immobilized on the working electrode, useful resources are used to recognize the purpose analyte. Catalytic interest of which also can moreover purpose each electron transfer, thereby producing a modern or contributing to deliver a voltage (Figure 10.2(A)). Enzymes are best bio-recognition molecules, because of the fact they provide first-rate Precise for their substrate targets and function immoderate catalytic interest [16].

CNTs were diagnosed very promising substances for reinforcing electron switch, way to their electric and electrochemical properties, which lead them to appropriate for integration into electrochemical biosensors. Their small size, big floor area, excessive conductivity, excessive chemical balance and sensitivity, excessive electro-catalytic effect, and rapid electron-switch charge lead them to extraordinarily properly ideal for that generate electro-active species and biosensing programs that's count on the enzymatic reactions. A considerable kind of electrochemical CNT biosensors become advanced to come across ions, metabolites, and protein biomarkers. For instance, several CNT-glucose biosensors are engineered based totally on the conjugation of glucose oxidase. Patolsky et al. noted glucose oxidase (GOx) having structural alignment on electrodes using SWNTs as electric powered connectors a few of the enzyme redox facilities and the electrode (Figure 10.2(B)). By using the SWNTs they proved that the surface-assembled GOx turned into electrically connected electrode, the enzyme redox-active site was electrically cord to the transducer floor by this electrically connected electrode, which acts as conductive nanoneedles. Cholesterol biosensors which include a changed display screen reveal electrodes with cholesterol esterase, oxidase, MWNTs yield and also peroxidase exceedingly touchy way of quantifying general cholesterol in blood. Electrochemical biosensors are used for detection of nitric oxide that is mostly based on functionalized CNTs – epinephrine sensing, and dopamine tracking in rat striatum. Detection of disease-related to glycoproteins in the blood is done by RNA aptasensor, changed into developed through manner of coating SWNTs grafted with protein-precise RNA aptamers present on an alumina electrode. Zhang et al. noted the selective detection of mobileular nitric oxide (NO) through the way of unmarried-stranded d(AT)15 DNA oligonucleotide which is adsorbed and wrapped round SWNTs (near-infrared fluorescent unmarried-walled carbon nanotubes. Jin et al. evolved SWNT-primarily based totally completely sincerely biosensors of H_2O_2 which have been performed to unmarried molecule imaging mostly in human epidermal cell carcinoma. Electronic tracking of electrochemical biosensors may be brilliant with the aid of using the mechanism of Potentiometric biosensors. The oxido-reduction capacity is measured by Potentiometric biosensors and used in transduction as voltametric, potentiometric, amperometric, conductometric or even or piezoelectric systems. An electrochemical reaction, and are primarily based on biological reactions that produce or take in hydrogen ions, inflicting a internet alternate in pH, which is measured as an electrical signal, capacity, on the floor of a pH-meter probe. Potentiometric biosensors employ ion-selective electrodes with a view to transduce the electric signal in organic reaction. Amperometric biosensors experience a modern-day produced whilst a capacity is implemented among electrodes and might consequently discover electro-active species found in biological samples, which can be most customarily produced way to enzymes. Piezo-electric powered biosensors are primarily based totally on piezo-electric powered crystals (inclusive of quartz) that vibrate beneath the effect with an electric powered field. This resonance frequency is proportional to the mass of adsorbed material and therefore it may changes as molecules adsorb or desorb material from the crystal surface. In present day years, a huge type of amperometric biosensors based mostly on CNT-modified electrodes has been engineered. Fei and co-people finished detection of cysteine on Pt/CNT electrodes with the useful resource of the usage of cyclic voltammetry. Antiochia et al. stated an amperometric CNT-biosensor developed with the useful resource like di-hydroxy benzaldehyde coating. Moreover, CNT-arrayed electrodes coated with antiPSA antibodies located internal a chamber were used to experience PSA toward a Pt twine counter electrode (Figure 10.2(C)). Biosensors based in combination with pneumatic micropumps on CNTs arrayed chip are engineered. The simultaneous detection of several biomarkers in combination with pneumatic micropumps (PSA-mAb and human chorionic gonadotropin hCG antibodies) [17].

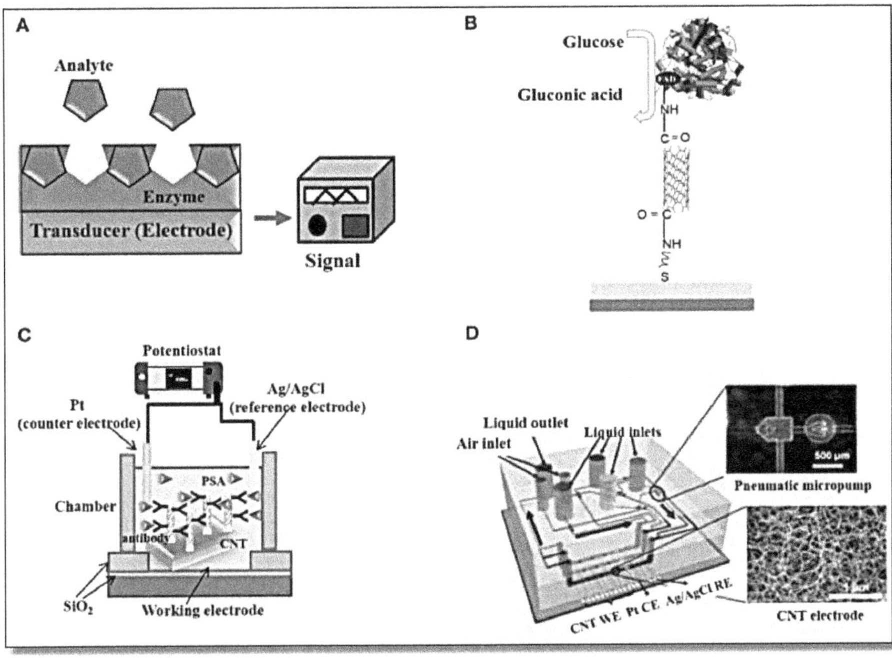

FIGURE 10.2 Electronic and electrochemical CNT biosensors.

Source: Carmen-Mihaela and Morris (2015) https://creativecommons.org/licenses/by/4.0/ [31]

Note: (A) An enzyme-based electrochemical biosensor with typical layout; (B) SWNT electrode with electrically-contacted glucose oxidase; (C) Simplified example amperometric biosensor that is of a label-free for PSA detection; and (D) simplified example of a microfluidic chip usually based on the CNT biosensor electrodes [12].

10.6 ELECTROCHEMICAL AND ELECTRONIC CNT BIOSENSORS FOR CANCER DETECTION

Feng et al. suggested a disposable paper-primarily based totally absolutely bipolar electrode (BPE) for the touchy electro chemiluminescent detection of prostate particular antigen (PSA) and confirmed that its response changed into notably superior after amendment of the BPE cathode with MWNTs.

Other than electro-deposition of CNTs. Their next functionalization with the right enzymes is used to make sure by sensitivity and specificity in electrochemical biosensing. Thus, MWNTs were used to make bigger biosensors based specifically on microsomal cytochrome P450 enzyme to electrochemically find tablets used withinside the treatment of breast cancer. The restriction of drug detection within healthy the healing variety even found in human serum thus it depends upon the deposition of the CNT-enzyme nanostructures onto the electrodes decreased the restriction of drug detection to healthy the healing variety even in human serum cells. Additionally, the identical group synthesized a multi-array sensor platform with the aid of using electrodeposition of chitosan/MWNTs to locate numerous various endogenous metabolites like glucose and lactate. Also drugs such as etoposide, mitoxantrone, and etodolac. Simultaneously, biosensing calibration are done while additionally tracking pH and temperature [18].

A screen-published carbon electrode used because the signal transducer of a dsDNA-primarily based totally biosensor turned into changed with the aid of using MWNTs and as that of colloidal gold nanoparticles (GNPs) for checking out berberine, as well as iso-quinoline plant alkaloid with considerable antimicrobial and anticancer activity. Detection of risky natural compounds (VOCs) in human breathing system to diagnose lung cancers is turning into an essential technique for sizable screening, because of its facility and coffee price advantages. Thus, tricosane ($C_{23}H_{48}$)-functionalized SWNTs biosensor confirmed stated sensitivity towards polar VOC molecules and that could donate electrons to the nanotubes after being completely absorbed. D-(+)-galactose conjugated SWNTs have been synthesized the usage of molybdenum electrodes for software as biosensors to come across most cancers marker galactin-3. Later, Zheng, and collaborators advanced folic acid functionalized polydopamine-covered carbon nanotubes for the electrochemical detection of HeLa and HL60 maximum cancers cells over-expressing the folate receptor (Figure 10.3(A)). Fayazfar et al. noted on a modern platform based mostly on aligned MWNTs for sensitive label-loose DNA detection based on the TP53 gene mutation (Figure 10.3(B)) generally depends on the growth of gold nanoparticles. The electrode with modified vertically aligned MWNTs and gold nanoparticles having superior density of the DNA probe further to the sensor sensitivity, They displayed reproducibility and also stability for two weeks, and can be regenerated through de-hybridization in heat water. Alternatively, the Au-Ag alloy-coated MWNTs were used as the sensing interface for the ultrasensitive detection of risky biomarkers of MGC-803 gastric maximum cancers cells detection [18].

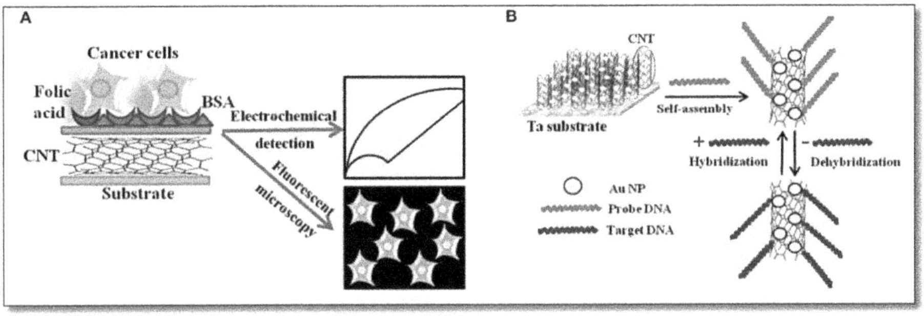

FIGURE 10.3 Electronic and electrochemical CNT biosensors used for detection of cancer.

Source: Carmen-Mihaela and Morris (2015) https://creativecommons.org/licenses/by/4.0/

Note: (A) Schematic example of the folic acid-targeted cytosensing approach for a more suitable electrochemical detection of most cancers cells the usage of polydopamine-coated carbon nanotubes; and (B) schematic illustration of a cancer detection based electrochemical DNA biosensor based on gold nanoparticles or aligned CNTs [13].

Recently, Shobba et al. evaluated and investigated the varied properties of every SWNTs and MWNTs for early-level detection of prostate cancers, by functionalization with DNA strands that come upon PSA discovered in blood samples. CNTs have moreover emerged as promising sensing systems for the detection of amphoteric and also quantification of the clinically relevant metabolites which incorporates substrate such as glucose, lactate, glutamate, and cholesterol. Incorporation of alpha-fetoprotein for detection of maximum cancers biomarkers are used. CEA, PSA, DNA, or micro-RNA biomarkers.

During the last couple of years, several, impedimetric, amperometric, and field-effect transistors (FET) CNT-biosensors are used that are advanced for detection of maximum cancers cells biomarkers. Thus a FET-CNT immunosensor become more superior for the detection of osteopontin (OPN). A biomarker of prostate maximum cancers with the useful resource of the use of attaching a genetically-engineered that is a single chain variable contains fragment protein having moderate binding affinity for OPN, This biomarkers are employed in a background of centered bovine serum albumin. A vertically aligned carbon nanotube-primarily based totally impedimetric biosensor turned into fabricated via a photolithography manner on Ni/SiO_2/Si the layers for the detection of SW48 cells, mainly remoted from grade IV human colon cancer cells.

Bareket et al. organized a rapid, touchy, selective, and cheaper CNT-changed screen-published electrode to reveal the amperometric reaction to formaldehyde launched from U251 human glioblastoma cells in reaction to remedy with formaldehyde-liberating anticancer prodrugs. More recently, a nanobiosensor turned into engineered technique for the detection of liver cancers cells (HepG2) with the aid of using the usage of actual time electric impedance sensing, due to meeting of CNT multilayers as well as antibodies to epithelial cell. It causes adhesion of molecules on an indium tin oxide electrode surface. Detection of tumor cell antibodies triggered growth of the electron-switch resistance and the electrochemical impedance improved in a linear style with the logarithm of most cancers cells concentration [19].

10.7 CNT IMMUNOSENSORS

Immunosensors rely upon recognition of antigens with the useful resource of the use of recombinant antibodies or antibody fragments. They constitute the receptor moiety of the biosensor that immobilized onto substrates. In 1983, Liedberg et al. developed and investigated the number one immunosensor through immobilization of antibodies onto a Chip, thus a precursor is designed that have been substantially used BIAcore system, which helps to transduces immuno-recognition of analytes with the useful resource of the use of floor plasmon resonance. Ever since, for selective reputation of biomarkers and goal analytes, a widespread kind of affinity reagents have become available, beginning from recombinant antibodies and antibody fragments (scFvs and Fabs). It can be determined on from phage display libraries. To date, a large amount of immunosensors they need to be engineered to probe HIV, hepatitis, and also the exclusive viral diseases, to test for tablets, and to display the presence of undesired or toxic effects of the compounds withinside the environment. Although, the larger amount of these is electrochemical, every piezoelectric immunosensors based mostly on antibody-ground through conjugation of antibodies to conductive nanomaterials coated quartz crystals are developed that have FET immunosensors. With the new generations of nano-immunosensors, with the useful resource of the also the use of immobilizing recombinant antibodies are developed or antibody fragments onto CNTs, a nanowires, as well as nanoparticles, and the quantum dots, therefore enhancing binding ability and sensitivity thresholds in evaluation to more traditional biosensors. Electrochemical immunosensors combine a sensing interface for intention detection with a sandwich-kind electrochemical immunoassay for amplification of the signal (Figure 10.4(A)). Electrochemical immunosensors have moreover been developed for cytosensing thru functionalization of SWNTs with RGDS peptides that understand mobileular ground integrin receptors (Figure 10.4(B)) [20].

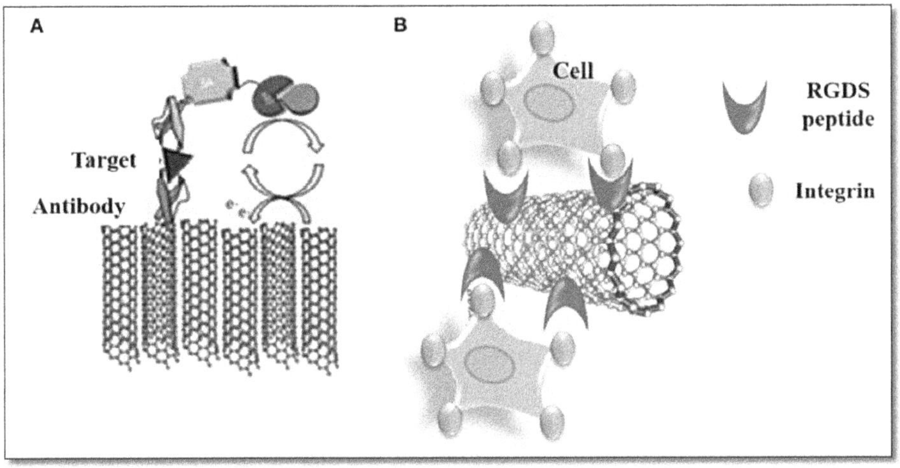

FIGURE 10.4 Immuno-CNT biosensors.

Note: (A) Schematic illustration of an electrochemical CNT-immunosensor that mixes a sensing interface for goal detection for amplification of the signal by using sandwich-type electrochemical immunoassay; and (B) based on functionalization of SWNTs and RGDS peptides, cytosensing immunosensor understand cell surface integrin receptors [14].

10.8 CNT IMMUNOSENSORS FOR CANCER DETECTION

A sizable shape of carbon-nanotube-based totally absolutely immunosensors have been developed to probe maximum cancers biomarkers. For instance, Rusling and coworkers developed an electrochemical immunosensor based totally mostly On SWNT forests for the affection of the enzymes or antibodies via way of manner of amidation. Squamous cell carcinomas of the top and neck have been detected a way to an ultrasensitive electrochemical immunosensor primarily based totally absolutely totally on SWNT forests incorporating antibodies to Interleukin-6 (Il-6) and horseradish peroxidase permitting detection of very low and accelerated degrees of Il-6. A multiplexing electrochemical immunosensor based totally mostly on screen-found out carbon electrodes modified into developed for synchronized recognition of PSA and Interleukin-8 (Il-8). A moment ago, an impedimetric immunosensor of human epidermal growth detail receptor 2 (HER2) modified into developed through manner of way of alternate of a gold nanoparticle-adorned MWNT-ionic liquid electrode. Gold nanoparticles were used to decorate the quantity of immobilization and to keep the immune activity of the HER2 antibody Herceptin at the electrode. This biosensor facilitates the uncovering of low concentrations of HER2 in serum samples of breast most cancers patients and display a linear boom in charge switch resistance with the awareness of HER2 [21].

10.9 OPTICAL CNT BIOSENSORS

As per the definition, optical biosensors account on finding of target biomolecules or analytes thru changes withinside the emission of light (UV, infrared, and visible) (Figure 10.5(A)). Following the quantity one fiber optic biosensor or "optode" explained thru manner of manner of Lubbers and Oppitz to degree carbon dioxide, alcohol, and oxygen, respectively, a vast character of optical biosensors have been made to check and report on dynamic biomolecular approaches *in vitro*, *in vivo* and in living cells [22].

Optical biosensors can be outstanding regular with the approach used to readout aim detection (floor Plasmon resonance, phosphorescence, absorbance, fluorescence, reflectance, wavelength depth, luminescence, anisotropy, lifetime, fluorescence strength transfer and quenching) or via their mechanism of acknowledgment (inquiring biosensors and reacting biosensors). Probing biosensors supervise versions withinside the interaction/affinity amongst analyte and recognition location of the sensor which bring about adjustments in optical response. Reacting biosensors exhibit awesome optical responses related to chemical tactics (chemisorption, catalytic reaction, formation of latest chemical bonds, etc.). Larger than the last decade, a amount of optical biosensors support mostly on floor plasmon resonance, waveguides, and resonant mirrors were developed to show label loose dreams *in vitro*. Colorimetric biosensors diploma adjustments in slight absorption as reactants are transformed to goods. Photometric slight depth biosensors stumble upon adjustments in fluorescent or bioluminescent techniques associated with adjustments withinside the spectral residences of probes involved right away or indirectly in aim detection. Fluorescence gives in particular appealing blessings for biosensing applications, along with its excessive inherent sensitivity and the possibility to photograph dynamic strategies in residing cells through fluorescence microscopy in a non-invasive style with excessive spatial and temporal resolution [23]. Target recognition is transduced via emission of a fluorescent sign which fluctuate from that of the biosensor in its liberated state. Fluorescent biosensors had been designed to apprehend and record at the presence, interest or conformation of a given goal in a selected and quantitative style, thereby offering approach to probe its dynamic molecular conduct via touchy modifications in fluorescence.

The first fluorescent biosensors had been advanced withinside the 1990s. Although they had been to start with primarily based totally on incorporation of synthetic probes which might be touchy to modifications of their surroundings into biosensor receptor moieties, the invention of the Green Fluorescent Protein (GFP) and its engineering into genetically-encoded journalists paved the manner for improvement of genetically-encoded fluorescent biosensors. This elegance of biosensors is predicated on ectopic expression of genetically-encoded auto fluorescent protein (AFP) fusions with receptor domain names that apprehend the goal of hobby in residing cells. For the bigger element those are single-chain biosensors which reply to enzymatic sports via fluorescence resonance electricity switch (FRET). For example genetically-encoded FRET biosensors of protein kinases, additionally called KARs (kinase interest newshounds) include a couple of genetically-encoded AFPs collectively with an enzyme-particular substrate collection and a phosphoaminoacid binding area (PAABD). When the substrate collection is phosphorylated through the kinase of hobby, it preferentially interacts with the PAABD, thereby inducing an intramolecular extrade which brings the AFPs nearer and promotes fluorescence electricity switch among the donor and the acceptor (Figure 10.5(A)) [24].

More latest efforts made via way of means of chemists have capitulate a palette of environmentally-sensitive synthetic fluorophores that reply to adjustments withinside the polarity in their environment, turning into greater fluorescent in non-polar solvents or upon interplay with a hydrophobic goal protein with superior spectral properties for *in vivo* imaging which may be conjugated to peptide/protein scaffolds, yielding appealing options to their genetically encoded counterparts. These structures are greater effortlessly relevant *in vitro* and might similarly be microinjected or added into dwelling cells via facilitated delivery. They have tested touchy and specifically properly ideal to screen protein kinase sports (Figure 10.5(B)). Fluorescent biosensors were broadly utilized by cell biologists to observe the spatio-temporal dynamics and behavior of enzymes in residing cells and in real-time in physiological and pathological framework, presenting records that couldn't be acquired via conventional biochemical approaches. But those gear have additionally been in large part carried out to biomedical applications, to focus on changes in pathological diseases, and in drug invention programs to display for, validate and signify the efficacy of newly recognized candidate drugs. Likewise, CNTs represent appealing biosensing gadgets for biomarker recognition and imaging. SWNTs are certainly characterized via way of means of inherent photoluminescence among 650 and 1,400 nm, which lets in for deep dissemination and imaging in organic tissues and organs with near and infrared light. Nonactivated SWNTs acquire low fluorescence constancy, concentration, and biocompatibility. In dissimilarity, surface functionalization, environmental adjustments, or interactions with goal biomolecules have an effect on SWNT fluorescence emission alerts significantly (wavelength and intensity), thereby making them properly ideal for fluorescence-primarily based totally sensing applications. Moreover, even though SWNTs reply to adjustments in neighborhood dielectric function, they continue to be solid to photo bleaching, consequently providing appealing possibilities for biomedical imaging applications [25].

For instance, SWNTs were coupled to beta-D-glucose. SWNT/luciferase conjugates were carried out for NIR detection of ATP in residing cells. A chaperone sensor for nitrosoaromatics became engineered way to peptides immobilized at the CNT surface and similarly carried out to picture adjustments in peptide conformation related to popularity of the molecular goal via NIR photoluminesence (Figure 10.5(C)). Stabilization of SWNTs with hereditarily make-up M13 phage has been applied for *in vivo* fluorescence imaging in lower tissues followed by IV injection. As well, non-covalent congregation of SWNTs with dye-applied oligonucleotide obtained an optical biosensor of single-stranded DNA (Single Stranded DNA), fluorescence of that is extinguish till the Single Stranded DNA goal binds and releases the categorized oligonucleotide from the SWNTs (Figure 10.5(D)). Heteropolymers of SWNTs lined with a corona phase designed to understand unique metabolites (riboflavin, L-thyroxine, and estradiol) had been used for NIR imaging of those compounds in area and in time in murine macrophages [26, 27].

More recently, a label-loose sensor of the troponin T became fabricated via way of means of immobilizing onto chitosan wrapped nanotubes and used to come across this cardiac biomarker of AMI via way of means of NIR fluorescence [28].

10.10 OPTICAL CNT BIOSENSORS FOR CANCER RECOGNITION

SWNTs-Indocyanine Green (ICG) combined with cyclic ArgGly-Asp (RGD) peptides to aim alpha (v) beta (3) integrins have been proven to function responsive photoacoustic distinction molecules subsequent IV administration in to tumor-bearing mice, accomplishing subnanomolar sensitivity and 300 instances better photoacoustic comparison in residing tissues than formerly mentioned SWNTs [29].

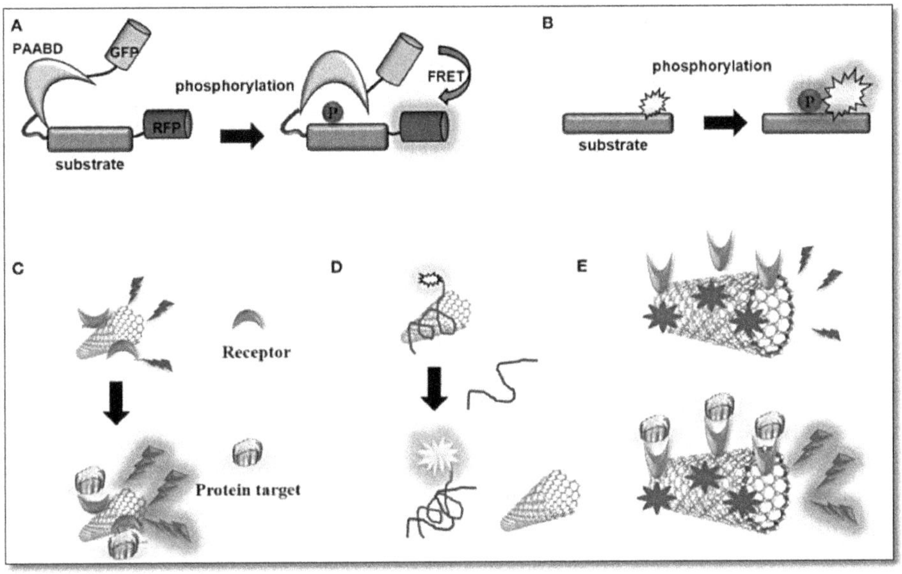

FIGURE 10.5 Optical CNT biosensors.

Note: (A) Schematic illustration of a FRET kinase biosensor that is genetically-encoded: acceptor (RFP) proteins and as well as to: the donor (GFP) proteins that are introduced in near proximity which allows phosphorylation-mediated intramolecular conformational change followed by FRET; (B) the schematic illustration of non-genetic, environmentally-touchy peptide-based biosensor: the phosphorylation of the substrate alters probe surroundings; (C) due to goal binding on a receptor that is conjugated into the SWNT, CNT-biosensors are used depending on wavelength shift of fluorescence; (D) optical biosensor used in single stranded DNA: fluorescence of a dye-categorize non-covalent assembly with SWNT that is quenched by oligonucleotide till the single Stranded DNA goal binds and the categorized oligonucleotide from the SWNT are released; and (E) photoacoustic detection pertaining integrins through indocyanine-categorized SWNT-biosensor conjugated with RGD peptides [15].

SWNTs were used to include a fluorescent cyclin a requisite motif resulting from p21WAF1. A easy, discriminating, and highly sensitive fluorescence assay turned into advanced for detection of cyclin A, a cell cycle regulator that is over expressed in certain human cancers. The fluorescence of cyclin A binding peptide turned into quenched through power switch and electron transfer strategies however displayed fluorescence enhancement upon popularity and attachment of cyclin A. Present method tested a nano-molar restrict of detection of cyclin A and turned into for that reason projected as a predictive indicator of early level cancer [30].

10.11 CONCLUSION

CNTs include flexible functions that integrate the capacity to supply for investigative and beneficial applications. While they will function as biosensors of most cancers biomarkers, they may be laden with anti-cancer API and applied as therapeutic systems in oncology. Although, CNTs-primarily based totally biosensors are promising it nonetheless has many practical issues in applications. For example, for the fabrication of biosensors generally wishes particular length and helicity, however it's far very tough to govern the length of CNTs whilst manufacturing. It is likewise very tough to make cost-powerful and excessive purity in mass manufacturing of CNTs this is the cause why the cutting-edge marketplace charges of CNTs is just too excessive for any sensible industrial applications. In CNT-primarily based totally biosensors, enzyme usually wishes to immobilize onto floor of CNTs. However, immobilization may also harm their bio-logical activity, biocompatibility, and structure stability and want to carry out their cytotoxicity. As it stated that, the structural stabilization and floor traits of CNTs are want to be standardized for the cytotoxicity determination. The continuous CNT fibers keep away from the leaching of CNT, implantable electrodes for *in-vivo* analysis. All the above-referred to problems need to be evaluated with the aid of using medical and systematic methods. It is obvious that a lot similarly development had to be addressed earlier than CNTs era may be carried out in carcinogenic treatments. The improvement of CNT-primarily based totally biosensors has many exclusive factors which want the cooperation among substances scientists, and engineers, who fabricates the brand new devices along with biosensors.

ACKNOWLEDGMENT

We thank MET's, Institute of Pharmacy, BKC, affiliated under Savitribai Phule Pune University, Nashik, Sandip Institute of Pharmaceutical Science and Divine College of Pharmacy Satana, for their constant support and providing all facilities to complete this work. We are also thankful to the Ministry of Tribal Affairs Government of India for providing financial assistance in the form of fellowship (Award No.: 202021-NFST-MAH-01235).

KEYWORD

- **applications of carbon nanotube**
- **biosensor**
- **carbon nanotube**
- **CNTs**

REFERENCES

1. Tîlmaciu, C. M., & Morris, M. C., (2015). Carbon nanotube biosensors. *Frontiers in Chemistry, 3*, 59.
2. Sireesha, M., Jagadeesh, B. V., Kranthi, K. A. S., & Ramakrishna, S., (2018). A review on carbon nanotubes in biosensor devices and their applications in medicine. *Nanocomposites, 4*(2), 36–57.
3. Feng, J., Chen, C., Sun, X., & Peng, H., (2021). Implantable fiber biosensors based on carbon nanotubes. *Accounts of Materials Research, 2*(3), 138–146.
4. Gergeroglu, H., Yildirim, S., & Ebeoglugil, M. F., (2020). Nano-carbons in biosensor applications: An overview of carbon nanotubes (CNTs) and fullerenes (C 60). *SN Applied Sciences, 2*(4), 1–22.
5. Yang, N., Chen, X., Ren, T., Zhang, P., & Yang, D., (2015). Carbon nanotube-based biosensors. *Sensors and Actuators B: Chemical, 207*, 690–715.
6. Zhu, Z., (2017). An overview of carbon nanotubes and graphene for biosensing applications. *Nano-Micro Letters, 9*(3), 1–24.
7. Huang, T. S., Tzeng, Y., Liu, Y. K., Chen, Y. C., Walker, K. R., Guntupalli, R., & Liu, C., (2004). Immobilization of antibodies and bacterial binding on nanodiamond and carbon nanotubes for biosensor applications. *Diamond and Related Materials, 13*(4–8), 1098–1102.
8. Laschi, S., Bulukin, E., Palchetti, I., Cristea, C., & Mascini, M., (2008). Disposable electrodes modified with multi-wall carbon nanotubes for biosensor applications. *IRBM, 29*(2, 3), 202–207.
9. Senthil Kumar, A., Gayathri, P., Barathi, P., & Vijayaraghavan, R. (2012). Improved electric wiring of hemoglobin with impure-multiwalled carbon nanotube/nafion modified glassy carbon electrode and its highly selective hydrogen peroxide biosensing. *J. Phys. Chem. C, 116*, 23692–23703.
10. Luo, X. L., Xu, J. J., Wang, J. L., & Chen, H. Y., (2005). Electrochemically deposited nanocomposite of chitosan and carbon nanotubes for biosensor application. *Chemical Communications, 16*, 2169–2171.
11. Heng, L. Y., Chou, A., Yu, J., Chen, Y., & Gooding, J. J., (2005). Demonstration of the advantages of using bamboo-like nanotubes for electrochemical biosensor applications compared with single walled carbon nanotubes. *Electrochemistry Communications, 7*(12), 1457–1462.
12. Tzeng, Y. H., Huang, T. S., Chen, Y. C., Liu, C., & Liu, Y. K., (2004). Hydration properties of carbon nanotubes and their effects on electrical and biosensor applications. *New Diamond and Frontier Carbon Technology, 14*(3), 193–201.

13. Poghossian, A., Schultze, J., & Schöning, M. J. (2003). Application of a (bio-) chemical sensor (ISFET) for the detection of physical parameters in liquids. *Electrochim. Acta, 48*, 3289–3297.
14. Trojanowicz, M., (2006). Analytical applications of carbon nanotubes: A review. *TrAC Trends in Analytical Chemistry, 25*(5), 480–489.
15. Patolsky, F., Timko, B. P., Yu, G., Fang, Y., Greytak, A. B., Zheng, G., & Lieber, C. M. (2006). Detection, stimulation, and inhibition of neuronal signals with high-density nanowire transistor arrays. *Science, 313*, 1100–1104.
16. Singh, C., Srivastava, S., Ali, M. A., Gupta, T. K., Sumana, G., Srivastava, A., Mathur, R. B., & Malhotra, B. D., (2013). Carboxylated multiwalled carbon nanotubes-based biosensor for aflatoxin detection. *Sensors and Actuators B: Chemical, 185*, 258–264.
17. Harper, A., & Anderson, M. R., (2010). Electrochemical glucose sensors—Developments using electrostatic assembly and carbon nanotubes for biosensor construction. *Sensors, 10*(9), 8248–8274.
18. Roy, S., & Gao, Z. (2009). Nanostructure-based electrical biosensors. *Nano Today, 4*, 318–334.
19. Pakchin, P. S., et al., (2018). Electrochemical immunosensor based on chitosan-gold nanoparticle/carbon nanotube as a platform and lactate oxidase as a label for detection of CA125 oncomarker. *Biosensors and Bioelectronics, 122*, 68–74.
20. Song, C. K., et al., (2018). Fluorescence-based immunosensor using three-dimensional CNT network structure for sensitive and reproducible detection of oral squamous cell carcinoma biomarker. *Analytica Chimica Acta, 1027*, 101–108.
21. Malhotra, R., et al., (2010). Ultrasensitive electrochemical immunosensor for oral cancer biomarker IL-6 using carbon nanotube forest electrodes and multilabel amplification. *Analytical Chemistry, 82*(8), 3118–3123.
22. Ferrier, D. C., & Kevin, C. H., (2021). Carbon nanotube (CNT)-based biosensors. *Biosensors, 11*(12), 486.
23. Hwang, H. S., et al., (2020). Carbon nanomaterials as versatile platforms for biosensing applications. *Micromachines, 11*(9), 814.
24. Majdinasab, M., Kohji, M., & Jean, L. M., (2019). Optical and electrochemical sensors and biosensors for the detection of quinolones. *Trends in Biotechnology, 37*(8), 898–915.
25. Balasubramanian, K. (2010). Challenges in the use of 1D nanostructures for on-chip biosensing and diagnostics: A review. *Biosens. Bioelectron., 26*, 1195–1204.
26. Divya, V., et al., (2021). Applications of carbon-based nanomaterials in health and environment: Biosensors, medicine and water treatment. *Carbon Nanomaterial Electronics: Devices and Applications* (pp. 261–284). Springer, Singapore.
27. Pindoo, I. A., & Sanjeet, K. S., (2020). Increased sensitivity of biosensors using evolutionary algorithm for bio-medical applications. *Radioelectronics and Communications Systems, 63*(6), 308–318.
28. Same, S., & Golshan, S., (2018). Carbon nanotube biosensor for diabetes disease. *Crescent J. Med. Biol. Sci., 5*, 1–6.
29. Hwang, J., Kim, H., Son, M., Oh, J., Hwang, S., & Ahn, D. (2008). Electronic transport properties of a single-wall carbon nanotube field effect transistor with deoxyribonucleic acid conjugation. *Phys. E Low-Dimens. Syst. Nanostructures, 40*, 1115–1117.
30. Antman-Passig, M., Tetyana, I., & Daniel, A. H., (2019). Carbon nanotube optical probes and sensors. *The Electrochemical Society Interface, 28*(4), 61.

CHAPTER 11

Carbon Nanotube: A Promising Role in Biomedical Imaging

PANKAJ AHER,[1] KHEMCHAND SURANA,[2] EKNATH AHIRE,[3] SWATI TALELE,[4] GOKUL TALELE,[5] SUNIL MAHAJAN,[6] and SANJAY KSHIRSAGAR[3]

[1]*Department of Pharmaceutical Chemistry, Loknete Dr. J. D. Pawar College of Pharmacy, Manur, Kalwan, India*

[2]*Department of Pharmaceutical Chemistry, Shreeshakti Shaikshanik Sanstha, Divine College of Pharmacy, Satana, Nashik, Maharashtra, India*

[3]*Department of Pharmaceutics, MET's Institute of Pharmacy, Affiliated to Savitribai Phule Pune University, BKC, Adgaon, Nashik, Maharashtra, India*

[4]*Department of Pharmaceutical Chemistry, Sandip Institute of Pharmacy, Nashik, Maharashtra, India*

[5]*Department of Pharmaceutical Chemistry, MGV's, Pharmacy College, Panchavati, Nashik, Maharashtra, India*

[6]*Department of Pharmaceutical Chemistry, Matoshri College of Pharmacy, Eklahare, Nashik, Maharashtra, India*

ABSTRACT

The most present generally molecular imaging embody molecular magnetic resonance imaging (MRI), optical bioluminescence/fluorescence, focused ultrasound, single photon emission computed tomography technique (SPECT), positron emission tomography technique (PET), and moreover single walled carbon nanotubes (SWCNTs) personal strong resonance Raman Scattering with especially extent scattering cross-section, and are

Carbon Nanotubes for Biomedical Applications and Healthcare.
Chin Hua Chia, Swati Gokul Talele, Ann Rose Abraham, and A. K. Haghi, (Eds.)

consequently excellent Raman probes useful in biological sensing and imaging. (CNTs) may be derivatized via way of means of both chemical reactions comprising covalent bonds at the ends and edges of nanotubes, or noncovalently with the assist of amphiphilic molecules through hydrophobic or different bodily interactions inclusive of π-π Stacking. Carbon nanotubes CNTs are promising nanomaterials with excessive capability withinside the biomedical sector. This consists of using CNTs now no longer handiest for diagnostic and therapeutic applications however additionally as substrates for cellular growth and tissue scaffolds, neural interfaces, stem cell differentiation and bone prosthetics. In the sector of biomedical imaging and drug delivery system, their needlelike form confers them advanced flow dynamics and an will increase ability to penetrate cellular membranes as compared to round nanoparticles. Among those modalities, fluorescence imaging withinside the first near-infrared region (NIR-I; 700–900 nm) has collect considerable interest in biomedical studies due to its excessive sensitivity, short feedback, non-dangerous radiation, low cost, and so forth. For quicker results, NIR-I fluorophores using rational layout techniques had been extensively used for biomedical applications, including correct real-time sentinel lymph nodes/tumor delineation, in addition to intra-operative image-guided surgical elimination of sentinel lymph nodes/tumor tissues. Hence carbon nanotubes have a massive quantity of applicability as biomedical and in field diagnostic [1–15].

11.1 INTRODUCTION

11.1.1 THE STANDARD X-RAY SOURCE: X-RAY IMAGING

A new biomedical imaging generation has emerged that broadly makes use of and applicability of carbon nanotubes (CNTs) because of the fact the electron emission (cathode) for the X-ray tube. Since the common general performance of the CNTs cathode is controlled through way of manner of easy voltage manipulation, CNT-enabled X-ray resets are perfect for the repetitive imaging steps applicable to capture three-dimensional medical information. As such, they have got be given the development of a gated micro-computed tomography (CT) scanner for small animal research similarly to stationary tomo-synthesis, an experimental approach for massive field-of-view human imaging. Roentgen determined X-rays whilst operating with a Crookes tube, a device to test fluorescence through producing a voltage ability among electrodes in a gas-filled or partially-evacuated tube. In order to enhance the X-ray output, Coolidge changed the tube withinside the early 1900s via heating the cathode. Today, virtually all X-ray devices authorized for affected person care heat a cathode filament to excite or energize electrons over the potential energy barrier of break out in a method referred to as thermionic emission (TE). Once released, the electrons are increased towards a metallic anode. A part of the energy released whilst electrons engage with atoms within-side the anode is over excited through X-ray photons, which might be directed toward the target and filtered. The long experience with TE due to the fact the approach of X-ray technology has produced the most reliable sources for a incredible type of diagnostic and therapeutic devices [16–20].

11.1.2 FIELD EMISSION AND THE CNT CATHODE

A new X-ray supply, based totally on CNTs technology and field emission (FE), has currently emerged. FE is a quantum phenomenon quite different from TE, in which the utility of an electric powered discipline allows electrons to 'tunnel' through the capacity power barrier. FE happens nearly at once and at room temperature. Attempts to gain an FE-primarily based completely X-ray supply date decrease returned to the 1960s. The earliest emitters had been metallic, and over the decades, checking out continued with many metal compounds. The cognizance become on figuring out substances from which electrons have to most without problems be extracted. However, with ongoing experience, the important significance of morphology on electron emission turn out to be recognized, highlighting the need for a high aspect ratio (length to width) and a sharp tip, as this shape concentrates the applied electric powered field. CNTs were found in the early 1990s. Their ability to obtain aspect ratios of >10, excessive thermal conductivity, and low chemical reactivity led short to FE testing, and internal a decade, CNT emitters had been integrated into numerous nonmedical gadgets, along with flat panel displays. Both single walled CNTs (SWNTs) and multi-walled CNTs (MWNTs) have been used to construct field emitters. SWNTs have smaller diameters and in desired fewer structural defects than MWNTs, each of which are appropriate abilities for a field emitter. However, SWNTs also are more reactive and thermally tons much less stable than MWNTs. Although the potential benefit of a compact electron supply with fast on–off times for clinical imaging become recognized early, fabricating a likely CNT-primarily based totally X-ray tube for biomedical use proved challenging. Cathodes powering clinical imaging devices must generate a high and incredibly uniform electron flux. Additionally, they must possess a long-term stability under excessive voltage and in a non-ideal vacuum environment. For those reasons, MWNTs are normally used as electron field emitters in excessive-strength X-ray tubes, even though experimental devices have moreover been built the use of SWNTs.

11.1.3 CNT-ENABLED PRECLINICAL IMAGING

Animal mouse models of human disease are ubiquitous, and research using the murine version of 10 involves CT scanning to evaluate anatomy in three dimensions. However, imaging the mouse thorax can be problematic, given movement blur as a result of the rapid heart and respiration rates. Continuous imaging at the same time as recording the respiratory and cardiac cycle permits for retrospective image selection, however involves a excessive radiation dose, frequently representing a great fraction of the lethal dose for a small animal. As such, the capacity to perform longitudinal scanning is limited. Intubation and mechanical ventilation can be used to control the animal's respiratory and thereby prospectively gate imaging, however this invasive approach affects lung morphology and physiology. Capturing prospectively-gated cardiac images has shown to be even more difficult. The responsiveness of the CNT cathode provided a way to imaging the anesthetized however free-respiration animal, due to the fact the capacity to pulse X-rays rapid over a short period allows for monitoring the respiration and cardiac cycles and triggering imaging simples ton the desired physiologic phase. With this reason in mind, CNT-enabled micro-CT scanners have been developed. Noninvasive pneumatic or optical sensors of chest expansion and electrocardiogram electrodes record the respiratory and cardiac cycles, respectively. The electronic signals are analyzed and interfaced with the X-ray supply to coordinate pulse generation. Specific physiologic time factors may be selected, including systole at cease expiration, and an image is collected while those conditions are present (Figure 11.2). Gantry rotation takes place and the tool and device awaits the same physiologic state to collect the next image. This method continues until the essential projections for Field lamp reconstruction are acquired. Depending on the animal's coronary heart and respiratory rates, a experiment time of 8–15 minutes is usually required to acquire a full image set, restrained primarily through gantry rotation speed. As an end result of the small focal spot size, excessive dose rate, and brief pulse width of 5–10 milliseconds, the attainable resolution is excellent, and given the restricted exposure of about 11 cGy per scan, repeated longitudinal imaging will become possible (Figure 11.1).

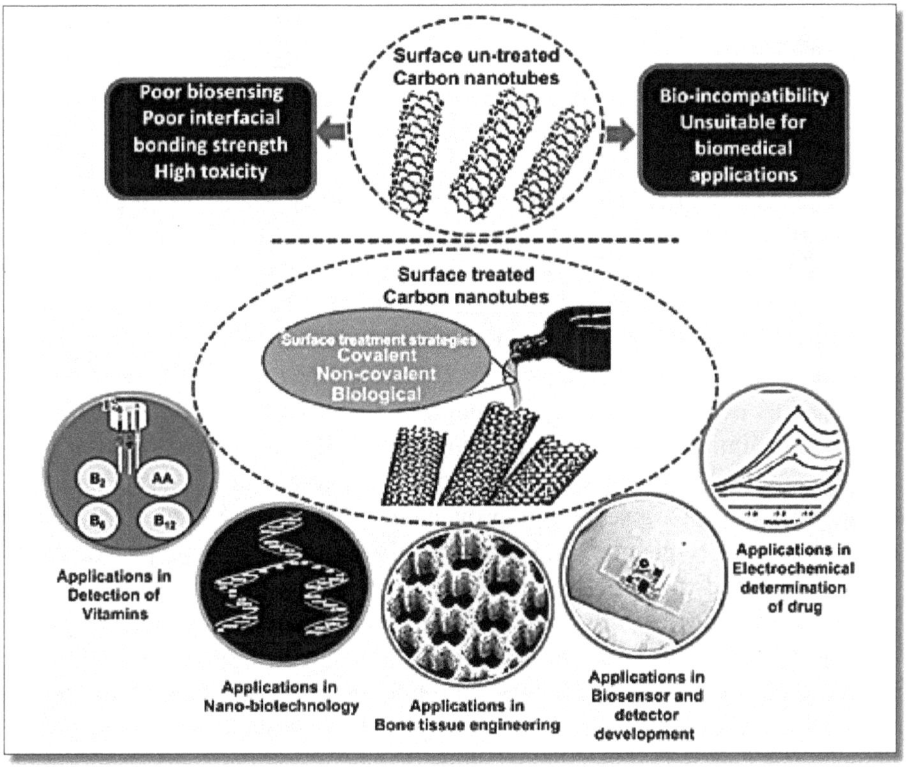

FIGURE 11.1 Surface treated strategies covalent non-covalent biological.

11.1.4 CNT-ENABLED CLINICAL IMAGING: MINIATURE X-RAY TUBES

CNT-enabled sources have been introduced into miniature X-ray tubes. There are many potential applications for small tubes, typically described as having diameters <1 cm, including hand-held devices and devices connected to scopes and catheters for get access into the body. Two CNT-enabled sources able to produce X-rays with enough power to penetrate biologic tissue had been developed. Both use SWNTs. The deliver tubes have outer diameters and lengths of 7 × 47 mm and 10 × 50 mm, generating maximum photon energies of 50 and 70 kV, respectively. The former has been included right into a dental imaging tool designed to be inserted in the mouth for capacity human applicability. Work keeps to optimize the stability of the CNT cathode on this settings.

11.1.5 CNT-ENABLED CLINICAL IMAGING: STATIONARY DIGITAL TOMOSYNTHESIS

11.1.5.1 THE EVOLUTION OF DIGITAL TOMO-SYNTHESIS AND ITS LIMITATIONS

Tomo synthesis (tomo) a term to an imaging method wherein planar projections are acquired from particular angles relative to the target. The end result is a chain of images that may be shifted and superimposed to bring into cognizance structural details present in the identical anatomic plane. In other way, it is a method which could be a few three-dimensional (three-D) statistics from a restricted number of two-dimensional (2D) projections. First introduced withinside the past due 1930s, tomo changed into the earliest strive to triumph over the primary limitation of planar imaging, especially the superposition of overlying detail. Tomo underwent a series of modifications in the direction of the subsequent 50 years, involving improvements in projection styles and viewing devices. It grew to become into adapted to many medical settings, along with angiography and remains used at some point of intravenous pyelography to assess the intensity of pathology withinside the kidney and gathering system. However, hobby in tomo waned thru the 1980s with the advent of CT. CT rotates the X-ray supply and detector throughout the target, taking into account the mathematical reconstruction and digital display of 3-Ddata with greater depth detail than tomo. Without question, CT scanning has been confirmed to be dramatically a hit and might be considered a major advance of present day medicine. However, in comparison to tomo, CT is expensive, every in terms of dollars and radiation dose. With the improvement of digital X-ray detectors in the late 1990s, interest in tomo returned, on the grounds that the software of picture processing and mathematical reconstruction greatly improved the ease of reader use and diagnostic accuracy of the displayed tomo picture stack. Digital tomo (DT) quickly determined niches in which the cost and radiation dose of CT regarded excessive, but planar imaging became regularly inadequate, maximum generally breast cancer screening and chest imaging for nodules.

11.2 RECENT ADVANCES FOR BIOMEDICAL IMAGING

11.2.1 FLUORESCENCE IMAGING

Fluorescence imaging plays an important feature within-side the clinical research and scientific diagnosis. However, the limited penetration depth of slight turns into the primary hurdle for the further software of fluorescence imaging. To overcome this problem, researchers had been that specialize in developing and enforcing fluorescent probes with excitation and emission wavelengths falling into the natural obvious NIR win do. The classical NIR window, or NIR window, is described to be from 700 nm to ~900 nm, internal which neither hemoglobin nor water well-known massive moderate absorbance. Currently, various probes, collectively with natural dyes, similarly to semiconducting quantum dots (QDs) lie internal this place. Recently, it is been exposed that moderate with even longer wavelength within-side the type of 1,100–1,400 nm, despite the fact that is probably barely absorbed with the aid of the usage of water, shows further decreased tissue absorbance, and in addition importantly, remarkably decreased scattering with the useful resource of the usage of herbal tissues, permitting *in vitro* assay and *in vivo* fluorescence imaging with advanced tissue penetration and lots higher spatial resolutions. SWNTs are quasi one dimensional quantum wires with electricity degrees become split due to the quantum confinement effect. The density of states (DOS) are characterized with the useful resource of the usage of the so referred to as van Hoff singularities (VHSs), which define narrow energy stages in which the DOS intensity may be very high. The band-hole amongst every semiconducting SWNTs is within-side the order of 1 eV, which permits for the fluorescence within-side the NIR-II location below the excitation within-side the NIR-I region. Furthermore, the massive Stoke-shift most of the excitation at 550–850 nm and emission at 900–1,600 nm might also additionally need to dramatically decrease the auto fluorescence of biological tissues in the course of imaging, imparting better *in vivo* imaging sensitivity.

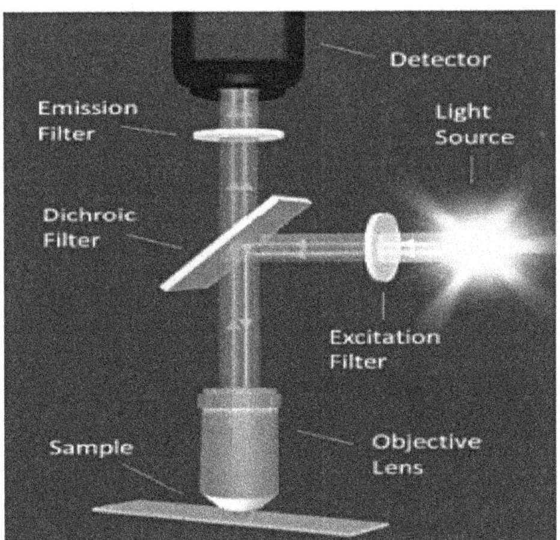

FIGURE 11.2 Diagram illustrating the optical filters and light path of a fluorescence microscope.

Source: Reprinted with permission from Alluxa.com. https://www.alluxa.com/optical-filter-applications/fluorescence-filters-microscopy-imaging/

11.2.2 RAMAN IMAGING

Unlike fluorescence, Raman scattering also involves the emission of photons with shifted wavelengths in the presence of light excitation, is a photon scattering process instead of photo luminescence. The inherent Raman scattering signals of molecules without related to enhancement mechanism inclusive of SERS are normally rather weak. However, the scattering efficiency gets large even as the laser power fits the power wanted for the electron transition from the valence to the conduction bands, and this enhancement of Raman signals is additionally named resonance Raman scattering. Typically, SWNTs have more than one Raman peaks, which includes the radical respiration mode (RBM, 100 cm^{-1}–300 cm^{-1}) and tangential G band (~1,580 cm^{-1}), which correspond to the vibration of carbon atoms with-inside the radical direction and with-inside the tangential direction, respectively. The resonance Raman scattering for SWNTs is determined through a such way that of method of the DOS available for the optical transition (e.g., E11 and E22 transition), which is closely determined by their diameters and chirality indices. When the Raman spectrum of SWNTs is taken, those SWNTs with E ii in resonance could provide strong resonance Raman scattering useful for organic sensing and imaging. The intrinsic Raman residences of SWNTs have been first adopted by Heller et al. for live cellular imaging in 2005. In their paintings, SWNTs wrapped through DNA oligonucleotide were used as markers for live cellular monitoring. Without including any extra fluorescent labels, the RBM height of SWNTs was recorded inside stay 3T3 cells beneath the excitation of a 785-nmlaser. Compared with organic dyes and quantum dots that may be step through step quenched or photo-bleached over time, SWNTs confirmed as a substitute strong Raman scattering indicators with none big quenching or photo bleaching, allowing them to be used for long-time period monitoring in natural samples over months. Taking advantage of the inherent Raman G band of carbon nanotubes, Lamprecht et al. had been capin a function to map and tune the intracellular distribution of carbon nanotubes after centered shipping to carcinoma cells. In some other current study, Kang et al. used high-velocity confocal Raman imaging to have a take a observe the mobile uptake of SWNTs. In their work of cellular-intrinsic and nine nanotube-derived Raman indicators in RAW 264.7 macrophage were taken to solve SWNTs with one-of-a-kind indices and aggregation states, further to their respective positions in the cells. This work highlighted the usefulness of Raman spectroscopy for molecular imaging of live cells. *In vivo* Raman imaging of tumors on mice has additionally been tested through the utilization of targeting ligand conjugated SWNTs. Raman scattering commonly well-known shows instead sharp peaks with various conditions for one-of-a-kind molecules, and for that reason is good for multiplexed sensing and imaging. The frequency of carbon-carbon bond vibration in the G band Raman heightening of SWNTs is decided through the carbon atom mass. By converting the carbon isotope from 12C to 13C, the G band peaks of SWNTs will be altered accordingly. The first multiplexed Raman imaging of live cells was identified through Liu et al. In this study, three types SWNTs with varied 13C doping ratio and for that reason, unique Raman G-band peaks have been conjugated with one-of-a-kind targeting ligands to understand the corresponding cellular lines. By method of spectrum immixing, multiplexed Raman imaging become found out simultaneously. A later work through the identical group went a similar step to recognize the five color Raman imaging of cells through conjugating SWNTs with different targeting molecules, for both multiplexed *in vitro* cellular imaging and *ex vivo* tissue slice staining.

11.2.3 PHOTOACOUSTIC IMAGING

Photoacoustic (PA) imaging is a presently developed imaging modality, which has been widely used in the biological field. The principle of PA imaging is as follows: the laser pulses can be absorbed with the useful resource of the use of mild-absorbing molecules, each endogenous molecules or evaluation sellers, with-inside the biological pattern to create heat, inducing short thermo-elastic growth and therefore most important to wide band ultrasonic emission, which can be detected with the useful resource of the use of an ultrasound microphone to bring together 2D or 3D images. Compared with traditional optical imaging, PA imaging detects sound in preference to mild, and therefore shows a number of obvious advantages along with notably improved tissue penetration and advanced spatial resolutions, with the useful resource of the use of maintaining off absorbance and scattering of the emission mild in fluorescence imaging, respectively. Various nanomaterials which have strong absorbance with-inside the NIR region are useful evaluation retailers in PA imaging. Both MWNTs and SWNTs have been observed as a photo-thermal agent due to its sturdy NIR absorbance. On the other hand, its strong NIR absorbance moreover makes nanotubes perfect comparison agents for photo-acoustic imaging. For cell imaging, Avti et al. observed photo-acoustic microscopy to detect, map, and quantify the trace amount (nanograms to micrograms) of SWNTs in numerous histological tissue specimens. The outcomes showed that the noise-equal detection sensitivity changed into as low as about 7 picograms, which allowed similarly software program in tissue analysis. For *in vivo* PA imaging, Gambhir et al. for the first time observed RGD conjugated SWNTs as PA evaluation agent. In their strong PA signs may be decided from the tumor in SWNT-RGD injected group, even as simplest prone signs were decided in the obvious SWNTs injected group (Figure 11.3).

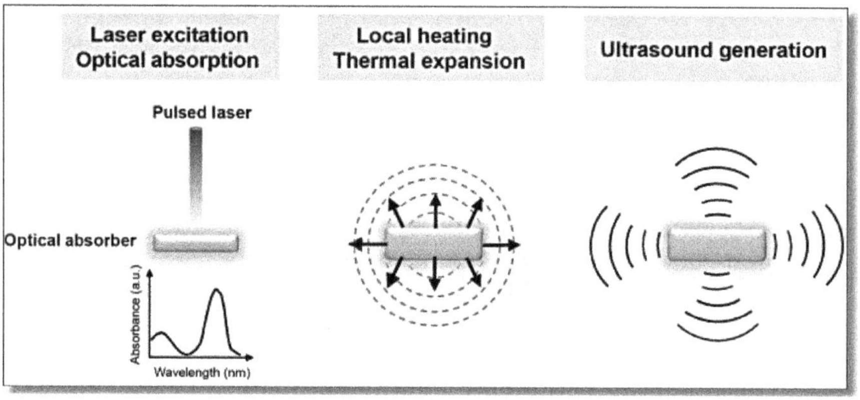

FIGURE 11.3 Illustration of PA signal generation.

Source: Liu and Li (2020). http://creativecommons.org/licenses/by/4.0/

11.2.4 MAGNETIC RESONANCE IMAGING

Magnetic resonance (MR) imaging is one of the only and noninvasive modalities of imaging. Annually, about 60 millions of MR imaging times are achieved withinside the health center worldwide, and 30% of them use assessment retailers. Generally, the contrast agents are comprised of T1-shortening agents (containing Gd^{3+}, Mn^{2+}, etc.) and T2-shortening retailers (e.g., iron oxide nanoparticle). A considerable amount of research has been accomplished to find out the ability software program of CNTs for MR imaging. For T1 weighted MR imaging, Sitharaman et al. first stated the nanoscale loading and confinement of aquated Gd^{3+}-ion clusters inside ultra-short SWNTs (US-tubes), obtaining Gd^{3+}@US-tube with strong T1-assessment useful in MR imaging. Richard et al. stated a noncovalent method to conjugate MWNTs with an amphiphilic gadolinium (III) chelate (GdL), making them useful to offer T1-evaluation in MR imaging. For T2 weighted MR imaging, Strano, and coworkers first stated that SWNTs with iron oxide nanoparticles connected at the quilt of nanotubes may be used as T2 assessment retailers for MR imaging, without the need of more labeling. Wu et al. stated MWNTs/cobalt ferrite synthesized via a solvothermal method. The acquired nanocomposite exhibited a large terrible assessment enhancement in T2-weighted MR imaging of most cancers cells. Metal catalysts (e.g., Fe, Co) are usually used for the duration of the synthesis of CNTs. Taking benefits of the impurities of iron contained in SWNTs, Faraj et al. studied the bio-distribution of SWNTs via measuring MR signals *in vivo*. Even after purification to cast off the bulk of catalyst metal nanoparticles withinside the nanotube sample, the purified SWNTs with trace amount of iron content material have been observed to be despite the fact that effective to provide strong T2-assessment in MR imaging. Stem cells have verified great ability in regenerative medicine and attracted notable interests in latest years. Sensitive and dependable techniques for stem mobile labeling and *in vivo* tracking are hence urgently needed. Carbon nanotubes have moreover been used for stem cellular labeling and tracking with the resource of the usage of numerous groups. Vittorrio et al. stated that MWNTs labeled mesenchymal stem cells (MSC) may be correctly tracked after being administrated into animals beneath neath T2-weighted MR imaging. Many organization nowadays used SWNTs to label human MSCs (hMSCs) for *in vivo* monitoring based mostly on triple modal imaging. PEG functionalized SWNTs were conjugated with protamine, which remarkably greater appropriate the mobile uptake of SWNTs for tremendously inexperienced stem cellular labeling. SWNT-labeled hMSCs showed unaffected differentiation and proliferation skills in comparison to un-labeled cells. The strong inherent resonance Raman scattering of SWNTs modified into carried out for *in vitro* and *in vivo* Raman imaging of SWNT-labeled hMSCs, allowing ultrasensitive *in vivo* detection of as few as 500 stem cells administrated proper right into a mouse. On the alternative hand, the metal catalyst nanoparticles related on nanotubes can be carried out due to the fact the T2-assessment agent in magnetic resonance (MR) imaging of SWNT-labeled hMSCs. Moreover, *in vivo* photoacoustic imaging of hMSCs in mice is also demonstrated. This paintings famous that SWNTs with appropriate ground functionalization must function multifunctional nano-probes for stem cellular labeling and multi-modal *in vivo* tracking.

11.2.5 NUCLEAR IMAGING

Besides adopting the intrinsic characteristics of SWNTs, outside labels together with radio-isotopes additionally may be introduced to increase the power of SWNT-based totally imaging probes. Wang et al. for the primary time stated the 125 is probably used to track the biodistribution of SWNTs in animals. The modality of micro-single photon emission automated tomography (micro-SPECT) become successfully obtained via labeling CNTs with 111In. Subsequently, McDevitt and coworkers labeled SWNTs with 86Y for position emission tomography (PET) imaging. *In vivo* tumor imaging in mouse models through radionuclide labeled SWNTs has moreover been stated through numerous groups. Conjugation through a 1,4,7,10-tetraazacyclododecane-1,4,7,10-tetraacetic acid (DOTA) chelator *in vivo* tumor-targeted PET imaging of U87MG tumors using 64Cu/DOTA-labeled SWNT–PEG–RGD have become determined out because of the right binding amongst RGD peptide and integrin avβ3 overexpressed on U87MG tumor cells in addition to tumor vasculatures. In addition to RGD peptide, anti-CD20 antibody have become significantly applied to purpose human Burkitt lymphoma through conjugating them with 111In labeled SWNTs. Besides using traditional chelation chemistry to achieve radiolabeled CNTs, radioisotopes will also be inserted into nanotubes for radiolabeling. Hong et al. said that Na125I may be sealed withinside the hole form of SWNTs, obtaining 125I-labeled SWNTs useful for SPECT/CT imaging. Compared with the modalities cited above, radio-labeled SWNTs show off numerous advantages, together with no tissue penetration intensity trouble and immoderate sensitivity. However, the improvement of using CNTs for nuclear imaging has come to be pretty slow withinside the present day 2–3 years, without showing lots substantial enhancement to our excellent knowledge. Nevertheless, the combination of nuclear imaging with distinct imaging techniques may additionally though be of tremendous hobbies withinside the development of CNT-based totally bio-imaging probes.

11.3 FUTURE PROSPECTS AND CHALLENGES

Different imaging modalities of SWNTs have their respective advantages similar to limitations. The fluorescence imaging withinside the NIR-II biological obvious window with SWNTs permits *in vivo* optical imaging with deep tissue penetration and immoderate spatial resolution, due to the low indigenous tissue scattering and the lots reduced photon scattering withinside the NIR-II location in comparison to that for fluorescence imaging in visible (400–700 nm) and traditional NIR-I region (700–900 nm). However, the QY of SWNTs remains now not excessive enough. Developing easy synthesis and purification strategies to get SWNTs with herbal chirality could be of extremely good importance to collect new SWNT-based definitely NIR-II imaging probes with brilliant and multi-colored fluorescence. SWNTs have a big scattering cross-phase and show strong resonance Raman scattering. Raman imaging through SWNT-probes has extremely good sensitivity, and is evidence towards photo bleaching and quenching. Relying on the SERS effect, noble metal covered SWNTs display in addition more Raman indicators, permitting Raman mapping with a much faster speed. However, no matter SERS enhancement, it although takes ~10 min to collect a Raman photo with the useful resource of the usage of conventional Raman mapping. The advances in instruments may be had to make SWNT-primarily based definitely Raman imaging a possible tool in actual biological research. Moreover, the usage of chirality-purified SWNTs with the majority of nanotubes in resonance to the excitation laser may moreover drastically boom the Raman signs of SWNTs on a consistent with mass basis. Other imaging techniques the use of CNTs, which include PA imaging, MR imaging, and nuclear imaging, have moreover demonstrated excellent functionality in biomedical imaging. The integration of a couple of imaging modalities has to enlarge the advantages of each single imaging modality and conquer their inherent limitations. The real splendor of the use of CNTs due to the fact the imaging probe is for that reason their multi-functionalities. Unlike many distinctive nanomaterials applied in bio-imaging, CNTs with tremendously enriched optical and magnetic properties are intrinsic multimodal imaging probes, without the need to engineer complicated nanostructures to afford a couple of capabilities. Moreover, the recovery capabilities of CNTs (e.g., drug and gene delivery, photothermal therapy) in mixture with imaging may want to in addition motive them to great theragnostic nano-platforms. Besides the regulations of each modality mentioned above, one primary task for the clinical utility of CNTs is the concern of their functionality long-term toxicity. CNTs without appropriate floor functionalized had been discovered to be toxic *in vivo*, inducing a huge sort of toxicity to animals. On the other hand, researchers have moreover evidenced that CNTs with well format ground coatings collectively with PEGylation exhibit no obvious *in vitro* and *in vivo* toxicity, and may be grade by grade excreted from animals through renal and/or facial excretion pathways. Several organizations moreover claimed the possibility of biodegradation of CNTs under enzyme induced oxidization. Nevertheless, it's far expected that on the equal time as CNT-based definitely biomedical imaging have to certainly have the wonderful capability in easy biomedical research similarly to *in vitro*/*ex vivo* scientific diagnosis, there may want to although be huge annoying conditions within-side the route of the usage of those nanomaterials for real *in vivo* scientific applications.

11.4 APPLICATIONS OF CARBON NANOTUBES

11.4.1 GENE DELIVERY

CNTs additionally may be used as a service for gene delivery, specially plasmid DNA, small interfering RNA (siRNA), small hairpin RNA (shRNA), and micro-RNA with the intention to overexpress or inhibit the expression of purpose proteins. The main approach for complexation of negatively charged nucleic acids is based on the functionalization of CNTs with cationic organizations which incorporates ammonium capabilities or virtually charged polymers which incorporates poly(ethylene imine). It has been validated that ammonium-MWCNTs display superior ability in assessment to cationic liposomes for the delivery of an apoptotic siRNA in competition to the cancer-related gene polo-like kinase (PLK1) in human lung carcinoma Calu6 xenograft mouse model after direct intratumoral administration. Currently, remedies based mostly on single treatments are nevertheless unsatisfying, hence combining recuperation strategies allows overcoming the contemporary limitations of each single therapy. In this context, CNTs were performed for combined drug and gene shipping in human gastric maximum cancers cells. In this study, a mixture of shRNA mediated gene silencing approach with chemotherapy the usage of very low cognizance of doxorubicin delivered approximately synergistic antitumor activity, while mitigating toxic aspect consequences of the drug (Figure 11.4).

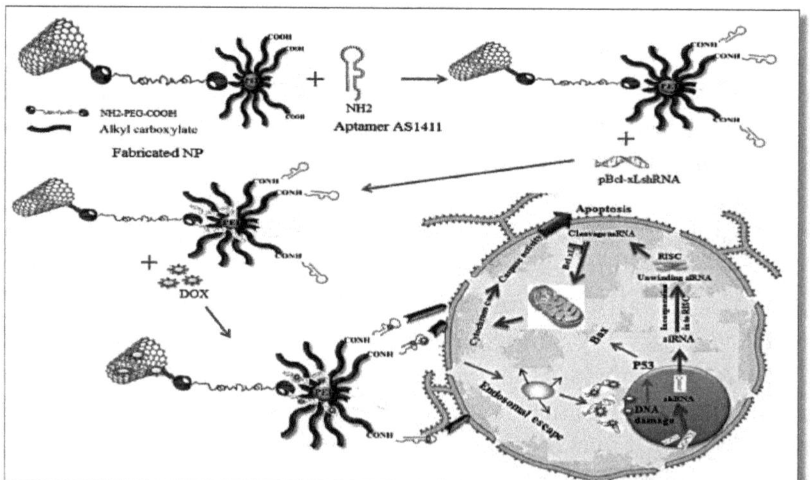

FIGURE 11.4 Illustration of the codelivery of shRNA and doxorubicin by functionalized CNTs into gastric cancer cells.

Source: Sahar et al. 2017

11.4.2 PHOTOTHERAPIES

11.4.2.1 PHOTODYNAMIC THERAPY

Photodynamic therapy (PDT) relies on the generation of singlet oxygen and reactive oxygen species (ROS) through way of approach of photosensitizers upon exposure to mild of a specific wavelength, most important to cell death. The photosensitizer transfers the absorbed light energy to molecular oxygen in reality located in tissues. CNTs can each act as photosensitizers themselves or be functionalized with photosensitizer molecules. A smart method for the generation of cytotoxic ROS after exposure to a specific goal has been designed through way of approach of wrapping SWCNTs with a photosensitizer that turn out to be covalently associated with an aptamer recognizing thrombin. CNTs can strongly quench the fluorescence of fluorophores even as in close to proximity to the nanotube surface. In this study, it become proposed that the CNTs have to quench the nearby photosensitizer in a similar manner. Hence, the photosensitizer grow to be activated through a manner of approach of slight best upon binding of the conjugate to the aim thrombin. The release of the photosensitizer from the nanotube sidewall allowed the recovery of its photodynamic efficiency.

11.4.2.2 PHOTOTHERMAL THERAPY

Photothermal therapy (PTT) is a noninvasive technique using nanoparticles that convert near-infrared (NIR) mild into warmness for cell ablation. Compared to short-wavelength mild, NIR mild is not risky to the human body and might penetrate tissues deeply (up to a few centimeters). Due to their immoderate absorption cross-section of NIR mild and great mild-to-warmness energy conversion efficiency, CNTs have been widely exploited as PTT agents for thermal ablation of recurrent tumors or of these resistant to traditional cures beneath neath NIR light irradiation. For instance, *in vivo* eradication of strong malignant tumors in mice has been accomplished through CNT-mediated PTT. In this study, the handled mice displayed whole obliteration of the tumors without extreme element consequences or tumor recurrence over a duration of 6 months, at the same time as the tumors of control groups grew until the death of the mice (Figure 11.5).

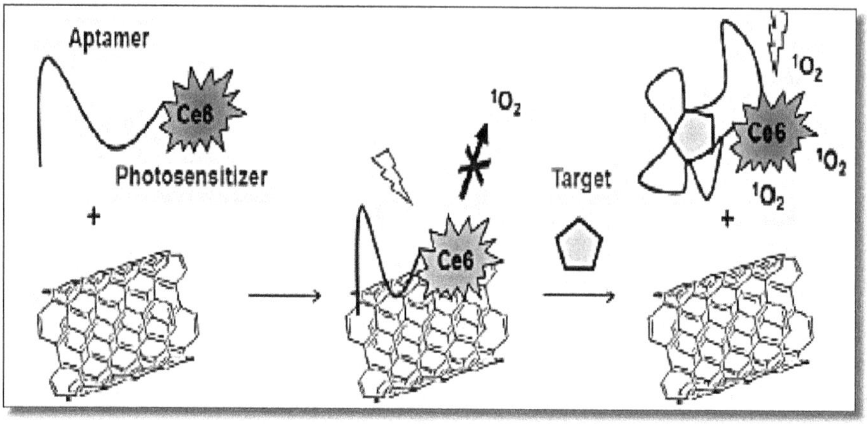

FIGURE 11.5 Illustration of the aptamer-photosensitizer-CNT complex and of the generation of ROS upon binding to the target molecule.

Source: Karunya and Hsu, 2016. Creative Commons CC BY License

11.4.3 BIOMEDICAL IMAGING

11.4.3.1 INTRINSIC PROPERTIES

The excellent physical properties of CNTs, especially SWCNTs, reason them to precise imaging probes with excellent ability in multimodal biomedical imaging. Several opinions have summarized progress on the applications of CNTs as multimodal contrast agents for biomedical imaging. The semi-conducting SWCNTs show a narrow band hollow allowing fluorescence emission withinside the NIR-I region (750–900 nm) and NIR-II region (1,000–1,700 nm) with greater tissue penetration and spatial resolution. Fluorescence imaging of SWCNTs withinside the NIRII region has made outstanding improvement for *in vivo* live animal imaging way to reduced scattering of photons, resulting in deeper penetration depths. Dai and coworkers have used semiconducting SWCNTs to visualize 3–4 μm extensive capillary blood vessels at a depth of ca. 3 mm. Meanwhile, the blood goes along with the waft tempo in a couple of person vessels modified into moreover imaged. Besides fluorescence imaging, SWCNTs had been exploited for Raman imaging. Indeed, they very own strong resonance Raman scattering with extraordinarily large scattering flow section. Gambhir and coworkers have used SWCNTs for whole-body Raman imaging to illustrate tumor targeting *in vivo*. The coating of SWCNTs with noble metallic nanoparticles, which include gold or silver nanoparticles, lets in developing their Raman scattering indicators and presenting opportunities for immediate Raman imaging of organic samples. CNTs have moreover been implemented for photoacoustic imaging due to their strong absorbance withinside the NIR region. Gambhir and coworkers need to localize SWCNTs functionalized with the RGD (Arg-Gly-Asp) peptide in tumor in mice after intravenous administration. RGD is recognized with the useful resource of the usage of a large sort of integrins expressed with the useful resource of the usage of every normal and tumor cells. Furthermore, the photoacoustic signal of CNTs can be dramatically stepped forward with the useful resource of the usage of coating with a gold shell or with the useful resource of the usage of conjugation of natural dyes.

11.4.3.2 LABELING OF CNTS

Besides taking gain of their intrinsic properties, CNTs can deliver imaging sellers for precise clinical modalities inclusive of MRI, positron emission tomography (PET), single photon emission computed tomography (SPECT), and X-ray computed tomography. For example, CNTs had been functionalized with T1 assessment agents (inclusive of gadolinium) or T2 assessment agents (collectively with iron oxide nanoparticles) for MRI. For nuclear imaging, they had been categorized with radioactive isotopes, namely, 64Cu for PET and 111In for SPECT. The use of multiple imaging modalities can enlarge the advantages of every single imaging approach and overcome their inherent limitations. The gain of the use of CNTs as imaging probe is their multifunctionality. For instance, SWCNTs have been utilized for stem cell labeling and *in vivo* multimodal monitoring the use of photoacoustic imaging, MRI, and Raman imaging. In addition, CNTs are endowed with healing functions combined with imaging, accordingly ensuing promising for theragnostic. Nevertheless, there are nevertheless some challenges towards the usage of CNTs for *in vivo* scientific applications, especially their capacity toxicity and the detection of hint quantity of nanotubes in complex biological media.

11.5 CONCLUSION

Carbon nanotubes open up a brand new technology for realistic packages and are beneficial in enjoyable the primary physics on the non-metric scale. They provide extremely good atypical packages to the approaching generations through their everlasting packages in electronics, chemical packages and nearly utterly with inside the biomedical field. The carbon nanotubes present genera of nanomaterials that own extraordinarily essential packages in diverse fields of therapeutics and biomedicine. Moreover, nanotechnology has been acted as a milestone in fixing the rules and regulations which have been there withinside the silicon microelectronics. CNTs can play a essential position in each attitude of discovery because of their particular structural, electrical, and mechanical properties. Established tumor-focused shipping the usage of CNTs is an answer for unresolved hurdles in cancer therapy. The capacity for transdermal drug shipping the usage of CNTs bucky-paper is likewise now known. The latest proof of BBB crossing with functionalized MWNTs extends its scope in drug shipping application. Further research are required to manufacture functionalized carbon nanotube as a provider device for green focused-mind therapy. The CNTs had been revolutionary for the established order of stem cellular healing procedures and additionally in divers e-mobile delivery systems. Even though the functionalization of CNTs is useful in supplying greater bioavailability and for deducting the cytotoxic effects, it's far essential to have a complete toxicological evaluation of this nanomaterial. Moreover, it additionally needs a deeper expertise of the underlying physiological mechanisms of CNT administration [21–26].

ACKNOWLEDGMENT

We thank MET's, Institute of Pharmacy, BKC, affiliated under Savitribai Phule Pune University, Nashik, Divine College of Pharmacy Satana and Sandip Institute of Pharmaceutical Science for their constant support and providing all facilities to complete this work. We are also thankful to the Ministry of Tribal Affairs Government of India for providing financial assistance in the form of fellowship (Award No.: 202021-NFST-MAH-01235).

KEYWORDS

- **biomedical imaging**
- **carbon nanotube**
- **positron emission tomography**
- **single photon emission computed tomography**

REFERENCES

1. Raphey, V., et al., (2019). Advanced biomedical applications of carbon nanotube. *Materials Science and Engineering: C, 100*, 616–630.
2. Puett, C., et al., (2018). An update on carbon nanotube-enabled X-ray sources for biomedical imaging. *Wiley Interdisciplinary Reviews: Nanomedicine and Nanobiotechnology, 10*(1), e1475.
3. Fairchild, S. B., et al., (2019). Carbon nanotube fiber field emission array cathodes. *IEEE Transactions on Plasma Science, 47*(5), 2032–2038.
4. Laszczyk, K. U., (2020). Field emission cathodes to form an electron beam prepared from carbon nanotube suspensions. *Micromachines, 11*(3), 260.
5. Cao, G., (2018). Biomedical X-ray imaging enabled by carbon nanotube X-ray sources. *Chinese Journal of Chemical Physics, 31*(4), 529–536.
6. Lee, K. S., & Chung, M. J., (2018). Limitations of detecting small solid lung nodules by using digital chest tomosynthesis. *Radiology, 287*(3), 1028–1029.
7. Horvat, J. V., et al., (2019). Calcifications at digital breast tomosynthesis: Imaging features and biopsy techniques. *Radiographics, 39*(2), 307–318.
8. Sobhani, Z., et al., (2020). Identification and visualization of microplastics/nanoplastics by Raman imaging (i): Down to 100 nm. *Water Research, 174*, 115658.
9. He, J., et al., (2019). Design of Raman tag-bridged core–shell Au@ $Cu_3(BTC)_2$ nanoparticles for Raman imaging and synergistic chemo-photothermal therapy. *Nanoscale, 11*(13), 6089–6100.
10. Vanden-Hehir, S., et al., (2019). Raman imaging of nanocarriers for drug delivery. *Nanomaterials, 9*(3), 341.
11. Hysi, E., et al., (2020). Photoacoustic imaging of kidney fibrosis for assessing pretransplant organ quality. *JCI Insight, 5*(10).
12. Geethanath, S., & Vaughan Jr. J. T., (2019). Accessible magnetic resonance imaging: A review. *Journal of Magnetic Resonance Imaging, 49*(7), e65–e77.
13. Zhou, Z., et al., (2019). Structure–relaxivity relationships of magnetic nanoparticles for magnetic resonance imaging. *Advanced Materials, 31*(8), 1804567.
14. Zanzonico, P., (2019). An overview of nuclear imaging. *Radiopharmaceutical Chemistry, 2019*, 101–117.
15. Iskandrian, A. E., (2018). The future of nuclear cardiac imaging: Reflection and a vision. *Journal of Nuclear Cardiology, 25*(1), 1–5.
16. Simon, J., Flahaut, E., & Golzio, M., (2019). Overview of carbon nanotubes for biomedical applications. *Materials, 12*(4), 624.
17. Ali, S., et al., (2019). Challenges and opportunities in functional carbon nanotubes for membrane-based water treatment and desalination. *Science of the Total Environment, 646*, 1126–1139.
18. Kassem, A., Ayoub, G. M., & Malaeb, L., (2019). Antibacterial activity of chitosan nano-composites and carbon nanotubes: A review. *Science of the Total Environment, 668*, 566–576.
19. Kinloch, I. A., et al., (2018). Composites with carbon nanotubes and graphene: An outlook. *Science, 362*(6414), 547–553.
20. Rahman, G., et al., (2019). *An Overview of the Recent Progress in the Synthesis and Applications of Carbon Nanotubes C, 5*(1), 3.

21. Wang, R., et al., (2018). Mechanisms and applications of carbon nanotubes in terahertz devices: A review. *Carbon, 132*, 42–58.
22. Ferreira, F. V., et al., (2019). Synthesis, characterization, and applications of carbon nanotubes. In: *Carbon-Based Nanofillers and Their Rubber Nanocomposites* (pp. 1–45). Elsevier.
23. Castro-Rojas, M. A., et al., (2021). Dental applications of carbon nanotubes. *Molecules, 26*(15), 4423.
24. Hasnain, M. S., & Nayak, A. K., (2019). Applications of carbon nanotubes. In: *Carbon Nanotubes for Targeted Drug Delivery* (pp. 33–36). Springer.
25. Iizumi, Y., et al., (2018). Oxygen-doped carbon nanotubes for near-infrared fluorescent labels and imaging probes. *Scientific Reports, 8*(1), 1–6.
26. Negri, V., et al., (2020). Carbon nanotubes in biomedicine. *Surface-modified Nanobiomaterials for Electrochemical and Biomedicine Applications*, 177–217.
27. Liu, WW., Li, PC. Photoacoustic imaging of cells in a three-dimensional microenvironment. J Biomed Sci 27, 3 (2020). https://doi.org/10.1186/s12929-019-0594-x
28. Taghavi, Sahar, Azadeh Hashem Nia, Khalil Abnous, and Mohammad Ramezani. "Polyethylenimine-functionalized carbon nanotubes tagged with AS1411 aptamer for combination gene and drug delivery into human gastric cancer cells." International journal of pharmaceutics 516, no. 1-2 (2017): 301–312.
29. Albert, Karunya, and Hsin-Yun Hsu. "Carbon-based materials for photo-triggered theranostic applications." Molecules 21, no. 11 (2016): 1585.

CHAPTER 12

Carbon Nanotubes for Bioimaging

BONY K. JOHN, NEENAMOL JOHN, JINCY MATHEW, and BEENA MATHEW

School of Chemical Sciences, Mahatma Gandhi University, Kottayam, Kerala, India

ABSTRACT

Carbon nanotubes (CNTs) exhibit a number of unique characteristics that make them promising carbon nanomaterial for various applications. The interaction of these moieties with the cell membrane receptors leads to their incorporation into the cell. However, pure CNTs are toxic, and their invasion into the living cells may damage during bioimaging. The performance of CNTs can be considerably improved by surface modification and incorporation of elements into the CNTs structure. Since surface-modified CNTs possess high aqueous dispersibility, excellent biocompatibility, and minimal cytotoxicity, they are widely used in fluorescent bioimaging applications. CNTs-based bioimaging is recognized to be a next-generation building block for *in vivo* and *in vitro* imaging purposes and that can generate high-resolution images of cells, organs, tissues, and even the entire bodies of animals or humans. Fluorescence imaging, Raman imaging, photoacoustic imaging, and magnetic resonance imaging (MRI) are four fundamental approaches that may be used in CNTs-based bioimaging. This chapter discusses the most recent advancements in the application of CNTs, including single-walled carbon nanotubes (SWNTs) and multi-walled carbon nanotubes (MWNTs) as multi-functional bioimaging nanoprobes. Fluorescence imaging (NIR imaging) region with excellent tissue penetration and spatial resolution originated from the intrinsic band-gap fluorescence of semiconducting SWNTs. Raman imaging based on the resonance Raman scattering of SWNTs is beneficial for *in vitro* and *in vivo* imaging of biomaterials. The extraordinary

Carbon Nanotubes for Biomedical Applications and Healthcare.
Chin Hua Chia, Swati Gokul Talele, Ann Rose Abraham, and A. K. Haghi, (Eds.)

absorption in the NIR range can be exploited for photoacoustic imaging. The photoacoustic signals can be further amplified by adding organic dyes or coatings with various metallic shells. CNTs can also be used as a T2-contrast agent in magnetic resonance imaging by using metal nanoparticle impurities attached to nanotubes.

12.1 INTRODUCTION

CNTs are allotropes of carbon consisting of a hexagonal layer of carbon atoms stacked to form a cylindrical tubular structure. Because of their broad absorption spectrum, large surface area, high signal-to-noise ratio, high biocompatibility, label-free detection, easy monitoring, excellent sensitivity, easy preparation, excitation dependent emission, photochemical stability, and easy solubility in the aqueous medium, CNTs have recently emerged as a new class of novel and eco-friendly fluorescent carbon-based nanomaterials [1–4]. CNTs have been utilized widely in electrochemical [5], theranostics [6], tissue engineering [7], composite material [8], drug delivery, bioimaging [4, 9, 10], and biomedical science [11–16] areas. The CNTs are classified into two based on their structure: single-walled carbon nanotubes (SWCNTs) and Multi-walled carbon nanotubes (MWCNTs). Carbon nanotubes formed from a single graphene sheet with a diameter between 0.4 and 2.5 nm. is commonly called SWNTs. They exhibit distinct chemical, optical, electrical, and physical properties and have the ability to load multiple molecules via π-π stacking interactions. Functionalized single-wall carbon nanotubes have high optical absorption in the near-infrared (NIR) band, making them suitable for *in vivo* and *in vitro* bioimaging. They are a good option for biological imaging because of their photoluminescence in the NIR range and Raman scattering characteristics [17]. Multi-walled carbon nanotubes (MWNTs) are made up of two or more graphene sheets stacked one over the other to build concentric carbon cylinders with diameters of up to 100 nm. MWCNTs generally exhibit low stability and weak optical properties than SWCNTs due to their surface defect [18, 19]. However, due to the weak van der Waal's force of attraction, both MWCNTs and SWCNTs can cause toxicity in living cells when used for bioimaging. This is due to their propensity to aggregate to form a cluster or bundle form due to the weak van der Waal's force of attraction. Several attempts have been made to minimize the toxic effect and enhance the biocompatibility of CNTs in living systems to make them more desirable for practical applications. The surface modification of CNTs is the best technique to improve their solubility and biocompatibility [20].

Fabrication of CNTs from carbonaceous materials employing various methods such as arc discharge, laser ablation, chemical vapor deposition, and pyrolysis [21–26] has become well established in recent years. The bioimaging applications using fluorescence emitting CNTs in the near infrared II (NIR-II) area with outstanding tissue penetration and spatial resolution have received much attention in recent years. However, the toxicity, limited dispersibility and solubility of CNTs have been the key problems for their usage in bioimaging applications. Several attempts were made to ensure the biocompatibility of CNTs by surface functionalization, conjugated with organic compounds and metallic nanoparticles. This chapter explicitly discusses the various synthetic methods of CNTs and their recent advancements in bioimaging applications.

12.2 SYNTHESIS OF CARBON NANOTUBES

Depending on the technique through which CNTs are synthesized, they have a wide range of applications today. The arc discharge, chemical vapor deposition (CVD), and laser ablation are the three frequently employed procedures for the fabrication of CNTs.

12.2.1 ARC DISCHARGE

Arc discharge is the first method used to synthesize nanotubes and is the perfect method for the synthesis of MWCNTs. In this method, DC current is allowed to pass between two electrodes kept in vacuum in an inert atmosphere chamber [27]. During this process rapid deposition of carbon on the electrode took place as the plasma inside the chamber helps in the deposition. The parameters such as arc current and inert gas pressure should be controlled during this process. The CNT deposition occurs when the positive electrode comes closer to the negative electrode and they collide, as a result, an arc is formed. During this process, the electrodes become red hot, and a plasma is formed between the electrodes with the deposition of CNTS on the negative electrodes. Both SWCNTs and MWCNTs are synthesized using this process. However, this process requires a suitable catalyst for SWCNTs synthesis, while no catalysts are necessary for MWCNTs synthesis. This technique can develop the CNTs having a diameter of 2–20 nm with a length of several microns. Lijima et al. successfully conducted arc discharge method to fabricate MWCNTs for the first time in 1991. Later in 1993 they have developed the first SWCNTs by modifying the synthetic method using iron as the catalyst [28, 29].

12.2.2 LASER ABLATION

Laser ablation is another technique for the synthesis of CNTs. In this method, laser treatment is used for the fabrication of CNTs, and this method can overcome the difficulties in the arc charge method of synthesis [30]. Both SWCNTs and MWCNTs can be manufactured by this method in a larger amount. For the synthesis of CNTs, a pulsed laser is applied on the precursors in the presence of a catalyst and inert gas [31]. The nanotubes developed by these methods have 5–20 nm in diameter and a 100 to several microns in length. The factors affecting the fabrication of CNTs by this technique include catalyst, inert gas selection, temperature, laser power, wavelength, pressure, and the fluid dynamics near the carbon target. All these parameters should be controlled for the successful synthesis of CNTS. However, the high temperature of the products obtained after the synthesis is one of the flaws of this method. Thess et al. applied laser-ablation technique for fabricating CNTs using graphite SWNTs at 1200°C [32].

12.2.3 CHEMICAL VAPOR DEPOSITION

The endless efforts by the scientists for a better method for the development of CNTs finally led to the introduction of the chemical vapor deposition method (CVD). This is the most efficient and effective synthesis method for CNTs, which involves the use of a suitable catalyst and carbon source for the successful preparation. In the CVD method, CNTs are generally fabricated from hydrocarbons such as methane, ethylene, and acetylene with the help of energy source, such as electron beam or resistive heating. Reactive radicles are formed from the hydrocarbons by receiving energy from the energy sources at the temperature range of 550–750°C. CNTs are formed by diffusing these reactive species to the substrate, followed by binding in a first row transition metal catalyst such as Ni, Fe, or Co.

The CVD technique was first used by Yacamán et al. to develop the catalytic growth MWCNTs with fullerene structure by passing acetylene gas over iron particles supported on graphite at 700°C [33]. Khan et al. reported the fabrication of cobalt (Co) catalyzed multi-walled carbon nanotube (Co-MWCNT) films on silicon oxide grown silicon substrate, which acts as a sensor for CO detection [34]. Several studies have shown that pristine or unfunctionalized CNTs are highly hydrophobic in nature and are insoluble in an aqueous solution and organic solvents. This limits their importance in biomedical applications. Hence, surface functionalization of CNTs was carried out to reduce its hydrophobic nature, improve the solubility in both aqueous and organic solvents and amalgamate into different biological systems [35]. Three main methods have been reported to modify CNT structures: the covalent functionalization, the non-covalent adsorption of many biomolecules, and the endohedral filling of CNT's inner empty cavity [36].

However, TEM analysis showed that CNTS developed through this method exhibits very poor crystallinity compared to the other two methods [37]. In addition to that, the requirement of too many precursors and high temperatures are other disadvantages of this method. To overcome this issue inductively coupled chemical vapor deposition (ICP-CVD) method was introduced. Here, the nanotubes are developed in the plasma atmosphere created by the ICP system. In this method, the CNTs in the crystalline form were developed even at the temperature of 500°C. This low-temperature synthesis is essential for the microstructures of CNTs. Another method called plasma enhanced chemical vapor deposition (PECVD) is most effective technique for the synthesis of nanotubes by generating a glow discharge in the chamber [38]. Compared with thermal CVD, PECVD required very low temperature for the crystalline CNT synthesis [39, 40]. PECVD technique is of interest due to the fabrication of CNTs as electron emission sources. These electron emitters are very useful in displays, bioimaging, and parallel electron-beam lithography [41].

12.3 BIOIMAGING APPLICATION OF CNTS

Bioimaging is an excellent tool for obtaining high-resolution images of cells, tissues, organs, and even the whole body of animals or humans. The unique physicochemical properties of CNTs enables them to be used in different biomedical imaging applications [42]. Fluorescence emission, photoacoustic imaging, Raman imaging, magnetic resonance imaging (MRI) and bioimaging associated with drug delivery are three fundamental approaches that can be executed on CNTs to bioimaging the living cells [43]. It is reported that CNTs can be directed using an external magnetic source toward a specific organ

[44]. Surface modification and the addition of elements to CNT structure can provide a new perspective of the analysis of their performance. For example, assembling different nanoparticles, including gold nanoparticles, quantum dots, up conversion nanoparticles, PET imaging nanoprobes, and iron oxide nanoparticles into CNTs enhancing their properties and wider applications [45]. As a result, biomedical imaging offers a promising and simple platform for imaging living cells in tissue engineering and biomedical engineering.

12.3.1 FLUORESCENCE IMAGING

Fluorescence imaging has a vital role in medical diagnosis and scientific research. The insufficient penetration capacity of fluorescent light into living organism's cell walls is considered the key impediment to its further application in fluorescence imaging [46]. To solve this problem, researchers have been working on creating and implementing fluorescent probes with excitation and emission wavelengths that lie within the biologically transparent NIR window [47]. The typical NIR window is described as a range of wavelengths between 700 and 900 nm in which neither hemoglobin nor water absorbs a considerable amount of light. Various probes, such as organic dyes [48–50] and semiconducting quantum dots (QDs) [51], are currently used in this area. Recently it has been reported that light with even longer wavelengths in the range of 1,100–1,400 nm, despite being slightly absorbed by water, shows further diminished absorbance and, more notably, impressively reduced scattering by biological tissues, allowing *in vitro* assay [52] and *in vivo* fluorescence imaging with better tissue penetration and much better spatial resolutions [53–56]. SWNTs are quasi-one-dimensional quantum wires with split energy levels caused by the quantum confinement effect. The density of states (DOS) is defined by van Hoff singularities (VHSs), which define narrow energy ranges with a high DOS intensity [57]. The band-gap between each semiconducting SWNT is in the order of 1 eV, allowing for fluorescence in the NIR-II region under NIR-I stimulation [58]. Furthermore, the substantial Stoke-shift between excitation at 550–850 nm and emission at 900–1,600 nm will significantly diminish biological cell autofluorescence during imaging, improving sensitivity for *in vivo* imaging. Despite the encouraging results of employing SWNTs in NIR fluorescence, the low QY of SWNTs made imaging challenging and remained the key challenge in developing SWNTs for *in vivo* imaging. Although the modified SWNTs had a high QY, they appeared to be harmful to biological tissues.

Although non-covalent PEGylation of SWNTs has advantages such as enhanced water solubility and biocompatibility, it is not recommended the QY of the reaction obtained was very low.

SWNTs were used as an NIR-II contrast agent by Welsher et al. to study the anatomy of mice using a high frame rate fluorescence video imaging technique [52]. SWNTs were initially injected into the mice, and they discovered that SWNTs first entered the lungs a few seconds after injection, followed by the spleen and liver at a later time. The anatomic resolution of organs was greatly enhanced by principal component analysis (PCA). After PCA analysis of NIR-II, fluorescence images of mice with SWNT injection, even the pancreas, which could not be resolved from real-time raw images, could be distinguished. As a consequence of this study, it was discovered that when NIR-II fluorescence imaging is paired with PCA, it can act as a powerful tool for a wide range of applications, including biomedical research and disease diagnostics in the future. Robinson et al. used a new type of PEGylated amphiphilic polymer, poly(maleic anhydride-alt-1-octadecene)-polyethylene glycol (C18PMH-PEG), to prepare a well functionalized SWNTs formulation with long blood circulation (half-life of 30 h) *in vivo* to achieve ultrahigh accumulation of 30% inject dose in 4T1 murine breast cancer bearing Balb/c mice [53]. They employed high-resolution fluorescent video rate imaging with PCA for the first time to track fluorescent signals from tumors and other organs. The tumor produced a rapid fluorescent signal after only 20 sec of injection, which lasted for up to 72 h.

In 2009, Dai and workers devised a coating exchange approach for developing biocompatible SWNTs with good QY [59]. The SWNTs were unbundled and solubilized in a sodium cholate solution, which was then substituted in their method with phospholipid–PEG (PL–PEG). The modified method is more effective and efficient than the traditional method, involving sonicating SWNTs in PL-PEG solutions for 15 min. For the first time, *in vivo* whole-body, NIR-II fluorescence imaging of mice with intravenously (i.v.) injected SWNTs was achieved using PEGylated SWNTs with high QY obtained by this method. In addition, after injecting SWNTs, high-resolution *in vivo* intravital microscopy imaging was achieved after injecting SWNTs, revealing tiny tumor arteries behind the thick skin.

Hong et al. introduced a dynamic contrast-enhanced NIR-II imaging technique for arterial and venous vessels imaging in mice in addition to tumor imaging [60]. One disadvantage of this approach is the generation of SWNTs with different chiralities. As a result, only a tiny portion of fabricated SWNTs are stimulated by the laser to produce fluorescence, while the remainder is not in resonance with the excitation laser wavelength and hence cannot give any images. Therefore, using chirality-purified SWNTs for NIR-II fluorescence imaging can reduce the amount of CNTs needed for bioimaging. For the purification and isolation of chiral SWNTs from a racemic mixture, various procedures such as dielectrophoresis, density gradient centrifugation [61], DNA wrapping chromatography [62], and gel filtration [63–65] are widely used. Diao et al. proposed a simple gel separation approach to enrich semiconducting (12,1) and (11,3) SWNTs with similar resonance absorption at 808 nm and emission at 1,200 nm based on this concept. The chiral separated SWNTs showed 5 times more fluorescence intensity under the resonant excitation at 808 nm than unseparated SWNTs on a per mass basis, resulting in a substantial reduction in the SWNT injection dosage required for *in vivo* imaging [66].

Welsher and his team developed NIR fluorescent SWCNTs for biological imaging applications. They showed negligible autofluorescence and profound tissue penetration capability in the NIR region beyond 1 μM [68]. They subsequently sonicated the SWCNTs with sodium cholate and phospholipid–polyethylene glycol to produce phospholipid–polyethylene glycol coated nanotubes via a surfactant exchange process. The exchange-SWNT conjugates were found to be highly fluorescent, biocompatible, and capable of *in vivo* imaging. The conjugates were successfully used as an NIR photoluminescence contrast agent for cell imaging, tumor vessel identification, and *in vivo* NIR photoluminescence imaging utilizing high-resolution intravital microscopy in live mice. Imaging tumor vessels in mice beneath thick skin was achieved by injecting a reasonably low dose (17 mg/l) of modified SWCNTs [67]. Hong et al. developed high-pressure CO conversion (HiPCO) single-walled fluorescent carbon nanotube IRDye800 conjugates (SWNT–IRDye800) and investigated their potential as a brain imaging agent in the visible and near-infrared regions. They have allowed SWNT–IRDye800 to penetrate into the skull of mouse for imaging the cerebral vasculature without craniotomy. It is a non-invasive brain imaging technique with high spatial resolution. The non-invasive and dynamic imaging ability of SWNT–IRDye800 conjugate is particularly useful for assessing a blood flow anomaly in the cerebral artery of a mouse and to observe biological processes in the brain at the molecular level. Yudasaka and his team fabricated PMB-CNTs by covering CNTs with a biocompatible polymer called poly(2-methacryloyloxyethyl phosphorylcholine-co-n-butyl methacrylate (PMB), which has unique NIR-PL imaging ability. The synthesized PMB-CNTs have a non-invasive and high resolution imaging ability towards brown fat. They injected PMB-CNTs into the mice, and the selective imaging of capillary endothelial cells of adipose tissue was performed [69].

Danné and his group developed luminescent SWCNTs suspended in phospholipid polyethylene glycol (pl-PEG) for imaging brain tissues. As a bioimaging agent, pl-PEG-coated SWCNTs were permitted to penetrate into the lateral cerebroventricles of rat brain [70]. This method helps to reduce tissue inflammation and conserves the most native structure and integrity of brain tissues. Singh et al. designed MWCNTs from chickpea peel at 400°C through the pyrolysis method. They exhibited 7.0 nm diameter and 0.28 nm graphitic spacing. The fabricated MWCNTs with a consistent fluorescence was developed as a potential candidate for bioimaging in the cytoplasm of 22RV1 human prostate carcinoma cell line without exerting any sign of cytotoxicity. The MWCNTs also exhibited remarkable cytocompatibility in human immortalized prostate epithelial RWPE1 cells [71]. For multimodal bioimaging applications, Choi and co-workers designed a heterostructured complex combining magnetic iron oxide nanoparticles and NIR-SWNT. With a magnetic relaxation time scale ratio (T1/T2) of around 12, this compound is super magnetic in nature and exhibits a magnetic moment larger than pure Fe_2O_3. Imaging of macrophage cells that engulf the DNA-wrapped complexes were carried out using both MRI and NIR methods. Thus SWNT/iron oxide found application as a multimodal biomedical imaging agent. SWNT/iron oxide can be further functionalized using monoclonal antibodies to image cancer cells and atherosclerotic regions [72]. Mandal et al. designed phospholipid-polyethylene glycol-encapsulated p-nitroaryl functionalized SWCNTs that can be used in bioimaging. The developed SWCNTs allowed for high signal-to-noise ratio imaging in live brain tissues using ultra-low excitation intensities. Their NIR emissions of 1,160 nm assure that they will perform well *in vivo* fluorescence imaging experiments [73].

SWCNT coupled M13 bacteriophage carrying modified peptide binding to the SPARC protein was developed by Ceppi et al. for the fluorescence imaging of debulking surgery in an ovarian cancer mouse model [74]. The developed system allows detection in the NIR region with a pixel-limited resolution of 200 μm, indicating potential fluorescence imaging applications for guided surgeries in ovarian cancer patients. SWCNTs functionalized with amphiphilic C18-alkylated polymer combined with bright perylene bisimide fluorophores was fabricated by Katharina et al. and used for *in vitro* heLa cells imaging applications [75]. The polymer coating enables increased water solubility and biocompatibility to the SWCNTs. The potential for the developed system was confirmed from fluorescence emission of the SWCNT and the direct imaging of the cellular updake of SWCNTs through perylene bisimide by the heLa cells using microscopic studies. Park et al. used mussel adhesive proteins to modify CNTs for targeted imaging of malignancies in tissues. To achieve NIR fluorescence imaging, they chose CNTs combined with the ZW800 NIR fluorophore [76]. The proposed CNT-protein probes bind to a specific tumor in less than an hour and are easily eliminated through urine, indicating that they could be used for tumor imaging and detection. They investigated the effect of the CNT-NIRF hybrid carriers by intravenously injected on a specific tumor in mice, and the bioimaging was done through NIR fluorescence as given in Figure 12.1. Kaeriyama et al. introduced the folic acid (FA) treated carboxyl functional SWCNTs containing a copolymer poly(para-phenylene) (PPP) with polystyrene (PSt) and poly(ε-caprolactone) (PCL) side chains (PPP-g-PSt-PCL) through π-π stacking reactions. The developed system exhibits excellent potential to imaging HeLa cells [77].

Hassan et al. proposed a new approach for *in vivo* imaging of the biodistribution of SWCNTs labeled recombinant thermo-stable Luciola cruciate luciferase (LcL) [78]. For the first time, they showed that the strong binding of LcL to the SWCNTs helped for the imaging applications. Furthermore, they demonstrated that drug-loaded CNTs did not interfere with the chemiluminescence of LcL. Banerjee and group have fabricated a highly versatile multi-functional nanosystem for both *in vitro* and *in vivo* fluorescence bioimaging [79]. They have modified CNTS with combined covalently assembling Fe_3O_4 nanoparticles, polyethylene glycol (PEG), and fluorescein isothiocyanate (FITC) dye. Confocal microscopic examination during *in vitro* imaging revealed that the Fe_3O_4-PEG-FITC-CNT nanosystem was more concentrated at the perinuclear area of MCF7 cells than free FITC. Furthermore, the CNT nanosystem showed no signs of toxicity on cell growth. As a result, this system provides *In vitro* multi-components based enhanced FITC cellular uptake, site-specific targeting capability, and zero toxicity. Nagai and his group reported synthesis of brighter NIR emitting PNIPAM/lf-SWCNTs from *N*-isopropyl acrylamide (NIPAM) and local functionalized SWCNTs (lf-SWCNTs) [80]. They compared *E*11*, *E*112* and *E*11 excitation using radical polymer grafting on the SWCNT surface. The micelle polymerization during the process facilitates the formation of emissive sp^3 defects through local functionalization (If). A cross-linker added during the process allows the formation of polymer cross-linking, which resulted in the development of a very stable coating layer on the SWCNT surface, with a bright PL emission. The obtained PNIPAM/lf-SWCNTs was made into a biocompatible polymer gel and biological imaging applications were developed.

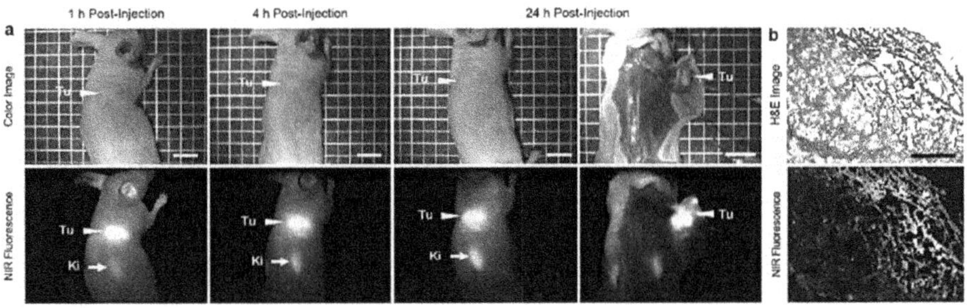

FIGURE 12.1 *In vivo* tumor targeting performance of the CNT-NIRF hybrid carriers for 24 h after injection. (a) Mouse was injected intravenously with CNT-NIRF hybrid carriers 24 h before imaging and resection. The arrowhead and arrow show tumor tissue (TU) and kidneys (Ki), respectively; and (b) H&E histology and NIR fluorescence microscopy of resected tumor targeted by CNT-NIRF hybrid carriers at 24 h after injection.

Source: Reprinted with permission [76], Copyright 2019, Springer.

12.3.2 Photoacoustic Imaging

Photoacoustic imaging (PAI) is a more advanced imaging technique frequently employed in the biological field [81–83]. In this imaging technique, a laser beam is allowed to incident on either endogenous molecules or contrast agents in the biological sample, followed by the light absorption by these molecules, resulting in the formation of heat energy. This causes a transient thermoelastic expansion within the molecules and leads to wideband ultrasonic emission. An ultrasound microphone can detect the sound emitted by the molecules to construct 2D or 3D images. Thus compared with traditional imaging techniques, PA imaging detects sound rather than light for bioimaging applications. This approach has various advantages over other conventional methods, including significantly enhanced tissue penetration and superior spatial resolutions, by avoiding absorbance and scattering of the emission light in fluorescence imaging, respectively. Nanomaterials with a high absorbance in the NIR region can be employed as contrast agents in PA imaging [84–86]. As a result of the strong NIR absorbance, both MWNTs and SWNTs can act as excellent photothermal as well as an ideal contrast agent in PA imaging [87–89].

Photoacoustic microscopy was used by Avti et al. to detect, map, and quantify the trace amounts of SWNTs for cell imaging in various histological tissue specimens. The results revealed that the noise-equivalent detection sensitivity was as low as 7 picograms, allowing for future tissue analysis applications [90]. Gambhir et al. employed RGD conjugated SWNTs as a

PA contrast agent for the first time in *in vivo* PA imaging. In their investigation, the SWNT–RGD injected group exhibited high PA signals from the tumor, whereas the pure SWNTs injected group produced only weak signals [91]. A gold layer or some organic molecules with NIR absorbance were coupled with SWNTs to enhance their absorbance in the NIR region, which can further improve the sensitivity of the photoacoustic signal of SWNTs. To improve the intrinsic PA signals of SWNTs, Zharov and co-workers developed 'golden nanotubes' (GNTs) by coating CNTs with gold [92]. The researchers employed a thin coating of gold encapsulated on the surface of SWNTs to improve their optical density in the NIR range, then combined the GNTs with antibodies that specifically target the endothelium of murine lymphatic vessels. Using extremely low laser fluency levels of a few mJ/cm^2, the generated GNTs provided increased NIR PA imaging contrast (102 fold) for targeting lymphatic arteries in mice. The lymphatic endothelial receptor was also mapped using antibody-conjugated GNTs. GNTs were later used to detect circulating tumor cells (CTCs) under PA imaging in a later study by the same group. Folate conjugated GNTs were employed as the PA contrast agent to image CTCs *in vivo* after being captured by an external magnetic field [93], by taking advantage of the strong PA signals of GNTs. Gambhir et al. [94] used π-π stacking to load indocyanine green (ICG) molecules on PEGylated SWNTs for dye enhanced PA imaging with SWNTs, which raised the optical density of the nanoprobe by 20 fold at 780 nm. When compared to the sensitivity of plain SWNTs (50 nM) in PA imaging, SWNT–ICG had sub-nanomolar detection sensitivity in PA imaging.

They also developed multiplexed PA imaging probes based on the same principle, employing PEGylated SWNTs to load five types of NIR dyes with shifted absorbance peaks [95]. The SWNTs loaded with QSY21 (SWNT–QSY) or indocyanine green (SWNT–ICG) in particular have prominent and distinct absorbance spectra, enabling sensitive multicolor *in vivo* PA imaging. As a result, CNTs with a high NIR absorbance could be useful contrast agents in photoacoustic imaging. In addition to their intrinsic optical absorbance, CNTs could be employed as a versatile nano-platform by combining them with other light-absorbing nano-structures or molecules for improved or multiplexed photoacoustic imaging. Although SWNTs are used in the majority of CNT-based photoacoustic imaging probes currently published, MWNTs should also be beneficial in this imaging modality. RGD-conjugated silica-coated gold nanorods on the surface of MWCNTs were introduced by Cui et al. for *in vivo* targeted photoacoustic imaging of gastric cancer cells [96]. The modified probe has enhanced water solubility and minimal toxicity, allowing for *in vivo* imaging of gastric cancer cells using powerful photoacoustic imaging. The binding of small optical dyes to SWCNTs (SWCNT dye) as a photoacoustic contrast for bioimaging has been described by Gambhir's group [97]. The dyes such as QSY21 (SWCNT-QSY) or indocyanine green (SWCNT-ICG coated SWCNTs shows more than 100 times phctivity otoacoustic ability in living tissues with greater selectivity and sensitivity compared to plain SWCNTs. Further conjugation of SWCNT-dye with cyclic Arg-Gly-Asp peptides to molecularly target the αvβ3 integrin enables targeted tumor imaging in mice. The comparison of results showed that the mice injected with the targeted contrast agent produced a relatively higher photoacoustic signal than in mice injected with the untargeted contrast agent. They also demonstrate the possibility of multiplexing *in vivo* experiments by carefully separating SWCNT-QSY and SWCNT-ICG photoacoustic signals from living animals.

Zerda et al. prepared cyclic ArgGly-Asp (RGD) peptides conjugated SWCNTs and employed as a contrast agent for photoacoustic tumor imaging. The proposed technique was extremely selective, with a significant photoacoustic signal after intravenous administration in mice. Raman microscopy was used to confirm the results obtained. The modified system has no negative effects on the targeted tissues and can efficiently bind with the targeted molecule. The research on malignant cells in mice implies that 3D photoacoustic images with deep penetration into the cells could be obtained [98]. A photoacoustic contrast agent based on bis-carboxylic acid derivative of indocyanine green (ICG) covalently conjugated to single-wall carbon nanotubes (ICG/SWCNT) was developed by Zanganeh and his group for the *in vivo* imaging of tumor in mouse. Separate intravenous administration of ICG and ICG/SWCNT in to mice demonstrates a 196% enhancement in photoacoustic signal strength in ICG/SWCNT and two times more postinjection contrast compared to ICG [99]. Kim et al. fabricated carbon nanotubes coated gold nanotubes (GNT), which were then conjugated with the lymphatic endothelial receptor antibody to target specific lymphatic vessels by PAI [100]. The functional composite materials displayed enhanced contrast in lymphatic arteries after NIR irradiation, which could lead to more efficient PA imaging as well as biocompatibility and lower toxicity. Furthermore, after the bio-conjugation with the antibody (anti-LYVE-1) that is specific to the lymphatic endothelial hyaluronan receptor-1 (LYVE-1), the resultant materials permitted mapping of the lymphatic endothelial cells (LECs); this could lead to a useful alternative to the current fluorescent labeling method which is limited in its *in vivo* applications due to potential cytotoxicity, immune response, photobleaching, and signal interference. Figure 12.2 represents *in vivo* molecular targeting of murine lymphatics with GNTs using PA/PT technique. Xie et al. albumin/Ce6 loaded E.B./carbon nanotube-based system (ACEC), from SWCNTs, Chlorin e6 (Ce6) and evans blue (EB). In mice, the developed method demonstrated excellent photoacoustic imaging of tumors [101].

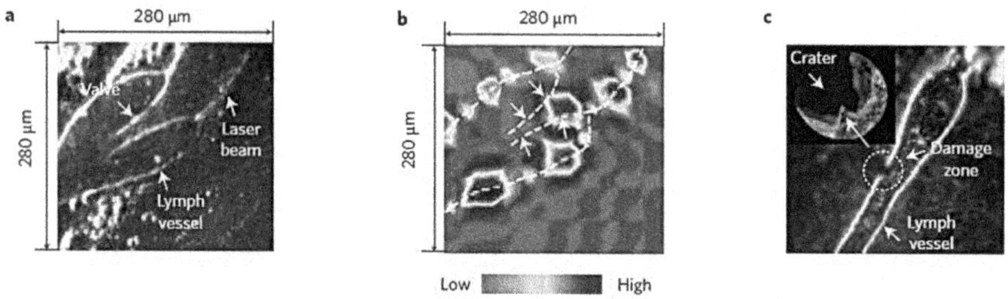

FIGURE 12.2 *In vivo* molecular targeting of murine lymphatics with GNTs guided by an integrated PA/PT technique: (a) fragment of mouse mesentery with mapping area; (b) enlarged version; and (c) laser-induced localized lymphatic wall destruction.

Source: Reprinted with permission [92], Copyright 2009, Nature.

12.3.3 MAGNETIC RESONANCE IMAGING

Magnetic resonance imaging (MRI) is a strong diagnostic tool used in the medical research field today. It is one of the most potent non-invasive imaging modalities offering high-quality images [102]. MRI is essentially a clinical imaging procedure to generate detailed images of the cells, tissues, and organs in the body. This imaging method uses a magnetic field and computer-engendered radio waves for imaging purposes. The MRI technique has developed as a powerful tool because of its exceptional temporal and spatial resolution. This technique has additional advantages of the absence of radiation exposure and the quick *in vivo* attainment of images. The extended effective imaging window also benefits the MRI tool [103, 104].

In a year, 30% of the total 60 million MRI cases conducted globally use MRI contrast agents (CA). Contrast agents play a crucial role in clinical magnetic resonance imaging to enhance illness recognition by improving sensitivity and diagnostic sureness. T1-shortening agents and T2-shortening agents are the significant constituents of contrast agents. Usually, the more prominent effect on T1 relaxation time is caused by paramagnetic chelating ions (like Mn^{2+}, Gd^{3+}, etc.) containing contrasting agents. Superparamagnetic iron oxide nanoparticle is commonly used as a T2-shortening agent

[105]. The incomparable structure and unique properties of carbon nanotubes (CNTs) contribute to the increased attraction of CNTs in biomedical fields. Carbon nanotubes have great potential for numerous applications in diagnostics and therapeutics. Nano-probes based on carbon nanotubes are extensively used and investigated in magnetic resonance imaging [106]. MRI active, carbon nanotube-based contrasting agents are fabricated mainly by incorporating paramagnetic agents like Mn^{2+}, Gd^{3+} or iron oxide nanoparticles like superparamagnetic agents within the CNT skeleton [107]. In 2005, Sitharaman et al. reported the first MRI CA based on CNT encompassing Gd^{3+} ions [108, 109]. This CA was entitled the 'Gadonanotubes' or GNTs. In GNT, ultra-short SWCNTs were internally loaded with clusters of Gd^{3+} ions. The relaxivity values exhibited by GNTs were remarkably superior to other CAs used clinically. GNTs show outstanding performance as T1-weighted CAs. In addition to this, the cluster of Gd^{3+} ions contained within the CNTs are so tightly held and do not get out under any biological circumstances [110]. This property is essential for the clinical application of GNTs because of the extreme toxicity of free Gd^{3+} ions [111]. Better sensitivity and spatial resolution of GNTs for cellular imaging and visualization in clinical MRI systems at 9.4 T were reported because of their extremely large transverse relaxations. Further studies revealed the application of GNTs for labeling macrophage cells [112], mesenchymal stem cells [113], and HeLa cells [114]. GNTs are restricted in the cell cytoplasm in all these labeling processes, distributing almost 109 Gd^{3+} ions for each cell. In an alternative study, water-soluble ser-GNTs were formulated by Hassan et al. via the derivatization of GNTs with substituents of serine amino acid [115]. Ser-GNTs find excellent application in intra-cellular magnetic labeling of human breast cancer cells with no cytotoxicity or morphological effects.

A further advanced study by Law et al. successfully fabricated GNTs of ultra-short SWCNTs loaded with different Gd chelate compounds such as $Gd(acetylacetone)_3 \cdot 2H_2O$, $Gd(hexafluoroacetylacetone)_3 \cdot 2H_2O$, and $Gd(2,2,6,6,\text{-tetramethyl-}3,5\text{-heptanedione})_3$ [116]. In this way, three novel Gd-based CAs were formulated. This study was carried out to observe the relation between nanoconfinement and relaxivity of Gd-based CA for MRI. The number of water molecules coordinatively bonded to the central Gd^{3+} ion is represented by a value called q, which is directly related to the relaxivity of the CA. A better value for q was obtained for free non-chelated Gd^{3+} ions than chelated ones. Crucial information regarding the structure around Gd^{3+} ions encapsulated within ultra-short CNTs was obtained from the X-ray absorption spectroscopic study by Ma et al. [117]. The exceptional performance of Gd^{3+} ion encapsulated GNT than chelated Gd-based GNT is due to the higher q value and the shorter Gd-H bond length. Another attempt to prepare an extremely water-dispersible GNT CA was made by fabricating a high-performing, functionalized Gd^{3+} ion-containing GNT by a surfactant-free strategy. This GNT developed by Gizzatov et al. was proven effective for labeling stem cells [118]. The issue with the leaking of Gd^{3+} ions under acidic functionalization conditions has been addressed by encapsulating chelates like Gd(acetylacetone)$_3$·2H$_2$O or Gd(hexafluoroacetylacetone)$_3$·2H$_2$O in the ultra-short SWCNTs followed by the surface functionalization of the resulting product. Nanoparticles of Gd_2O_3 were used to catalyze the chemical vapor deposition strategy preparation of a Gd-SWCNT CA. The developed CA was used for T1-weighted MRI and this was demonstrated by Sitharaman and co-workers [119, 120]. The final product has 6.2% Gd^{3+} content and better dispersion in water. It was obtained by a phospholipid polymer-based non-covalent functionalization. The usefulness of the CA for cell labeling was tested on the NIH/3T3 fibroblast cells. When compared with the phantom studies of the unlabeled cells, the signal intensity at a T1 weighted MRI showed four times increase for the labeled cells at 3 T. Avti et al. has come up with a continuation study assessing the *in vivo* pharmacokinetics of the synthesized Gd-SWCNTs after the intravenous administration of non-toxic amount into male Wistar rats [121]. In the rats, the uptake of Gd-SWCNT was shown in the liver, spleen, lungs, brain, and kidneys. The assessment using bright-field optical microscopy revealed the exit of Gd-SWCNT materials after 24 h from the circulatory system and accumulation in various other organs. The genetic and molecular response study also confirmed the complete removal of Gd-SWCNT materials within 10 days. But, in all the studies of Gd-SWCNTs discussed above, there is no sign of their *in vivo* MRI data.

Marangon et al. reported the diethylenetriaminepentaacetic dianhydride (DTPA) functionalized oxidized MWCNTs, followed by chelation to Gd^{3+} [122]. About 2.5 mg/kg and 12.5 mg/kg doses of this CA were administered intravenously on female C57/Bl6 mice, and the *in vivo* MRI studies were conducted. The massive uptake of the Gd-based CA was seen in the MRI studies on the bladder of the mice, followed by its spleen and liver after five hours and this MRI contrast signal enhancement is shown in Figure 12.3. The renal clearance of a substantial amount of Gd-DTPA functionalized MWCNTs was confirmed by various studies, including MRI. Studies on CAs developed for MRI by encompassing nanoparticles of superparamagnetic iron oxide in CNTs were also reported. Wu et al. investigated the *in situ* packing of Fe_3O_4 on the MWCNT surface [123]. Using diethylene glycol and diethanolamine solvents, a solvothermal strategy was adopted to prepare MWCNT/Fe_3O_4

composite material as a water-soluble CA At room temperature, the developed CA show superparamagnetic features and a higher T2-relaxivity value. In the MWCNT/Fe_3O_4 system, about 41.3% covered Fe_3O_4. The *in vitro* studies using MWCNT/Fe_3O_4 hybrid were done in both human and mice cells by Al Faraj et al. [124, 125]. The results produced excellent cell viability. The *in vivo* MRI studies were conducted in mice via i.v. administration of the MWCNT/Fe_3O_4 hybrid and exhibited uptake in the liver, spleen, and lungs. The treatment of SWCNTs with H_2SO_4 and HNO_3 produced oxidized nanotubes. The oxidized SWCNTs were incorporated with iron salts after suspending them in water. These Fe-labeled SWCNT materials were efficient MRI CA and drug-delivering magnetic agents. Peci et al. developed a theranostic agent comprising MWCNTs encapsulated with iron nanowire as a ferromagnetic material [126]. The Fe-MWCNTs with high coercivity were used as magnetic hyperthermia agents for cancer treatment. The metallic impurity in CNTs was utilized for T2-weighted MRI in a study conducted by Al Faraj and co-workers [127]. CNTs, when modified appropriately, can be used as CAs for T1 and T2-weighted MRI. For T2-weighted MRI, the metallic impurities in CNTs can be utilized for MR contrast. Therefore, no additional treatments are required. MRI is a more relevant clinical imaging technique that provides whole-body imaging deprived of depth limit. The MRI with CNTs, upon integration with other imaging methodologies, will offer new prospects in bioimaging.

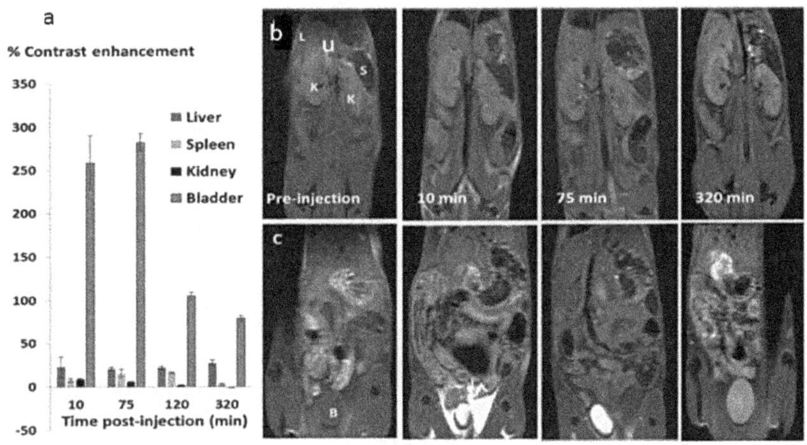

FIGURE 12.3 (a) A comparison of the MRI contrast improvement in liver, spleen, kidneys, and bladder before and after intravenous injection of Gd-CNT 5 (5 mg/mL, 100 μL); (b) and (c) MR portions indicating liver (L), spleen (S) and kidney (K), or bladder (B) at different-time points prior and post Gd-CNTs injection.

Source: Reprinted with permission [122], Copyright 2014, Wiley.

12.3.4 RAMAN IMAGING

Raman scattering is a process of photon scattering. Resonance Raman scattering is the Raman scattering with more significant scattering efficiency. The intrinsic signals of Raman scattering of molecules are generally weaker than the enhanced signals resulting from enhancement mechanisms like surface-enhanced Raman scattering (SERS) [128]. Usually, SWCNTs possess various Raman peaks corresponding to carbon atoms vibration in the radical and tangential directions. The SWCNT Raman peaks include the radical breathing mode (RBM) at 100 cm^{-1} to 300 cm^{-1} and the tangential G band at approximately 1,580 cm^{-1}. The resonance Raman scattering of SWCNTs depends on their diameters and chirality axes [129].

In 2005, the characteristic Raman properties of SWCNTs were utilized for living cell imaging by Heller et al. for the first time [130]. Heller and co-workers wrapped SWCNTs with DNA nucleotides and used them for live-cell tracking. Inside live 3T3 cells, the SWCNTs RBM peak was recorded under a 785 nm laser excitation. Strong Raman scattering signals were obtained for SWCNTs without any substantial quenching. This property allows SWCNTs to use for long-term biological sample tracking [131]. Lamprecht et al. took advantage of the characteristic Raman G band of CNTs for subsequent mapping and tracking the intracellular CNTs supply in carcinoma cells after targeted drug transport [132]. The significance of Raman spectroscopy for live-cell bioimaging was highlighted by Kang et al. [133]. This work utilized confocal Raman imaging of more incredible speed for studying the SWCNTs cellular uptake. The *in vivo* Raman imaging studies were carried out by taking Raman images of mice tumors, and it was demonstrated by Zavaleta et al. using conjugated SWCNTs with targeting ligands [134]. The raster-scan images of the mice tumors are given in Figure 12.4. Raman scattering exhibited sharp peaks with diverse locations for different molecules. This feature is perfect for imaging [135, 136].

Appropriate alterations in the Raman G band peaks of SWCNTs were done by changing the ^{12}C isotope to ^{13}C [137]. Liu et al. acknowledged the multiplexed Raman imaging of live cells for the first time [138]. Different targeting ligand conjugated three different SWCNTs with varying ratios of ^{13}C doping, and diverse Raman G band peaks were used for corresponding cell line recognition in this study. The same research group carried out a study on the five color Raman imaging of cells [108]. The five-color Raman imaging of cells was achieved by conjugating SWCNTs with diverse targeting groups. Amongst all single molecules, the SWCNTs are likely to show robust intrinsic Raman signals. But the Raman image acquisition time is longer for the SWCNTs labeled biological samples. The Raman signals of Raman tags greatly influence the Raman image acquisition time. The effective shortening in the imaging time can be achieved by improving the Raman signals of those Raman tags. Enhancement in the Raman signals of SWCNTs was done using SERS by coating the nanotube surface with nanoparticles of noble metals [98, 100]. The noble metal nanoparticles can be deposited on the nanotube surface by diverse methods. A widely used strategy is on-substrate deposition [67]. The incorporation of gold nanoparticles to covalently functionalized SWCNTs will result in the weakening of Raman signals because of the impairment of nanotube structure caused by functionalization [31].

A new SERS nanoprobe based on non-covalently functionalized SWCNTs coated with noble metals was reported recently by Wang et al. for the biological samples Raman imaging [19]. In the solution, SWCNTs coated with gold particles showed outstanding SERS effects, achieving strong Raman scattering and shorter imaging time. The specific cell labeling and Raman imaging were done by conjugating the gold nanoparticle-covered SWCNTs with folic acid. In this way, quick mapping of bio-samples can be done. Compared to organic Raman dyes, SWCNTs possess numerous advantages as an innovative Raman tag. SWCNTs provide simple Raman peaks which are intense and narrow. The SWCNT Raman signals are strong and do not undergo quenching or bleaching. This feature allows their long-term usage for both imaging and tracking. The Raman shifts can be introduced by variations in isotope compositions within SWCNTs. This technique enables multiplexed Raman imaging. SERS method can be integrated into the resonance Raman signals of CNTs to enhance the sensitivity of detection and reduce the time for imaging.

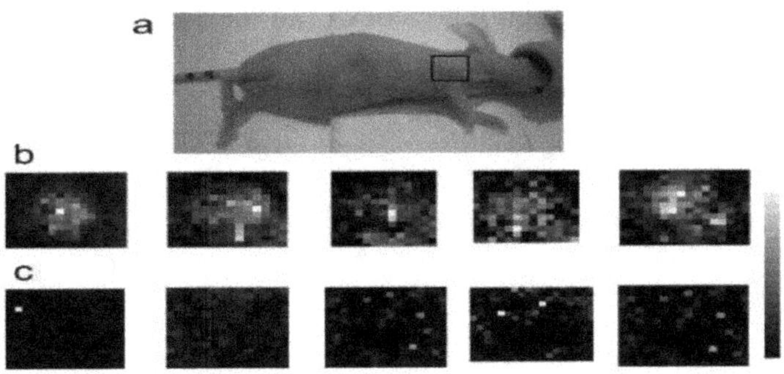

FIGURE 12.4 (a) Digital image of the mice with Raman spectroscopically scanned tumor area is highlighted in the black box. Raman mapped images of the tumor area from mice at different time intervals after injection of (b) conjugated SWCNTs with targeting ligands; and (c) plain SWCNTs.

Source: Reprinted with permission [134], Copyright 2008, ACS.

12.4 CONCLUSIONS

Presently, CNTs are widely used for the real-time and high-resolution imaging of living cells based on NIR-II fluorescence, photoacoustic imaging, Raman imaging, and magnetic resonance imaging. Most of the synthetic procedures for CNTs result in very low QY, but it can be increased by modifying the synthetic conditions and introducing chiral SWCNTs. The CNT-based NIR-II fluorescence imaging has exhibited more significant advantages over other methods due to their *in vivo* optical imaging with deep tissue penetration, negligible photon scattering, and excellent image resolution. The scattering cross-section of SWNTs is large, and they exhibit strong resonance Raman scattering. Raman imaging with SWNT-probes has excellent sensitivity and is photobleaching and quenching resistant. Noble metal coated SWNTs provide considerably amplified Raman signals owing to the SERS effect, allowing for much faster Raman mapping. Even with SERS augmentation, conventional Raman mapping takes around 10 min. to acquire a Raman image. Instrument advancements may be required to make SWNT-based Raman imaging a practical tool in biological research. Furthermore, using chirality-purified SWNTs with the majority of nanotubes in resonance with the excitation laser would considerably boost the Raman signals of SWNTs per mass. Other CNT-based imaging approaches, such as PA imaging, MR imaging, have also demonstrated considerable promise in biological imaging.

However, further research is needed to increase the QY, biocompatibility, and biodegradation ability of CNTs. The development of SWNTs with purified single chirality and distinct excitation and emission wavelengths can improve imaging efficiency. The long-term toxicity of CNTs further limits their applications in living cells. CNTs with proper surface functionalization have been reported to be non-toxic *in vitro* and *in vivo* and may be eliminated from animals gradually via renal and/or fecal excretion pathways. More investigation is needed for the development of CNTs for real *in vivo* therapeutic applications.

KEYWORDS

- **bioimaging**
- **carbon nanotubes**
- **fluorescence imaging**
- **magnetic resonance imaging**
- **photoacoustic imaging**
- **Raman imaging**

REFERENCES

1. Jorio, A., Dresselhaus, G., & Dresselhaus, M. S., (2008). Carbon nanotubes. *Top. Appl. Phys.,* 101.
2. Tuaev, X., Paraknowitsch, J. P., Illgen, R., Thomas, A., & Strasser, P., (2012). Nitrogen-doped coatings on carbon nanotubes and their stabilizing effect on Pt nanoparticles. *Phys. Chem. Chem. Phys., 14,* 6444–6447.
3. Hatton, R. A., Miller, A. J., & Silva, S. R. P., (2008). Carbon nanotubes: A multi-functional material for organic optoelectronics. *J. Mater. Chem., 18,* 1183–1192.
4. Wen, J., Xu, Y., & Li, H., (2015). Recent applications of carbon nanomaterials in fluorescence biosensing and bioimaging. *Chem. Commun., 51,* 11346–11358.
5. Lota, G., Fic, K., & Frackowiak, E., (2011). Carbon nanotubes and their composites in electrochemical applications. *Energy Environ. Sci., 4,* 1592–1605.
6. Liang, C., Diao, S., Wang, C., Gong, H., Liu, T., Hong, G., Shi, X., et al., (2014). Tumor metastasis inhibition by imaging-guided photothermal therapy with single-walled carbon nanotubes. *Adv. Mater., 56,* 5646–5652.
7. Harrison, B. S., & Atala, A., (2007). Carbon nanotube applications for tissue engineering. *Biomaterials, 28,* 344–352.
8. Hammel, E., Tang, X., Trampert, M., Schmitt, T., Mauthner, K., Eder, A., & Pötschke, P., (2004). Carbon nanofibers for composite applications. *Carbon, 42,* 1153–1158.
9. Iizumi, Y., Yudasaka, M., Kim, J., Sakakita, H., Takeuchi, T., & Okazaki, T., (2018). Oxygen-doped carbon nanotubes for near-infrared fluorescent labels and imaging probes. *Sci. Rep., 8,* 6272.
10. Boghossian, A. A., Zhang, J., Barone, P. W., Reuel, N. F., Kim, J. H., Heller, D. A., Ahn, J. H., et al., (2011). Near-infrared fluorescent sensors based on single-walled carbon nanotubes for life sciences applications. *Chem. Sus. Chem., 4,* 848–863.
11. Shi, W., & Plata, D. L., (2018). Vertically aligned carbon nanotubes: Production and applications for environmental sustainability. *Green. Chem., 20,* 5245–5260.
12. Arnold, M. S., Green, A. A., Hulvat, J. F., Stupp, S. I., & Hersam, M. C., (2006). Sorting carbon nanotubes by electronic structure using density differentiation. *Nat. Nanotechnol., 1,* 60–65.
13. Zhou, J., Wang, C., Qian, Z., Chen, C., Ma, J., Du, G., Chen, J., & Feng, H., (2012). Highly efficient fluorescent multi-walled carbon nanotubes functionalized with diamines and amides. *J. Mater. Chem., 22,* 11912–1914.
14. Liu, Z., Tabakman, S. M., Chen, Z., & Dai, H., (2009). Preparation of carbon nanotube bioconjugates for biomedical applications. *Nat. Protoc., 4,* 1372–1381.
15. Schnorr, J. M., & Swager, T. M., (2011). Emerging applications of carbon nanotubes. *Chem. Mater., 23,* 646–657.
16. Mohammadinejad, R., Karimi, S., Iravani, S., & Varma, R. S., (2015). Plant-derived nano-structures: Types and applications. *Green Chem., 18,* 20–52.
17. Liu, Z., Tabakman, S., Welsher, K., & Dai, H., (2009). Carbon nanotubes in biology and medicine: *In vitro* and *in vivo* detection, imaging and drug delivery. *Nano Res., 2,* 85–120.
18. Das, S., Mitra, S., Khurana, S. M. P., & Debnath, N., (2013). Nanomaterials for biomedical applications. *Frontiers in Life Science, 7,* 90–98.
19. Saleh Ahammad, A. J., Lee, J.-J., & Rahman, M. A. (2009). Electrochemical sensors based on carbon nanotubes. *Sensors, 9,* 2289–2319.

20. Nalwa, H. S., (2014). A special issue on reviews in biomedical applications of nanomaterials, tissue engineering, stem cells, bioimaging, and toxicity. *J. Biomed. Nanotechnol., 10*, 2421–2423.
21. Journet, C., Maser, W. K., Bernier, P., Loiseau, A., Lamy De La, C. M., Lefrant, S., Deniard, P., et al., (1997). Large-scale production of single-walled carbon nanotubes by the electric-arc technique. *Nature, 388*, 756–758.
22. Maser, W. K., Muñoz, E., Benito, A. M., Martínez, M. T., De La Fuente, G. F., Maniette, Y., Anglaret, E., & Sauvajol, J. L., (1998). Production of high-density single-walled nanotube material by a simple laser ablation method. *Chem. Phys. Lett., 292,* 587–593.
23. Che, G., Lakshmi, B. B., Martin, C. R., Fisher, E. R., & Ruoff, R. S., (1998). Chemical vapor deposition-based synthesis of carbon nanotubes and nanofibers using a template method. *Chem. Mater., 10*, 260–267.
24. Cheng, H. M., Li, F., Su, G., Pan, H. Y., He, L. L., Sun, X., & Dresselhaus, M. S., (1998). Large-scale and low-cost synthesis of single-walled carbon nanotubes by the catalytic pyrolysis of hydrocarbons. *Appl. Phys. Lett., 72*, 3282–3284.
25. Singh, V., Rawat, K. S., Mishra, S., Baghel, T., Fatima, S., John, A. A., Kalleti, N., et al., (2018). Biocompatible fluorescent carbon quantum dots prepared from beetroot extract for *in vivo* live imaging in *C. elegans* and BALB/c mice. *J. Mater. Chem. B, 6,* 3366–3371.
26. Lara-Romero, J., Ocampo-Macias, T., Martínez-Suarez, R., Rangel-Segura, R., López-Tinoco, J., Paraguay-Delgado, F., Alonso-Nuñez, G., et al., (2017). Parametric study of the synthesis of carbon nanotubes by spray pyrolysis of a biorenewable feedstock: α-pinene. *ACS sustain. Chem. Eng., 5*, 3890–3896.
27. Sinha, N., Ma, J., & Yeow, J. T. W., (2006). Carbon nanotube-based sensors. *J. Nanosci. Nanotechnol., 6*, 573–590.
28. Iijimaa, S., (1991). Helical microtubules of graphitic carbon. *Nature, 354*, 56–58.
29. Iijima, S., & Ichihashi, T., (1993). Single-shell carbon nanotubes of 1-nm diameter. *Nature, 363*, 603–605.
30. Vajtai, R., Wei, B. Q., & Ajayan, P. M., (2004). Controlled growth of carbon nanotubes. *Philos. Trans. R Soc. Lond. Ser. A Math. Phys. Eng. Sci., 362*, 2143.
31. Yogeswaran, U., Thiagarajan, S., & Chen, S.-M. (2008). Recent updates of DNA incorporated in carbon nanotubes and nanoparticles for electrochemical sensors and biosensors. *Sensors, 8*, 7191–7212.
32. Zeng, Q., Li, Z., & Zhou, Y., (2006). Synthesis and application of carbon nanotubes. *J. Nat. Gas Chem., 15,* 235–246.
33. Khan, Z. H., Ansari, M. S., Salah, N. A., Memic, A., Habib, S., & Shahawi, M., (2011). Cobalt catalyzed-multi-walled carbon nanotubes film sensor for carbon mono-oxide gas. *Dig. J. Nanomater. Biostructures, 6*, 1947–1956.
34. Sano, N., Wang, H., Chhowalla, M., Alexandrou, I., & Amaratunga, G. A. J., (2001). Synthesis of carbon onions in water. *Nature, 414*, 506, 507.
35. Tasis, D., Tagmatarchis, N., Bianco, A., & Prato, M., (2006). Chemistry of carbon nanotubes. *Chem. Rev., 106*, 1105–1136.
36. Honda, S., Katayama, M., Lee, K. Y., Ikuno, T., Ohkura, S., Oura, K., Furuta, H., & Hirao, T., (2003). Low temperature synthesis of aligned carbon nanotubes by inductively coupled plasma chemical vapor deposition using pure methane. *J. Appl. Phys. Part 2 Lett., 42*, 441–443.

37. Daenen, M., De Fouw, R. D., Hamers, B., Janssen, P., & Schouteden, K., (2003). *The Wondrous World of Carbon Nanotubes* (pp. 1–35). Eindhoven University of Technology.
38. Bingshe, X., Li, T., Liu, X., Lin, X., & Li, J., (2007). Growth of well-aligned carbon nanotubes in a plasma system using ferrocene solution in ethanol. *Thin Solid Films, 515*, 6726–6729.
39. Point, S., Minea, T., Besland, M. P., & Granier, A., (2006). Characterization of carbon nanotubes and carbon nitride nanofibers synthesized by PECVD. *Eur. Phys. J. Appl. Phys., 34*, 157–163.
40. Teo, K. B. K., Lee, S. B., Chhowalla, M., Semet, V., Binh, V. T., Groening, O., Castignolles, M., et al., (2003). Plasma enhanced chemical vapor deposition carbon nanotubes/nanofibers-how uniform do they grow? *Nanotechnology, 14*, 204.
41. Gong, H., Peng, R., & Liu, Z., (2013). Carbon nanotubes for biomedical imaging: The recent advances. *Adv. Drug Deliv. Rev., 65*, 1951–1963.
42. Tong, L., Liu, Y., Dolash, B. D., Jung, Y., Slipchenko, M. N., Bergstrom, D. E., et al., (2012). Label-free imaging of semiconducting and metallic carbon nanotubes in cells and mice using transient absorption microscopy. *Nat. Nanotechnol., 7*, 56–61.
43. De La Zerda, A., Zavaleta, C., Keren, S., Vaithilingam, S., Bodapati, S., Liu, Z., et al., (2008). Carbon nanotubes as photoacoustic molecular imaging agents in living mice. *Nat. Nanotechnol., 3*, 557–562.
44. Li, J., Chang, X., Chen, X., Gu, Z., Zhao, F., Chai, Z., et al., (2014). Toxicity of inorganic nanomaterials in biomedical imaging. *Biotechnol. Adv., 32*, 727–743.
45. He, X., Gao, J., Gambhir, S. S., & Cheng, Z., (2010). Near-infrared fluorescent nanoprobes for cancer molecular imaging: Status and challenges. *Trends Mol. Med., 16*, 574–583.
46. Chance, B., (1998). Near-infrared images using continuous, phase-modulated, and pulsed light with quantitation of blood and blood oxygenation. In: Alfano, R. R., (ed.), *Advances in Optical Biopsy and Optical Mammography* (pp. 29–45).
47. Ishizawa, T., Fukushima, N., Shibahara, J., Masuda, K., Tamura, S., Aoki, T., Hasegawa, K., et al., (2009). Real-time identification of liver cancers by using indocyanine green fluorescent imaging. *Cancer, 115*, 2491–2504.
48. Sekijima, M., Tojimbara, T., Sato, S., Nakamura, M., Kawase, T., Kai, K., Urashima, Y., et al., (2004). An intraoperative fluorescent imaging system in organ transplantation. *Transplant. Proc., 36*, 2188–2190.
49. Morimoto, S., (2007). *In-vivo* imaging of tumors with protease activated near-infrared fluorescent probes. *Tanpakushitsu Kakusan Koso, Protein, Nucleic Acid, Enzyme, 52*, 1774–1775.
50. Kim, S., Lim, Y. T., Soltesz, E. G., De Grand, A. M., Lee, J., Nakayama, A., Parker, J. A., et al., (2004). Near-infrared fluorescent type II quantum dots for sentinel lymph node mapping. *Nat. Biotechnol., 22*, 93–97.
51. Iizumi, Y., Okazaki, T., Ikehara, Y., Ogura, M., Fukata, S., & Yudasaka, M., (2013). Immunoassay with single-walled carbon nanotubes as near-infrared fluorescent labels. *ACS Appl. Mater. Interfaces*, 7665–7670.
52. Welsher, K., Sherlock, S. P., & Dai, H., (2011). Deep-tissue anatomical imaging of mice using carbon nanotube fluorophores in the second near-infrared window. *Proc. Natl. Acad. Sci., 108*, 8943–8948.

53. Robinson, J. T., Hong, G., Liang, Y., Zhang, B., Yaghi, O. K., & Dai, H., (2012). *In vivo* fluorescence imaging in the second near-infrared window with long circulating carbon nanotubes capable of ultrahigh tumor uptake. *J. Am. Chem. Soc., 134*, 10664–10669.
54. Lim, Y. T., Kim, S., Nakayama, A., Stott, N. E., Bawendi, M. G., & Frangioni, J. V., (2003). Selection of quantum dot wavelengths for biomedical assays and imaging. *Mol. Imaging, 2*, 50–64.
55. Diao, S., Hong, G., Robinson, J. T., Jiao, L., Antaris, A. L., Wu, J. Z., Choi, C. L., & Dai, H., (2012). Chirality enriched (12,1) and (11,3) single-walled carbon nanotubes for biological imaging. *J. Am. Chem. Soc., 134,* 16971–16974.
56. Yi, H., Ghosh, D., Ham, M. H., Qi, J., Barone, P. W., Strano, M. S., & Belcher, A. M., (2012). M13 phage-functionalized single-walled carbon nanotubes as nanoprobes for second near-infrared window fluorescence imaging of targeted tumors. *Nano Lett., 12,* 1176–1183.
57. Kuzmany, H., Burger, B., Fally, M., Rinzler, A. G., & Smalley, R. E., (1998). Effect of dimensionality in polymeric fullerenes and single-wall nanotubes. *Physica B, 244,* 186–191.
58. Jorio, A., Pimenta, M., Souza, F. A., Saito, R., Dresselhaus, G., & Dresselhaus, M., (2003). Characterizing carbon nanotube samples with resonance Raman scattering. *New J. Phys., 5*, 139.1–139.17.
59. Welsher, K., Liu, Z., Sherlock, S. P., Robinson, J. T., Chen, Z., Daranciang, D., & Dai, H., (2009). A route to brightly fluorescent carbon nanotubes for near-infrared imaging in mice. *Nat. Nanotechnol., 4*, 773–780.
60. Hong, G., Lee, J. C., Robinson, J. T., Raaz, U., Xie, L., Huang, N. F., Cooke, J. P., & Dai, H., (2012). Multifunctional *in vivo* vascular imaging using near-infrared II fluorescence. *Nat. Med., 18,* 1841–1846.
61. Ghosh, S., Bachilo, S. M., & Weisman, R. B., (2010). Advanced sorting of single-walled carbon nanotubes by nonlinear density-gradient ultracentrifugation. *Nat. Nanotechnol., 5*, 443–450.
62. Tu, X., Manohar, S., Jagota, A., & Zheng, M., (2009). DNA sequence motifs for structure-specific recognition and separation of carbon nanotubes. *Nature, 460*, 250–253.
63. Liu, H., Nishide, D., Tanaka, T., & Kataura, H., (2011). Large-scale single-chirality separation of single-wall carbon nanotubes by simple gel chromatography. *Nat. Commun., 2*, 1–8.
64. Miyata, Y., Shiozawa, K., Asada, Y., Ohno, Y., Kitaura, R., Mizutani, T., & Shinohara, H., (2011). Length-sorted semiconducting carbon nanotubes for high-mobility thin film transistors. *Nano. Res., 4*, 963–970.
65. Moshammer, K., Hennrich, F., & Kappes, M. M., (2009). Selective suspension in aqueous sodium dodecyl sulfate according to electronic structure type allows simple separation of metallic from semiconducting single-walled carbon nanotubes. *Nano Res., 2*, 599–606.
66. Diao, S., Hong, G., Robinson, J. T., Jiao, L., Antaris, A. L., Wu, J. Z., Choi, C. L., & Dai, H., (2012). Chirality enriched (12,1) and (11,3) single-walled carbon nanotubes for biological imaging. *J. Am. Chem. Soc., 134*, 16971–16974.
67. Vashist, S. K., Zheng, D., Al-Rubeaan Luong, J. H. T., & Sheu, F.-S. (2011). Advances in carbon nanotube based electrochemical sensors for bioanalytical applications. *Biotechnol. Adv., 29*, 169–188.

68. Hong, G., Diao, S., Chang, J., Antaris, A. L., Chen, C., Zhang, B., Zhao, S., et al., (2014). Through-skull fluorescence imaging of the brain in a new near-infrared window. *Nat. Photonics, 8,* 723–730.
69. Yudasaka, M., Yomogida, Y., Zhang, M., Tanaka, T., Nakahara, M., Kobayashi, N., Okamatsu-Ogura, Y., et al., (2017). Near-Infrared photoluminescent carbon nanotubes for imaging of brown fat. *Scientific Reports, 7,* 1.
70. Danné, N., Godin, A. G., Gao, Z., Varela, J. A., Groc, L., Lounis, B., & Cognet, L., (2017). Comparative analysis of photoluminescence and upconversion emission from individual carbon nanotubes for bioimaging applications. *ACS Photonics, 5,* 359–364.
71. Singh, V., Chatterjee, S., Palecha, M., Sen, P., Ateeq, B., & Verma, V., (2020). Chickpea peel waste as sustainable precursor for synthesis of fluorescent carbon nanotubes for bioimaging application. *Carbon Lett., 31,* 117–123.
72. Choi, J. H., Nguyen, F. T., Barone, P. W., Heller, D. A., Moll, A. E., Patel, D., Boppart, S. A., & Strano, M. S., (2007). Multimodal biomedical imaging with asymmetric single-walled carbon nanotube/iron oxide nanoparticle complexes. *Nano Lett., 7,* 861–867.
73. Mandal, A. K., Wu, X. J., Ferreira, J. S., Kim, M., Powell, L. R., Kwon, H., Groc, L., et al., (2020). Fluorescent sp(3) defect-tailored carbon nanotubes enable NIR-II single particle imaging in live brain slices at ultra-low excitation doses. *Sci. Rep., 10*(1), 5286.
74. Ceppi, L., Bardhan, N. M., Na, Y., Siegel, A., Rajan, N., Fruscio, R., Del Carmen, M. G., et al., (2019). Real-time single-walled carbon nanotube-based fluorescence imaging improves survival after debulking surgery in an ovarian cancer model. *ACS Nano, 13,* 5356–5365.
75. Huth, K., Glaeske, M., Achazi, K., Gordeev, G., Kumar, S., Arenal, R., Sharma, S. K., et al., (2018). Fluorescent polymer-single-walled carbon nanotube complexes with charged and noncharged dendronized perylene bisimides for bioimaging studies. *Small, 14,* 1800796.
76. Park, S., Kim, T., Jo, D., Jung, J. S., Jo, G., Park, Y., Kang, E. S., et al., (2019). Bioengineered short carbon nanotubes as tumor-targeted carriers for biomedical imaging. *Macromol., 27,* 833–838.
77. Ag, D., Seleci, M., Bongartz, R., Can, M., Yurteri, S., Cianga, I., Stahl, F., et al., (2013). From invisible structures of SWCNTs toward fluorescent and targeting architectures for cell imaging. *Biomacromolecules, 14,* 3532–3541.
78. El-Sayed, R., Eita, M., Barrefelt, Å., Ye, F., Jain, H., Fares, M., Lundin, A., et al., (2013). Thermostable luciferase from *Luciola* cruciate for imaging of carbon nanotubes and carbon nanotubes carrying doxorubicin using *in vivo* imaging system. *Nano Lett., 13,* 1393–1398.
79. Khandare, J. J., Jalota-Badhwar, A., Satavalekar, S. D., Bhansali, S. G., Aher, N. D., Kharas, F., & Banerjee, S. S., (2012). PEG-conjugated highly dispersive multi-functional magnetic multi-walled carbon nanotubes for cellular imaging. *Nanoscale, 4,* 837–844.
80. Nagai, Y., Nakamura, K., Yudasaka, M., Shiraki, T., & Fujigaya, T., (2020). Radical polymer grafting on the surface of single-walled carbon nanotubes enhances photoluminescence in the near-infrared region: Implications for bioimaging and biosensing. *ACS Appl. Nano Mater., 3,* 8840–8847.
81. Wang, X., Pang, Y., Ku, G., Xie, X., Stoica, G., & Wang, L. V., (2003). Noninvasive laser-induced photoacoustic tomography for structural and functional *in vivo* imaging of the brain. *Nat. Biotechnol., 21,* 803–806.

82. Ku, G., & Wang, L. V., (2005). Deeply penetrating photoacoustic tomography in biological tissues enhanced with an optical contrast agent. *Opt. Lett., 30*, 507–509.
83. Hoelen, C., De Mul, F., Pongers, R., & Dekker, A., (1998). Three-dimensional photoacoustic imaging of blood vessels in tissue. *Opt. Lett., 23*, 648–650.
84. Yang, K., Hu, L., Ma, X., Ye, S., Cheng, L., Shi, X., Li, C., et al., (2012). Multimodal imaging guided photothermal therapy using functionalized graphene nanosheets anchored with magnetic nanoparticles. *Adv. Mater., 24*, 1868–1872.
85. Ku, G., Zhou, M., Song, S., Huang, Q., Hazle, J., & Li, C., (2012). Copper sulfide nanoparticles as a new class of photoacoustic contrast agent for deep tissue imaging at 1064 nm. *ACS Nano, 6*, 7489–7496.
86. Agarwal, A., Huang, S., O'Donnell, M., Day, K., Day, M., Kotov, N., & Ashkenazi, S., (2007). Targeted gold nanorod contrast agent for prostate cancer detection by photoacoustic imaging. *J. Appl. Phys., 102*, 064701–064704.
87. Robinson, J. T., Welsher, K., Tabakman, S. M., Sherlock, S. P., Wang, H., Luong, R., & Dai, H., (2010). High performance *in vivo* near-IR (N1 μm) imaging and photothermal cancer therapy with carbon nanotubes. *Nano Res., 3*, 779–793.
88. Liu, X., Tao, H., Yang, K., Zhang, S., Lee, S. T., & Liu, Z., (2011). Optimization of surface chemistry on single-walled carbon nanotubes for *in vivo* photothermal ablation of tumors. *Biomaterials, 32*, 144–151.
89. Moon, H. K., Lee, S. H., & Choi, H. C., (2009). *In vivo* near-infrared mediated tumor destruction by photothermal effect of carbon nanotubes. *ACS Nano, 3*, 3707–3713.
90. Avti, P. K., Hu, S., Favazza, C., Mikos, A. G., Jansen, J. A., Shroyer, K. R., Wang, L. V., & Sitharaman, B., (2012). Detection, mapping, and quantification of single walled carbon nanotubes in histological specimens with photoacoustic microscopy. *PloS One, 7*, 35064.
91. De La Zerda, A., Zavaleta, C., Keren, S., Vaithilingam, S., Bodapati, S., Liu, Z., Levi, J., et al., (2008). Carbon nanotubes as photoacoustic molecular imaging agents in living mice. *Nat. Nanotechnol., 3*, 557–562.
92. Kim, J. W., Galanzha, E. I., Shashkov, E. V., Moon, H. M., & Zharov, V. P., (2009). Golden carbon nanotubes as multimodal photoacoustic and photothermal high-contrast molecular agents. *Nat. Nanotechnol., 4*, 688–694.
93. Galanzha, E. I., Shashkov, E. V., Kelly, T., Kim, J. W., Yang, L., & Zharov, V. P., (2009). *In vivo* magnetic enrichment and multiplex photoacoustic detection of circulating tumor cells. *Nat. Nanotechnol., 4*, 855–860.
94. Zerda, A. D. L., Liu, Z., Bodapati, S., Teed, R., Vaithilingam, S., Khuri-Yakub, B. T., Chen, X., et al., (2010). Ultrahigh sensitivity carbon nanotube agents for photoacoustic molecular imaging in living mice. *Nano Lett., 10*, 2168–2172.
95. De La Zerda, A., Bodapati, S., Teed, R., May, Y. S., Tabakman, S. M., Liu, Z., Khuri-Yakub, B. T., et al., (2012). Family of enhanced photoacoustic imaging agents for high-sensitivity and multiplexing studies in living mice. *ACS Nano, 6*, 4694–4701.
96. Wang, C., Bao, C., Liang, S., Zhang, L., Fu, H., Wang, Y., Wang, K., et al., (2014). HAI-178 antibody-conjugated fluorescent magnetic nanoparticles for targeted imaging and simultaneous therapy of gastric cancer. *Nanoscale Research Letters, 9*, 1.
97. Rafique, I., Kausar, A., Anwar, Z., & Muhammad, B. (2016). Exploration of epoxy resins, hardening systems, and epoxy/carbon nanotube composite designed for high performance materials: A review. *Polym. Plast. Technol. Eng.*, *55*, 312–333.

98. Nugent, J. M., Santhanam, K. S. V., Rubio, A., & Ajayan, P. M. (2001). Fast electron transfer kinetics on multiwalled carbon nanotube microbundle electrodes. *Nano Lett., 1*, 87–91.
99. Zanganeh, S., Li, H., Kumavor, P. D., Alqasemi, U., Aguirre, A., Mohammad, I., Stanford, C., et al., (2013). Photoacoustic imaging enhanced by indocyanine green-conjugated single-wall carbon nanotubes. *Journal of Biomedical Optics, 18*, 096006.
100. Prasek, J., Drbohlavova, J., Chomoucka, J., Hubalek, J., Jasek, O., Adam, V., & Kizek, R. (2011). Methods for carbon nanotubes synthesis—Review. *J. Mater. Chem., 21*, 15872–15884.
101. Xie, L., Wang, G., Zhou, H., Zhang, F., Guo, Z., Liu, C., Zhang, X., & Zhu, L., (2016). Functional long circulating single walled carbon nanotubes for fluorescent/photoacoustic imaging-guided enhanced phototherapy. *Biomaterials, 103*, 219–228.
102. Geraldes, C. F. G. C., & Laurent, S., (2009). Classification and basic properties of contrast agents for magnetic resonance imaging. *Contrast. Media Mol. Imaging, 4*, 1–23.
103. Schroeder, T., (2008). Imaging stem-cell-driven regeneration in mammals. *Nature, 453*, 345–351.
104. Herschman, H. R., (2003). Molecular imaging: Looking at problems, seeing solutions. *Science, 80*, 605–608.
105. Sitharaman, B., Kissell, K. R., Hartman, K. B., Tran, L. A., Baikalov, A., Rusakova, I., Sun, Y., et al., (2005). Superparamagnetic gadonanotubes are high-performance MRI contrast agents. *Chem., 31*, 3915–3917.
106. Wang, C., Ma, X., Ye, S., Cheng, L., Yang, K., Guo, L., Li, C., et al., (2012). Protamine functionalized single-walled carbon nanotubes for stem cell labeling and *in vivo* Raman/magnetic resonance/photoacoustic triple-modal imaging. *Adv. Funct. Mater., 22*, 2363–2375.
107. Al Faraj, A., Cieslar, K., Lacroix, G., Gaillard, S., Canet-Soulas, E., & Crémillieux, Y., (2009). *In vivo* imaging of carbon nanotube biodistribution using magnetic resonance imaging. *Nano Lett., 9,* 1023–1027.
108. Karousis, N., Tagmatarchis, N., & Tasis, D. (2010). Current progress on the chemical modification of carbon nanotubes. *Chem. Rev., 110*, 5366–5397.
109. Sitharaman, B., & Wilson, L. J., (2006). Gadonanotubes as new high-performance MRI contrast agents. *J. Nanomedicine, 1*, 291–295.
110. Hartman, K. B., Laus, S., Bolskar, R. D., Muthupillai, R., Helm, L., Toth, E., et al., (2008). Gadonanotubes as ultrasensitive pH-smart probes for magnetic resonance imaging. *Nano Lett., 8*, 415.
111. Broome, D. R., (2008). Nephrogenic systemic fibrosis associated with gadolinium-based contrast agents: A summary of the medical literature reporting. *Eur. J. Radiol., 66*, 230.
112. Tang, A. M., Ananta, J. S., Zhao, H., Cisneros, B. T., Lam, E. Y., & Wong, S. T., (2011). Cellular uptake and imaging studies of gadolinium-loaded single-walled carbon nanotubes as MRI contrast agents. *Contrast Media Mol. Imaging, 6*, 93.
113. Tran, L. A., Hernández-Rivera, M., Berlin, A. N., Zheng, Y., Sampaio, L., Bové, C., et al., (2014). The use of gadolinium-carbon nano-structures to magnetically enhance stem cell retention for cellular cardiomyoplasty. *Biomaterials, 35*, 720.

114. Holt, B. D., Law, J. J., Boyer, P. D., Wilson, L. J., Dahl, K. N., & Islam, M. F., (2015). Subcellular partitioning and analysis of Gd^{3+} loaded ultrashort single-walled carbon nanotubes. *ACS Appl. Mater. Interfaces, 7*, 14593–14602.
115. Hassan, A. A., Chan, B. T. Y., Tran, L. A., Hartman, K. B., Ananta, J. S., Mackeyev, Y., et al., (2010). Serine-derivatized gadonanotubes as magnetic nanoprobes for intracellular labeling. *Contrast Media Mol. Imaging, 5*, 34.
116. Law, J. J., Guven, A., & Wilson, L. J., (2014). Relaxivity enhancement of aquated tris(βdiketonate) gadolinium(III) chelates by confinement within ultrashort single-walled carbon nanotubes. *Contrast Media Mol. Imaging, 9*, 409–412.
117. Ma, Q., Jebb, M., Tweedle, M. F., & Wilson, L. J., (2013). The gadonanotubes: Structural origin of their high-performance MRI contrast agent behavior. *J. Mater. Chem. B, 1*, 5791.
118. Gizzatov, A., Hernández-Rivera, M., Keshishian, V., Mackeyev, Y., Law, J. J., Guven, A., et al., (2015). Surfactant-free Gd^{3+} ion-containing carbon nanotube MRI contrast agents for stem cell labeling. *Nanoscale, 7*, 12085–12091.
119. Sitharaman, B., Jacobson, B. D., Wadghiri, Y. Z., Bryant, H., & Frank, J., (2013). The magnetic, relaxometric, and optical properties of gadolinium-catalyzed single walled carbon nanotubes. *J. Appl. Phys., 113*, 134308.
120. Avti, P. K., Caparelli, E. D., & Sitharaman, B., (2013). Cytotoxicity, cytocompatibility, cell-labeling efficiency, and *in vitro* cellular magnetic resonance imaging of gadolinium catalyzed single-walled carbon nanotubes. *J. Biomed. Mater. Res. A., 101*, 3580–3591.
121. Avti, P. K., Talukdar, Y., Sirotkin, M. V., Shroyer, K. R., & Sitharaman, B., (2013). Toward single walled carbon nanotube–gadolinium complex as advanced MRI contrast agents: Pharmacodynamics and global genomic response in small animals. *J. Biomed. Mater. Res. B Appl. Biomater., 101*, 1039–1049.
122. Marangon, I., Ménard-Moyon, C., Kolosnjaj-Tabi, J., Béoutis, M. L., Lartigue, L., Alloyeau, D., et al., (2014). Covalent functionalization of multi-walled carbon nanotubes with a gadolinium chelate for efficient t1-weighted magnetic resonance imaging. *Adv. Funct. Mater., 24*, 7173–7186.
123. Wu, H., Liu, G., Zhuang, Y., Wu, D., Zhang, H., Yang, H., et al., (2011). The behavior after intravenous injection in mice of multi-walled carbon nanotube / Fe_3O_4 hybrid MRI contrast agents. *Biomaterials, 32*, 4867–4876.
124. Al Faraj, A., Shaik, A. P., & Shaik, A. S., (2014). Magnetic single-walled carbon nanotubes as efficient drug delivery nanocarriers in breast cancer murine model: Non-invasive monitoring using diffusion-weighted magnetic resonance imaging as sensitive imaging biomarker. *Int. J. Nanomedicine, 10*, 157–168.
125. Al Faraj, A., Shaik, A. S., & Al Sayed, B., (2015). Preferential magnetic targeting of carbon nanotubes to cancer sites: Non-invasive tracking using MRI in a murine breast cancer model. *Nanomed., 10*, 931–948.
126. Peci, T., Dennis, T. J. S., & Baxendale, M., (2015). Iron-filled multi-walled carbon nanotubes surface-functionalized with paramagnetic Gd (III): A candidate dual-functioning MRI contrast agent and magnetic hyperthermia structure. *Carbon, 87*, 226–232.
127. Al Faraj, A., Bessaad, A., Cieslar, K., Lacroix, G., Canet-Soulas, E., & Crémillieux, Y., (2010). Long-term follow-up of lung biodistribution and effect of instilled SWCNTs using multiscale imaging techniques. *Nanotechnology, 21*, 175103.

128. Martin, R., & Falicov, L., (1983). Resonant Raman scattering. *Light Scattering in Solids I*, 79–145. Springer.
129. Rao, A., Richter, E., Bandow, S., Chase, B., Eklund, P., Williams, K., Fang, S., et al., (1997). *Diameter-Selective Raman Scattering from Vibrational Modes in Carbon Nanotubes, 275*, 187–191.
130. Heller, D. A., Baik, S., Eurell, T. E., & Strano, M. S., (2005). Single-walled carbon nanotube spectroscopy in live cells: Towards long-term labels and optical sensors. *Adv. Mater., 17*, 2793–2799.
131. Liu, Z., Davis, C., Cai, W., He, L., Chen, X., & Dai, H., (2008). Circulation and long-term fate of functionalized, biocompatible single-walled carbon nanotubes in mice probed by Raman spectroscopy. *Proc. Natl. Acad. Sci., 105*, 1410–1415.
132. Lamprecht, C., Gierlinger, N., Heister, E., Unterauer, B., Plochberger, B., Brameshuber, M., Hinterdorfer, P., et al., (2012). Mapping the intracellular distribution of carbon nanotubes after targeted delivery to carcinoma cells using confocal Raman imaging as a label-free technique. *J. Phys. Condens. Matter, 24*, 164206–164216.
133. Heller, D., Kang, J. W., Lue, N., & Dasari, R. R., (2013). *Measuring Uptake Dynamics of Multiple, Identifiable Carbon Nanotube Species Via High-Speed Confocal Raman Imaging of Live Cells.* 223rd ECS Meeting, ECS.
134. Zavaleta, C., De La Zerda, A., Liu, Z., Keren, S., Cheng, Z., Schipper, M., Chen, X., et al., (2008). Noninvasive Raman spectroscopy in living mice for evaluation of tumor targeting with carbon nanotubes. *Nano Lett., 8*, 2800–2805.
135. Cao, Y. C., Jin, R., & Mirkin, C. A., (2002). Nanoparticles with Raman spectroscopic fingerprints for DNA and RNA detection. *Science, 297*, 1536–1540.
136. Keren, S., Zavaleta, C., Cheng, Z., De La Zerda, A., Gheysens, O., & Gambhir, S., (2008). Non-invasive molecular imaging of small living subjects using Raman spectroscopy. *Proc. Natl. Acad. Sci., 105*, 5844–5849.
137. Li, X., Tu, X., Zaric, S., Welsher, K., Seo, W. S., Zhao, W., & Dai, H., (2007). Selective synthesis combined with chemical separation of single-walled carbon nanotubes for chirality selection. *J. Am. Chem. Soc., 129*, 15770–15771.
138. Liu, Z., Li, X., Tabakman, S. M., Jiang, K., Fan, S., & Dai, H., (2008). Multiplexed multicolor Raman imaging of live cells with isotopically modified single walled carbon nanotubes. *J. Am. Chem. Soc., 130*, 13540–13541.
139. Liu, Z., Tabakman, S., Sherlock, S., Li, X., Chen, Z., Jiang, K., Fan, S., & Dai, H., (2010). Multiplexed five-color molecular imaging of cancer cells and tumor tissues with carbon nanotube Raman tags in the near-infrared. *Nano Res., 3*, 222–233.
140. Takagi, D., Homma, Y., Hibino, H., Suzuki, S., & Kobayashi, Y., (2006). Single-walled carbon nanotube growth from highly activated metal nanoparticles. *Nano Lett., 62*, 2642–2645.
141. Chen, Y. C., Young, R. J., Macpherson, J. V., & Wilson, N. R., (2011). Silver-decorated carbon nanotube networks as SERS substrates. *J. Raman Spectrosc., 42*, 1255–1262.
142. Chu, H., Wang, J., Ding, L., Yuan, D., Zhang, Y., Liu, J., & Li, Y., (2009). Decoration of gold nanoparticles on surface-grown single-walled carbon nanotubes for detection of every nanotube by surface-enhanced Raman spectroscopy. *J. Am. Chem. Soc., 131*, 14310–14316.
143. Chen, Z., Tabakman, S. M., Goodwin, A. P., Kattah, M. G., Daranciang, D., Wang, X., Zhang, G., et al., (2008). Protein microarrays with carbon nanotubes as multicolor Raman labels. *Nat. Biotechnol., 26*, 1285–1292.

144. Beqa, L., Fan, Z., Singh, A. K., Senapati, D., & Ray, P. C., (2011). Gold nano-popcorn attached SWCNT hybrid nanomaterial for targeted diagnosis and photothermal therapy of human breast cancer cells. *ACS Appl. Mater. Interfaces, 3*, 3316–3324.
145. Wang, X., Wang, C., Cheng, L., Lee, S. T., & Liu, Z., (2012). Noble metal coated single-walled carbon nanotubes for applications in surface enhanced Raman scattering imaging and photothermal therapy. *J. Am. Chem. Soc., 134*, 7414–7422.

CHAPTER 13

CNTs as Promising Adsorbents for Wastewater Purification

AVINASH V. BORGAONKAR[1] and SHITAL B. POTDAR[2]

[1]*Assistant Professor, Department of Mechanical Engineering, Pimpri Chinchwad College of Engineering (PCCOE), Pune, Maharashtra, India*

[2]*Department of Chemical Engineering, National Institute of Technology, Warangal, Telangana, India*

ABSTRACT

Water is the primary need of living organisms. However, increased population and industrialization cause severe water pollution. Hence to meet the water need, it is essential to find an environment friendly and cost-effective wastewater process. The application of nanomaterials in heavy metal and dye removal from wastewater is well-proven. Carbon-based materials have proved their ability as an adsorbent in wastewater treatment. In particular, CNTs have great potential as an adsorbent owing to their characteristic chemical, mechanical, electrical, thermal, and structural properties and its high potential in adsorption due to large specific surface area makes them more suitable as compared to conventional adsorbents in wastewater treatment. The present chapter overviews the various pollutants present in wastewater and the role of CNTs in wastewater treatment as a promising adsorbent. The mechanism of heavy metal ion absorption and the effect of adsorption are well illustrated.

Carbon Nanotubes for Biomedical Applications and Healthcare.
Chin Hua Chia, Swati Gokul Talele, Ann Rose Abraham, and A. K. Haghi, (Eds.)

13.1 INTRODUCTION

Around the world, there is still a lack of safe drinking water. The bacteria and other harmful components present in the wastewater leads to many diseases and many time results in death also. Hence to treat these bacterial disinfection processes are carried out which mainly consist of uses of ozone, chlorine or chlorine dioxide, etc. However, the use of disinfectants causes to formation of by-products (e.g., halophenols, trihalomethanes, aldehydes, and ketones) [1–3]. The chlorination process effects on taste and odor of drinking water. Therefore, after chlorination removal of generated by-products becomes essential [4]. Also water pollution causes due to other several sectors not limited to industrial sector, agricultural, and domestic sector, etc. The wastewater from industrial sector largely contains heavy metals, dyes. Beside in fact human body needs a certain amount of metal ions such as zinc, but their higher dosage often leads to many diseases like diarrhea, chronic asthma, coughing, and headaches as well as nausea, dermatitis, vomiting, liver or kidney damage, insomnia, Wilson disease and cancer [5, 6]. Hence, the removal of such metal ions from the wastewater is necessary. At present various wastewater treatment processes such as reduction, precipitation, adsorption, oxidation, and ion exchange are being used. The complete removal of these pollutants is not possible as well the cost of the process is very high. Out of these techniques, adsorption technique is most adoptable method due to its high efficiency and economic considerations [7–9]. The conventional adsorption technique possesses the ability to remove these heavy metal ions but have the limitation of low adsorption efficiency and capacity [10]. The development in wastewater process in the present time emphasizes on use of nanomaterials. The wide research is going on the use of various nanomaterials such as metals, meta-oxides, carbon based materials, wires tubes [11, 12]. The choice of nanomaterial as an adsorption depends on fulfillment of following properties to be an ideal adsorbent: The nanomaterial should have high efficiency and capacity for adsorption of heavy metal ion. The adsorbent should be non-toxic and recyclable; the desorption process of heavy metal ions from the adsorbent surface should be easy [13–15].

The present chapter overviews the various components of wastewater and associated health issues; the importance of Carbon nantubes as an adsorbent material; types of CNT membranes and their applications; functionalization of CNT for adsorption performance improvement; comparison of performance of CNTs based membrane with other conventional membranes and challenges for CNTs in water purification and need for further research.

13.2 CARBON NANOTUBES (CNTs) AS AN ADSORBENT FOR WASTEWATER TREATMENT

13.2.1 COMPONENTS OF WASTEWATER AND HEALTH ISSUES WITH WASTEWATER

The wastewater from various sectors have different types of pollutants which mainly constitutes of metal ions, organic pesticides used in agricultural sector, dyes, and pigments from textile industries and other pollutants such as oil radionuclides. The major concern associated with heavy metal ions like arsenic, chromium, cadmium, copper, mercury, lead zinc and nickel is that they cannot be decomposed and thus gets saturated in living organisms [16]. The toxicity and presence of non-biodegradable sites affect the living organisms. In many people the diseases observed due to high concentration of heavy metal ion are aggressive behavior, allergic reactions, autoimmune diseases, damage to the gastrointestinal tract, enzymes inhibition, fatigue, high blood pressure, lung disease, neurological disorder, renal dysfunction, irritability, vascular occlusion, memory loss [17].

The wastewater treatment methods are broadly categorized into primary (screening, filtrating, centrifuging, segregation, sedimentation, coagulating, and flocculation), secondary (aerobic and anaerobic treatments) and tertiary (distillation, crystallization, evaporation, extraction of solvents, oxidation, precipitation, ion exchange, reverse osmosis (RO), nano-filtration (NF), ultra-filtration (UF), micro-filtration (MF), adsorption, electrolysis, and electro-dialysis) levels water treatment methods [18, 19]. The selection of treatment method depends on the degree of concentration of initial heavy metals and the cost incurred. Also these techniques have pros and cons. For instance, the process of coagulation and flocculation produces a high quantity of sludge and flotation of this is costly. The ion exchange process possesses the advantage of removal of heavy metals, but the reproduction of the resins causes secondary contamination. Similarly, the chemical precipitation process is cheaper and easy to operate, but it produces hazardous by-products, and removal of the same requires additional operating cost. The electrodialysis treatment process needs high energy, which makes it more expensive [20, 21].

13.2.2 CARBON NANOTUBES (CNTS) AS AN ADSORBENT FOR WASTEWATER TREATMENT

Amongst many proposed adsorbent, carbon nanotubes (CNTs) are gaining attention in the field of wastewater treatment. Basically CNTs are a new and attractive member in the carbon family. CNTs are broadly classified based on their number of layers as a single walled CNTs (SWCNTs) and multi-walled CNTs (MWCNTs). CNTs are considered as an ideal adsorbent among carbon nanomaterials owing to their unique one-dimensional structure, extraordinary excellent electronic properties, mechanical properties, and potential applications.

Another striking advantage of CNTs is their high thermal (thermal resistance) and chemical stabilities (alkaline and acid stability). The structure of CNT provides it with large specific surface areas, excessive porous, hollow, and layered structures, light mass density, high reactivity. The intensive interaction between adsorbate molecules and CNTs and unique chemical and physical properties indicate CNTs as a promising candidate in adsorption for wastewater treatment [22, 23]. Other key features of CNTs are easy functionalization, high aspect ratio and high flux in water permeability [24]. CNTs can also be employed directly as filters to enhance the membrane performance because of their antifouling nature, high strength, and ability of disinfection, rejection, and permeability [25]. The inner hollow cavity of CNTs offers higher probability for desalinating the water. The smooth hydrophobic walls, high aspect ratios and inner pore diameter of CNTs provide smooth transport of water molecules [26].

The use of SWNTs in a membrane was effective for the elimination of microbial pathogens from the water. The study demonstrated that the SWNTs membrane has high anti-bacterial activity against *E. coli* [27]. In wastewater treatment, the adsorption of pollutants largely depends on the type and nature of an adsorbent. Bandaru et al. [28] synthesized thiol-derivatized SWCNTs by acid-cut reaction of SWCNTs with cysteamine hydrochloride employing carbodiimide coupling. As compared to Pristine SWCNTs, the acid functionalized CNTs exhibited three times higher adsorption capacity and four times higher in comparison with activated carbon. Veličković et al. [29] synthesized MWCNTs and functionalized them with oxidation and amino group. The performance of functionalized MWCNTs was evaluated in adsorption of pollutants with batch experiments. Sips isotherm model was found to be best for describing the performance of raw and oxidized-MWCNTs whereas for amino functionalized

MWCNTs Freundlich model was found to be more suitable. Sobhanardakani et al. [30] carried out the synthesis of oxidized MWCNTs for rejection of Cu^{2+} ions from the aqueous solutions. The Langmuir model was observed to be the best suitable to describe the experimental data than the Freundlich model.

13.3 TYPES OF CNT MEMBRANES AND THEIR APPLICATIONS IN WASTEWATER TREATMENT

According to fabrication methods CNT membranes are classified into different categories, the two broad classes are: (i) freestanding CNT membranes; and (ii) mixed (nano-composite) CNT membranes. The main two types of freestanding CNT membranes, usually employed in desalination and water treatment process are vertically aligned CNT (VACNT) membranes and bucky-paper membranes [31]. In case of VA-CNT membranes, CNTs are aligned as cylindrical pores that force the fluid to move through the hollow CNT interior or between the CNTs bundles. Whereas in bucky-paper CNT membranes, the CNTs are randomly arranged in an extremely large porous 3D network possessing large specific surface area [32]. The Mixed-CNT membranes possess structure equivalent to thin-film composite RO membranes, where the top layer is mixed with CNT and a polymer. The VA-CNT and mixed CNT membranes are shown in Figure 13.1.

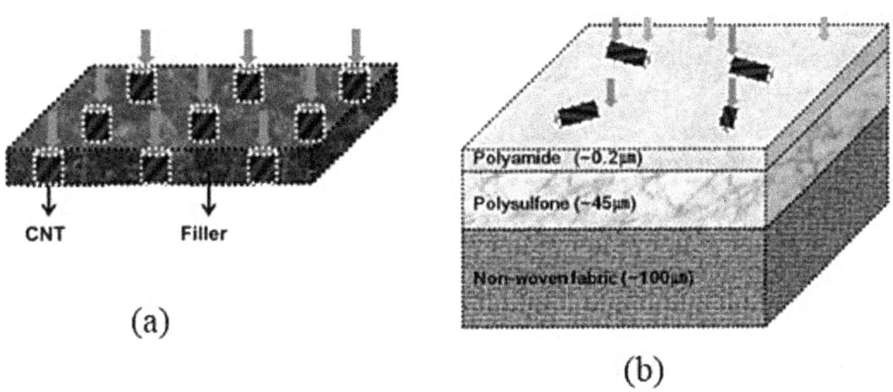

FIGURE 13.1 Representative structures of CNT membranes. (a) Vertically aligned (VA) CNT membranes; and (b) mixed CNT membranes.

Source: Reprinted with permission from Ref. [19].

13.3.1 VERTICALLY ALIGNED CARBON NANOTUBE MEMBRANES

Due to the compact nanotube forest and short nano-channel length, the VA-CNT membranes possess high water flux. In addition, because of the high flow rate, the VA-CNT membranes exhibit strong antibacterial characteristics and an outstanding performance for the removal of various salts. However, the complex fabrication methods are the biggest problem associated with the fabrication of these types of membranes for large-scale applications. Brady-Estevez et al. [33] introduced SWNT filter for the elimination of microbial pathogens from water. It was observed that this filter was demonstrated high antibacterial activity against *E. coli*. Lee et al. [34] fabricated and tested a thick ultrafiltration membrane and found it possess high water permeability. The anti-biofouling nature of the membranes was investigated employing Pseudomonas Aeruginosa (PA01) as a model bacterium. It was observed that the CNT membranes have good resistance against biofilm formation and prevent bacterial adhesion.

Du et al. [35] synthesized super long VA-CNT and epoxy composite membranes. They observed that these membranes demonstrated high flow rate for different liquids such as water, dodecane, and hexane. The iron nanoparticles have been attracted and removed from the membrane by using a magnetic field developed using magnetic coil. Kim et al. [36] fabricated VA-CNT/polymer composite films using *in-situ* bulk polymerization method. The VA-CNT array was penetrated using styrene monomer with a specific amount of polystyrene–polybutadiene (PS–PB) copolymer. The inclusion of PS-b–PB copolymer into the matrix helped to improve the elongation at break of the CNT/PS composite film which was ensured by the micro-indentation measurements. The prepared CNTs polymer composite exhibited high water and gas permeability compared to other VA-CNT composite membranes. Park et al. [37] synthesized VA-CNT membranes using CVD method. The developed VA-CNT membrane demonstrated high water permeability and a rapid irreversible fouling because of hydrophobic interactions between the membrane surface and foulants. The rejection capability of the developed VA-CNT membranes observed similar to the commercial polymeric UF membranes. The surface modification of methacrylic acid (MA) by graft polymerization helped to enhance the features of VA-CNT and UF membranes. The introduction of carboxylic groups results into reduction in contact angle of the membranes. The modified CNT membrane demonstrated enhanced rejection of bovine serum albumin (BSA) and reduced fouling propensity.

Despite of the tremendous fluid transport properties of VA-CNTs, the alignment control of CNTs in the membrane matrix and control of agglomeration of CNTs is still a big challenge.

13.3.2 BUCKY-PAPER CNTs MEMBRANES

In bucky-paper membranes CNTs are arranged arbitrarily in the form of a thin mat adhered together by van der Waals interactions. Due to Van der Waals interactions, the CNTs are strongly aggregated forming a cohesive bucky-paper structure. The bucky-paper CNT membranes possess large porous 3D network and specific surface area. The bucky-paper CNT membranes are synthesized using various methods such as electro-spinning, vacuum supported filtration and layer-by-layer (LBL) deposition.

The purification of CNTs is the most important step in the fabrication of bucky-paper CNT membranes. Commonly, in order to remove carbonaceous impurities oxidative treatment is used. However, implementation of such purification treatments may also shorten and damage the CNTs. But at the same time, this purification process assists in functionalizing the CNTs with carboxyl and hydroxyl groups. This makes the CNTs hydrophilic, which helps to disperse them into polar solvents like water [38]. Dumée et al. [39] demonstrated the fabrication of bucky-paper CNTs membranes and examined their potential and functioning in direct contact membrane distillation (DCMD). It was observed that CNTs membrane possesses highly porous and hydrophobic structure and high thermal conductivity. These CNTs membranes demonstrated superior desalination performance in DCMD. A bucky-paper CNT membrane developed employing a polymeric support was also found effective for desalination of seawater via DCMD [40]. Brady-Esétvez et al. [41] found that a SWNT bucky-paper demonstrated excellent performance for elimination of the model virus (MS_2 bacteriophage) because of depth filtration and was also found effective for retaining *E. coli* cells.

13.3.3 MIXED (NANOCOMPOSITE) CNTs MEMBRANES

The mixed (nano-composite) CNT membrane was developed with the primary purpose to enhance the performance of existing polymeric membranes by incorporation of CNTs. As the CNTs offer several fascinating features like mechanical and thermal stability, surface hydrophilicity, antifouling, and antimicrobial properties as well as better salt rejection capability. Due to van der Waals interactions, CNTs tend to agglomerate, which confines their applications in some of the cases [42]. However, acid treated CNTs exhibited enhanced dispersion in the polymer matrix in comparison with pristine CNTs. The CNTs can be integrated with the polymer matrix by several ways. The most commonly used methods are phase inversion [43], interfacial polymerization [44], layer-by-layer [45] and solution-casting [46].

13.4 FUNCTIONALIZATION OF CNT FOR ADSORPTION PERFORMANCE IMPROVEMENT

13.4.1 CNTs WITH DIFFERENT MORPHOLOGIES AND SURFACE MODIFICATION

The functionalization of CNTs is carried out in order to implant different functional groups that offer additional adsorption sites. Out of the reported functionalization techniques, oxidation is a simple technique for introducing carbonyl and hydroxyl groups to the sidewalls of CNTs [47]. Oxidized MWCNTs were observed to be highly efficient in the removal of methylene blue (MB) and methylene red (MR) from the aqueous solutions.

Other functionalization techniques include surfactant treatment, where the closed tips are opened. In addition, the CNT surfaces are connected by metals, metal oxides or organic ligands to enhance dispersibility and reactivity for its improved performance in wastewater treatment. The acid functionalization of CNTs is carried out for adsorption of divalent metal ions on the modified CNTs surface is depicted in Figure 13.2. The increase in the pH, results in negative surface charge of the functionalized CNT. Hence an electrostatic attraction takes place between positively charged metal ions and negatively surface charged CNTs resulting in the cations-ions absorption. In contrast, at lower pH values, the surface charge of the adsorbent turns positive due to which less cation adsorption takes place, eventually resulting in large Coulombic repulsion of metal ions. In acidic media, the adsorption sites of adsorbent are inhibited and protonated by reacting with metallic ions. Figure 13.2 shows the three forms of functionalization.

The closed tip ends of CNTs can be opened with the suitable wet chemical process for faster water permeability. However, the choice of oxidizing agents should be done carefully to open up the closed tips of CNT, and it was followed by the addition of hydrophilic functional groups along with high affinity for water molecules in CNT.

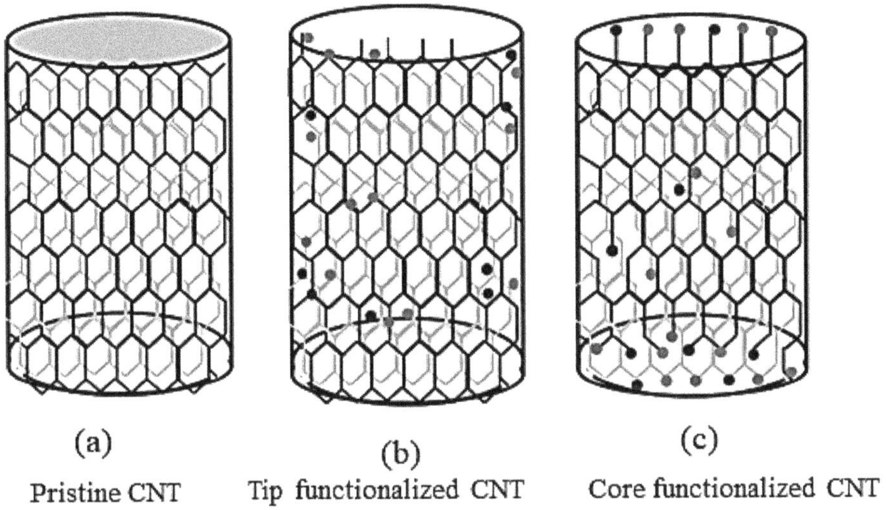

FIGURE 13.2 Functionalization of CNT membrane. (a) Pristine CNT; (b) tip functionalized CNT; and (c) core functionalized CNT.

Source: Reprinted with permission from Ref. [12] (AAP).

Corry [48] has demonstrated the 100% removal of Na^{++} and Cl^{-} ions employing CNTs functionalized with –COOH, $–NH_3$ and –OH groups with molecular dynamic simulations. Recently, Yang et al. [49] observed that functionalization of CNTs with plasma treatment improves the adsorption capacity compared to activated carbon based materials. Chan et al. [50] reported that the functionalization of CNT membranes done by attaching two zwitter ions with tip ends helped to achieve 100% ion rejection. Elmi et al. [51] observed that Fe_3O_4-functionalized, non-oxidative graphene/CNT helps to filter out arsenic in a Couette-Taylor flow. The enhanced arsenic elimination efficiency was observed in batch methods due to 3D structure, which improves the water permeability and helps to increase the contact area with Fe_3O_4. Gupta et al. [52] performed the synthesis of MWCNTs functionalization with three different functional groups namely, oxide (OX), iodide (I) and sulfur (S). The mercury adsorption capacity for the synthesized adsorbents was found to be higher for sulfur followed by iodide and then oxide.

Farghali et al. [53] synthesized MWCNTs with chemical vapor deposition (CVD) approach and functionalized using an acid functional group. These MWCNTs exhibited the higher surface area and porous structure. The adsorption efficiency of the functionalized MWCNTs was found to be superior.

13.4.2 MECHANISM OF HEAVY METAL ADSORPTION WITH CNT AND SITES OF ADSORPTION ON CNT

Many investigations are carried out to understand the underlying phenomenon of adsorption by CNT. The adsorption efficiency of CNTs is the function of site density, surface area, purity, porosity, functional groups and kind of CNTs. In practice, many adsorption sites are present on the CNTs to eliminate the contaminants from wastewater like inner sites, interstitial channels, grooves, and outside surface as depicted in Figure 13.3. It has been observed that the adsorption takes rapidly on the external sites as compared to internal sites, as external sites were easily accessible for adsorbing material [12]. For further adsorption, always the unblocked CNTs sites are useful. Some research studies observed that by opening the CNTs caps increases the number of adsorption sites and thus adsorption ability of CNT increases.

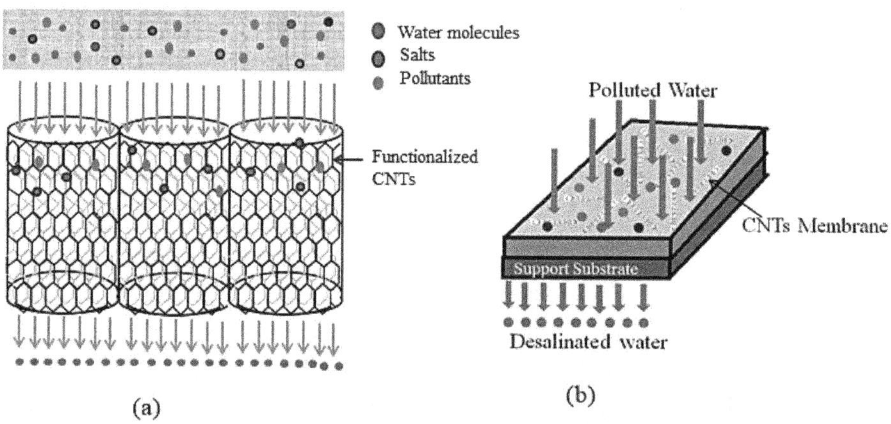

FIGURE 13.3 Prototype CNT membranes. (a) Vertically aligned CNT membrane; and (b) mixed matrix CNT membranes.

Source: Reprinted with permission from Ref. [12] (AAP).

The adsorption of pollutants from wastewater using CNT is largely depends upon the pH values of the solution, adsorbent mass, temperature of the system, contact time and metal ion concentration present in the wastewater source [54]. The adsorption efficiency is also a function of ionic strength, surface charge, agitation speed, competition among metal ions and isoelectric point. To enhance the performance of CNTs in adsorption, it is required to optimize these parameters.

13.4.3 COMPARISON OF PERFORMANCE OF CNTs-BASED MEMBRANE WITH OTHER CONVENTIONAL MEMBRANES IN WASTEWATER TREATMENT

In order to implement the CNTs as an adsorption agent in wastewater treatment, it will be desirable to compare the performance and economic aspect with conventional membrane performance and economy.

RO and NF techniques have the requirement of pressure for passing the water through it which consumes more energy. On the other hand, UF and MF membranes require less energy to pass the water, but only suspended particles retains on the membrane surface and micro- and nano-sized pollutants are passed through the membrane. Interestingly CNT membranes have the potential to substitute both RO and UF, the CNT process requires less amount of energy for the filtration process. Because hydrophobic hollow structure of CNT attracts the polar water molecules and nano-sized pore structure rejects salts and retains ions.

The performance of aligned CNT membrane in water permeability and salt rejection was observed to be superior over conventional RO membranes. It can be concluded from the literature that low energy burning, functionality, self-cleaning ability, robustness, water permeability and superior contaminant rejection capability are the major parameters that need to be considered in the selection of membrane. The salt rejection and water permeability of CNT membrane is well proved in water desalination process. Also it is observed that armchair structured CNT exhibits good performance in water permeability and salt rejection. It was reported that decorated membrane demonstrates a superior ability to overcome the constraints of traditional wastewater treatment approaches. Cohen-Tanugi and Grossman [55] reported that CNT membranes have wide scope to substitute RO for salt rejection in wastewater and gives equivalent performance as that of commercial NF membrane. The CNT membrane with pore diameter lesser than 2 nm was synthesized by Holt et al. [56] and their study reported that improved performance of the synthesized membrane for salt rejection and water permeability. Thus it is observed that research nowadays is focusing on the synthesis of CNT with pore diameter in nanoscale which will facilitate the elimination of small metal ion components from wastewater.

13.5 CHALLENGES FOR CNTS IN WATER PURIFICATION AND NEED FOR FUTURE RESEARCH

The CNT membranes demonstrated an outstanding capacity to be the next generation technology for wastewater treatment. However, it is worth observing that CNT have not yet been used in commercial scale. This section tends to summarize the hurdle that restricts the commercial use besides having several advantages over conventional membranes available for wastewater treatment.

- The uneven alignment affects the performance of membrane and properties like flux and salt rejection. It is difficult to grow CNTs with appropriate alignment in VA-CNT membranes.
- The CNT synthesis methods developed till now are complicated.
- The fabrication of CNTs with suitable uniform pore size distribution is not well developed in order to employ it on a commercial scale.
- Efficient methods for the CNTs tip functionalization by retaining the properties of CNT need to develop.
- The CNTs atomic structural networks are highly responsive to different wet chemical treatments and thus it tends to change the structural properties of CNTs as well as destroys the CNT walls, reduces water flux and solute retention capacities.
- A standard terminology should be defined and outlined to evaluate the performance of CNTs as an adsorbent because the dimensions and experimental conditions used by various researchers differ; hence it is difficult to compare the performance and reproduce the results.
- Majority of CNT based membranes have been produced using polymeric or ceramic membrane that leads to weaken the CNT properties.
- Majority of the current research focused on the investigation of the performance of VA-CNT based on the simulation and modeling results. Hence there is a need to validate the result experimentally.
- Commercial availability, large scale production, and cost minimization are the major issues that need to be addressed.
- Evaluation of potential toxic effects of CNT is needed to be considered and addressed.
- SWCNT and DWCNT used as an adsorbent in wastewater treatment are costly and hence their use for large scale wastewater treatment is limited. Instead, MWCNT are low in cost and have the ability to substitute the UF membranes but are not suitable candidate to substitute NF membranes because of synthesis limitation of MWCNT at nanoscale.

- The cost of CNTs can be reduced by its use by recycling. However, the mechanism of separation of adsorbed hazardous compounds needs to be investigated properly.

13.6 CONCLUSION

The existence of hazardous heavy metals in wastewater is a primary concern for water source. The conventionally wastewater treatment methods like RO, NF, MF, UF are used to fulfill the demand of safe drinking water. In the recent years, CNTs have been widely researched and applied as an adsorbent for the elimination of various pollutants and heavy metals from wastewater. CNTs based membranes proved an extraordinary performance relating to water permeability, desalination capacity, energy savings and antifouling. The CNTs have extraordinary physical, chemical, and mechanical properties with large specific area which makes it a suitable candidate for wastewater treatment. The energy consumption in applying the pressure in conventional membrane techniques can be reduced to a great extent with the application of CNTs. The different types of CNTs (SWCNT, DWCNT MWCNT and VA-CNT) are in wide research focus owing to their uniform pore size distribution and large surface area. The metal ion rejection and water permeability performance of CNTs can be improved significantly by functionalizing with suitable agent like hydroxyl and carbonyl groups plasma treatment. Despite having tremendous potential of CNTs to substitute conventional membranes, the use of CNTs is limited as an adsorbent in wastewater treatment because of a lack of scalable synthesis techniques. However, it is believed that commercial synthesis of CNTs can greatly reduce the production cost and can come up as modern age technique in wastewater treatment.

KEYWORDS

- **adsorbent**
- **anti-fouling**
- **carbon nanotube (CNT)**
- **CNT functionalization**
- **CNT membranes**
- **wastewater treatment**

REFERENCES

1. Sadegh, H., Ali, G. A., Gupta, V. K., Makhlouf, A. S. H., Shahryari-Ghoshekandi, R., Nadagouda, M. N., & Megiel, E., (2017). The role of nanomaterials as effective adsorbents and their applications in wastewater treatment. *Journal of Nanostructure in Chemistry, 7*(1), 1–14.
2. Zwiener, C., Richardson, S. D., De Marini, D. M., Grummt, T., Glauner, T., & Frimmel, F. H., (2007). Drowning in disinfection byproducts? Assessing swimming pool water. *Environ. Sci. Technol., 41*(2), 363–372.
3. Karnik, B., Davies, S., Baumann, M., & Masten, S., (2005). The effects of combined ozonation and filtration on disinfection by-product formation. *Water Res., 39*(13), 2839–2850.
4. Zhang, Y., An, Y., Liu, C., Wang, Y., Song, Z., Li, Y., Meng, W., et al., (2019). Catalytic ozonation of emerging pollutant and reduction of toxic by-products in secondary effluent matrix and effluent organic matter reaction activity. *Water Research, 166*, 1–11.
5. Bansal, R. C., & Goyal, M., (2005). *Activated Carbon Adsorption.* CRC Press, Boca Raton.
6. Khlifi, R., & Hamza-Chaffai, A., (2010). Head and neck cancer due to heavy metal exposure via tobacco smoking and professional exposure: A review. *Toxicol. Appl. Pharmacol., 248*(2), 71–88.
7. Zare, K., Gupta, V. K., Moradi, O., Makhlouf, A. S. H., Sillanpa¨a, M., Nadagouda, M. N., Sadegh, H., et al., (2015). A comparative study on the basis of adsorption capacity between CNTs and activated carbon as adsorbents for removal of noxious synthetic dyes: A review. *J. Nanostruct. Chem., 5*(2), 227–236.
8. Sadegh, H., Shahryari-Ghoshekandi, R., Tyagi, I., Agarwal, S., & Gupta, V. K., (2015). Kinetic and thermodynamic studies for alizarin removal from liquid phase using poly-2-hydroxyethyl methacrylate (PHEMA). *J. Mol. Liq., 207*, 21–27.
9. Gupta, V., Moradi, O., Tyagi, I., Agarwal, S., Sadegh, H., Shahryari-Ghoshekandi, R., Makhlouf, A., et al., (2016). Study on the removal of heavy metal ions from industry waste by carbon nanotubes: Effect of the surface modification: A review. *Crit. Rev. Environ. Sci. Technol., 46*(2), 93–118.
10. Martínez, L. M. T., Kharissova, O. V., & Kharisov, B. I., (2019). *Handbook of Ecomaterials.* Springer.
11. Yaqoob, A. A., Parveen, T., Umar, K., & Mohamad, I. M. N., (2020). Role of nanomaterials in the treatment of wastewater: A review. *Water, 12*(2), 1–30.
12. Borgaonkar, A. V., & Potdar, S. B., (2022). CNTs as new emerging lubricant additives for enhancing energy efficiency. In: Haghi, A. K., et al., (eds.), *Carbon Nanotubes for Energy and Environmental Applications.* Apple Academic Press, CRC Press, Taylor and Francis group, Canada.
13. Ali, I., (2012). New generation adsorbents for water treatment. *Chem. Rev., 112*(10), 5073–5091.
14. Sharma, Y., Srivastava, V., Singh, V., Kaul, S., & Weng, C., (2009). Nanoadsorbents for the removal of metallic pollutants from water and wastewater. *Environ. Technol., 30*(6), 583–609.
15. Machida, M., Mochimaru, T., & Tatsumoto, H., (2006). Lead (II) adsorption onto the graphene layer of carbonaceous materials in aqueous solution. *Carbon, 44*(13), 2681–2688.

16. Garcia, F., Ortega, A., Domingo, J. L., & Corbella, J., (2001). Accumulation of metals in autopsy tissues of subjects living in Tarragona County, Spain. *Journal of Environmental Science and Health, Part A., 36*(9), 1767–1786.
17. Duruibe, J. O., Ogwuegbu, M. O. C., & Egwurugwu, J. N., (2007). Heavy metal pollution and human biotoxic effects. *International Journal of Physical Sciences, 2*(5), 112–118.
18. Crini, G., & Lichtfouse, E., (2019). Advantages and disadvantages of techniques used for wastewater treatment. *Environmental Chemistry Letters, 17*(1), 145–155.
19. Gautier, C., Lopez, I., & Breton, T. (2021). A post-functionalization toolbox for diazonium (electro)-grafted surfaces: Review of the coupling methods. *Mater. Adv.*, *2*, 2773–2810
20. Corry, B., (2008). Designing carbon nanotube membranes for efficient water desalination. *J. Phys. Chem. B., 112*(5), 1427–1434.
21. Cohen-Tanugi, D., & Grossman, J. C., (2012). Water desalination across nanoporous graphene. *Nano Lett., 12*(7), 3602–3608.
22. Mansourpanah, Y., Madaeni, S. S., Rahimpour, A., Adeli, M., Hashemi, M. Y., & Moradian, M. R., (2011). Fabrication new PES-based mixed matrix nanocomposite membranes using polycaprolactone modified carbon nanotubes as the additive: Property changes and morphological studies. *Desalination, 277*, 171–177.
23. Padaki, M., Surya, M. R., Abdullah, M. S., Misdan, N., Moslehyani, A., Kassim, M. A., Hilal, N., & Ismail, A. F., (2015). Membrane technology enhancement in oil-water separation. A review. *Desalination, 357*, 197–207.
24. Lee, J., Jeong, S., & Liu, Z., (2016). Progress and challenges of carbon nanotube membrane in water treatment. *Critical Reviews in Environmental Science and Technology, 46*(11, 12), 999–1046.
25. Li, Y. H., Zhao, Y. M., Hu, W. B., Ahmad, I., Zhu, Y. Q., Peng, X. J., & Luan, Z. K., (2007). Carbon nanotubes-the promising adsorbent in wastewater treatment. In: *Journal of Physics: Conference Series, 61*(140), 1–6.
26. Pendergast, M. M., & Hoek, E. M., (2011). A review of water treatment membrane nanotechnologies. *Energy Environ. Sci., 4*(6), 1946–1971.
27. Brady-Estévez, A. S., Schnoor, M. H., Kang, S., & Elimelech, M., (2010). SWNT – MWNT hybrid filter attains high viral removal and bacterial inactivation. *Langmuir, 26*(24), 19153–19158.
28. Bandaru, N. M., Reta, N., Dalal, H., Ellis, A. V., Shapter, J., & Voelcker, N. H., (2013). Enhanced adsorption of mercury ions on thiol derivatized single wall carbon nanotubes. *Journal of Hazardous Materials, 261*, 534–541.
29. Velicković, Z. S., Marinković, A. D., Bajić, Z. J., Marković, J. M., PerićGrujić, A. A., Uskokovic, P. S., & Ristic, M. D., (2013). Oxidized and ethylenediamine-functionalized multi-walled carbon nanotubes for the separation of low concentration arsenate from water. *Separation Science and Technology, 48*(13), 2047–2058.
30. Sobhanardakani, S., Zandipak, R., & Cheraghi, M., (2015). Adsorption of Cu^{2+} ions from aqueous solutions using oxidized multi-walled carbon nanotubes. *Avicenna Journal of Environmental Health Engineering, 2*(1), 1–6.
31. Das, R., Ali, E., Bee, S., Hamid, A., Ramakrishna, S., & Zaman, Z., (2014). Carbon nanotube membranes for water purification: A bright future in water desalination. *Desalination, 336*, 97–109.

32. Manawi, V. K., Hussein, M. A., Khaleel, M. A., Khraisheh, M., & Hilal, N., (2016). Can carbon-based nanomaterials revolutionize membrane fabrication for water treatment and desalination? *Desalination, 391*, 69–88.
33. Brady-Estevez, A. S., Kang, S., & Elimelech, M., (2008). A single-walled-carbon-nanotube filter for removal of viral and bacterial pathogens. *Small, 4*, 481–484.
34. Lee, B., Baek, Y., Lee, M., Jeong, D. H., Lee, H. H., Yoon, J., & Kim, Y. H., (2015). A carbon nanotube wall membrane for water treatment. *Nat. Commun., 6*(1), 1–7.
35. Du, F., Qu, L., Xia, Z., Feng, L., & Dai, L., (2011). Membranes of vertically aligned superlong carbon nanotubes. *Langmuir, 27*, 8437–8443.
36. Kim, S., Fornasiero, F., Gyu, H., Bin, J., Meshot, E., Giraldo, G., Stadermann, M., et al., (2014). Fabrication of flexible, aligned carbon nanotube/polymer composite membranes by in-situ polymerization. *J. Memb. Sci., 460*, 91–98.
37. Park, W. K., Yoon, Y., Kim, S., Yoo, S., Do, Y., Kang, J. W., Yoon, D. H., & Yang, W. S., (2016). Feasible water flow filter with facilely functionalized Fe_3O_4-non-oxidative graphene/CNT composites for arsenic removal. *Journal of Environmental Chemical Engineering, 4*(3), 3246–3252.
38. Sears, K., Dumée, L., Schütz, J., She, M., & Huynh, C., (2010). Recent developments in carbon nanotube membranes for water purification and gas separation. *Materials, 3*(1), 127–149.
39. Dumée, L. F., Sears, K., Schütz, J., Finn, N., Huynh, C., Hawkins, S., Duke, M., & Gray, S., (2010). Characterization and evaluation of carbon nanotube bucky-paper membranes for direct contact membrane distillation. *J. Memb. Sci., 351*, 36–43.
40. Dumée, L., Sears, K., Finn, N., Duke, M., Dumée, L., Sears, K., Finn, N., & Duke, M., (2010). Carbon nanotube based composite membranes for water desalination by membrane distillation. *Desalin. Water Treat., 17*, 72–79.
41. Kang, S., Pinault, M., Pfefferle, L. D., & Elimelech, M., (2007). Single-walled carbon nanotubes exhibit strong antimicrobial activity. *Langmuir, 23*, 8670–8673.
42. Choi, J. J., & Kim, W., (2006). Fabrication and characterization of multi-walled carbon nanotubes/polymer blend membranes. *J. Membr. Sci., 284*, 406–415.
43. Khalid, A., Al-Juhani, A. A., Al-Hamouz, O. C., Laoui, T., Khan, Z., & Atieh, M. A., (2015). Preparation and properties of nanocomposite polysulfone/multi-walled carbon nanotubes membranes for desalination. *Desalination, 367*, 134–144.
44. Inukai, S., Cruz-silva, R., Ortiz-medina, J., & Morelos-gomez, A., (2015). High-performance multifunctional reverse osmosis membranes obtained by carbon nanotube·polyamide nanocomposite. *Sci. Rep., 5*(1), 1–10.
45. Liu, L., Son, M., Chakraborty, S., & Bhattacharjee, C., (2013). Fabrication of ultra-thin polyelectrolyte/carbon nanotube membrane by spray-assisted layer-by-layer technique: Characterization and its anti-protein fouling properties for water treatment. *Desalin. Water Treat., 51*, 6194–6200.
46. Ahn, C. H., Baek, Y., Lee, C., Kim, S. O., Kim, S., Lee, S., Kim, S. H., et al., (2012). Carbon nanotube-based membranes: Fabrication and application to desalination. *Journal of Industrial and Engineering Chemistry, 18*(5), 1551–1559.
47. Sinnott, S. B., (2002). Chemical functionalization of carbon nanotubes. *Journal of Nanoscience and Nanotechnology, 2*(2), 113–123.
48. Corry, B., (2011). Water and ion transport through functionalized carbon nanotubes: Implications for desalination technology. *Energy & Environmental Science, 4*(3), 751–759.

49. Yang, S. T., Chen, S., Chang, Y., Cao, A., Liu, Y., & Wang, H., (2011). Removal of methylene blue from aqueous solution by graphene oxide. *J. Colloid Interface Sci., 359*(1), 24–29.
50. Chan, W. F., Marand, E., & Martin, S. M., (2016). Novel zwitterion functionalized carbon nanotube nanocomposite membranes for improved RO performance and surface anti-biofouling resistance. *Journal of Membrane Science, 509*, 125–137.
51. Elmi, F., Hosseini, T., Taleshi, M. S., & Taleshi, F., (2017). Kinetic and thermodynamic investigation into the lead adsorption process from wastewater through magnetic nanocomposite Fe_3O_4/CNT. *Nanotechnology for Environmental Engineering, 2*(1), 1–13.
52. Gupta, A., Vidyarthi, S., & Sankararamakrishnan, N., (2014). Enhanced sorption of mercury from compact fluorescent bulbs and contaminated water streams using functionalized multiwalled carbon nanotubes. *Journal of Hazardous Materials, 274*, 132–144.
53. Farghali, A., Tawab, H. A., Moaty, S. A., & Khaled, R., (2017). Functionalization of acidified multi-walled carbon nanotubes for removal of heavy metals in aqueous solutions. *Journal of Nanostructure in Chemistry, 7*(2), 101–111.
54. Abdullatif, J., Haleema, A., Yassine, M., Remi, M., Mohamed, B., & Aziz, F., (2021). Recent advances in the synthesis and applications of magnetic polymer nanocomposites. *Journal of Industrial and Engineering Chemistry, 99*, 1–18.
55. Cohen-Tanugi, D., & Grossman, J. C., (2012). Water desalination across nanoporous graphene. *Nano Lett., 12*(7), 3602–3608.
56. Holt, J. K., Park, H. G., Wang, Y., Stadermann, M., Artyukhin, A. B., Grigoropoulos, C. P., Noy, A., & Bakajin, O., (2006). Fast mass transport through sub-2-nanometer carbon nanotubes. *Science, 312*(5776), 1034–1037.
57. Hoon, C., Baek, Y., Lee, C., Ouk, S., Kim, S., Lee, S., Kim, S., Seek, S., Park, J., & Yoon, J., (2012). Carbon nanotube-based membranes: Fabrication and application to desalination. *J. Ind. Eng. Chem., 18*, 1551–1559.

CHAPTER 14

Carbon Nanotubes for Biomedical Applications and Health Care: New Horizons

CHIN HUA CHIA,[1] KAM SHENG LAU,[1] SIEW XIAN CHIN,[1,2] NURUL HAZWANI AMINUDDIN ROSLI,[1,3] JEI VINCENT,[1] and MD. SHAHARIAR CHOWDHURY[4]

[1]*Materials Science Program, Department of Applied Physics, Faculty of Science and Technology, Bangi, Selangor, Malaysia*

[2]*ASASIpintar Program, Pusat GENIUS@Pintar Negara, Universiti Kebangsaan Malaysia, Bangi, Selangor, Malaysia*

[3]*Physics Department, Center for Defense Foundation Studies, Universiti Pertahanan Nasional Malaysia, Kuala Lumpur, Malaysia*

[4]*Faculty of Environmental Management, Prince of Songkla University, Hat Yai, Songkhla, Thailand*

ABSTRACT

Carbon nanotubes have generated increasing interest in the scientific community due to their large surface area, excellent electrical and thermal conductivity, high thermal and chemical stabilities, high mechanical strength, etc. In this chapter, we have focused on five important biomedical applications of carbon nanotubes, i.e., (i) tissue engineering; (ii) biosensing; (iii) drug delivery; (iv) bioimaging; and (v) bioimaging, in which details on various preparation and modifications on the carbon nanotubes have also been covered. In addition, the toxicity issue of carbon nanotubes will also be briefly described.

Carbon Nanotubes for Biomedical Applications and Healthcare.
Chin Hua Chia, Swati Gokul Talele, Ann Rose Abraham, and A. K. Haghi, (Eds.)

14.1 INTRODUCTION

Carbon nanotubes (CNTs) have been receiving increasing attention over the years since its discovery in 1991 [1]. CNTs are one of the carbon allotropes in which the entire carbon atoms are arranged into hollow tube-like cylindrical nanostructures [2]. The carbon atoms in CNTs possess sp^2 hybridization, constructing delocalized electron clouds along the wall. There are two types of CNTs, i.e., single-walled (SWCNTs) and multi-walled CNTs (MWCNTs). The diameter of SWCNTs and MWCNTs can range from 0.5 to 2.5 nm and 2.5 to 100 nm, respectively, as shown in Figure 14.1 [3]. While the length of CNTs can be ranging from several centimeters to hundreds of centimeters [4].

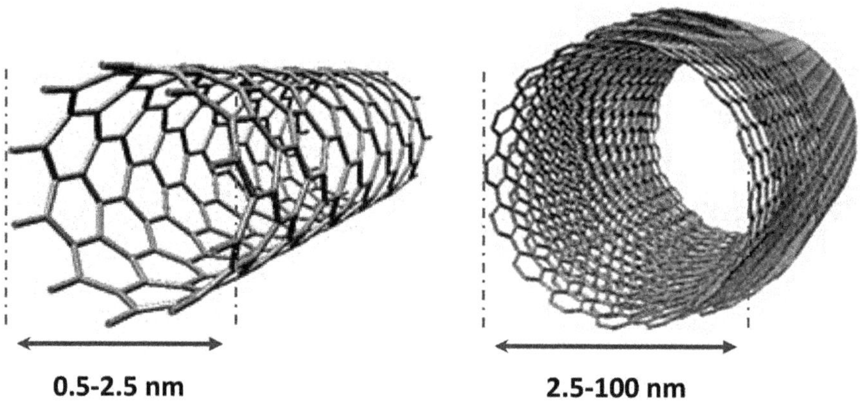

FIGURE 14.1 Schematic representation of CNTs: Single-walled (SWCNTs) and multi-walled (MWCNTs) carbon nanotubes.

Source: Adapted from Waseem et al, 2016

CNTs possess extremely high surface area and exhibit remarkable electrical and mechanical properties. They have both semi-metallic and metallic characteristics, and great chemical and thermal stability [5]. Besides these excellent properties, CNTs can also be further functionalized chemically to suit different applications, either by covalent attachment of chemical groups or wrapping of molecules non-covalently onto the tubes [3, 6]. In this chapter, we review several important biomedical applications of CNTs, including tissue engineering, bio-sensing, drug delivery, and bio-imaging. In the last section, we include the topic of toxicity of CNTs.

14.2 TISSUE ENGINEERING

In order to form a multicellular organism, a hierarchy of systems is required to be functioning from the scale of nano-through to macroscale [7]. Such sophisticating systems and processes from the smaller scales allow the biological systems formed to accomplish more intricate function in a macroscale. For example, The lipid bilayers that form the cell membranes are having thickness ranging from 3 to 10 nm [8]. Type I collagen, with the diameter less than 2 nm and length around 300 nm [9], is the most abundant protein that exists within human body which provides structural and mechanical scaffold or matrix for cornea, skin, blood vessel walls, bone, connective tissues with other tendons [10]. Diameters of human capillaries blood vessels are about 8 μm while for venules and arterioles, they are ranging from 20–30 μm [11]. For neuron, small or medium neuron's size ranges from 18–27 μm diameter while the large one is about 40 μm diameter and even larger [12]. However, axon, which is part and the output of neuron that carries impulse to another neuron is having diameter from 2 to 20 μm. Such minor size is vital in the successful function of the biological system. Minor changes within those nano-scale or primary cellular hierarchy will lead to a big impact to the biological system at the higher level. Such nanoscale properties had been found out to illustrate various biological functions and cellular responses like, cell-cell communication, immune system manipulation, cell adhesion, gene expression, differentiation, proliferation, migration, and protein production [13–16]. Therefore, artificial materials with nanoscale feature can give huge implication to the biological system thus be studied via numerous researchers on its biomedical applications.

Human bones are basically composite materials with nanoscale structure make up by hydroxyapatite ($Ca_{10}(PO_4)6(OH)_2$) as mineral phase, around 90% of type I collagen and 5% non-collagenous proteins as the organic phase, and finally around 2% lipids and water [17, 18]. Such compositions allow human bones to function as skeleton to support the weight of the human body while being a fulcrum for the movement of the human body as there are parts that allow the attachment of the muscle. There are several conditions that might lead to bone defection, including trauma, tumor, congenital etiology, surgery, and infection [19]. Although bones have the ability for self-regeneration spontaneously via producing marrow stroma cells as well as growth factors, if the bone defection is greater than the critical-size defects, such self-regeneration is limited and additional clinical treatment is vital [20, 21]. The current bone defection treatment including autografts, allografts, and xenografts. However, each method is suffered due to their own risk like infection, disease transmission, host rejection and more [22]. Hence, to overcome the drawback of current treatment, artificial bone substitutes that could be manipulated to mimic the actual bone properties can serve as both tissue engineering and regenerative purpose are now dragging tremendous attention from researchers as a novel route in bone defection treatment [20, 23, 24].

On the other hand, the heart, the organ that pumps the oxygenated and deoxygenated blood to cause circulation through the cardiovascular system within our body is the first organ to be active within an embryo [25]. Without it functioning, human body cell will not get oxygen and eventually lead to mortal. Unlike bone, the shortage of cardiomyocyte proliferation capacity results in the mammalian responds toward infarction are mainly on repair and not regeneration. After heart tissue injuries, there are no mitosis (only a limited number of rare and abnormal cases) occur at the injury sites. Instead, a scar is formed via the net-like extracellular matrix (ECM) to replace the injured muscle tissue. Such circumstance cause the contractility of myocardium reduce and even heart failure and death to the human [26, 27]. This phenomenon is even dire when the cardiovascular diseases (CVD) especially heart failure are the dominant sources for the mortality around the world and huge burden toward the government's healthcare system [26, 28]. Ditto as bone defection treatment, organ transplantation is the ultimate treatment for the CVD like heart failure with the same demerits with limitation of donor's availability and surgical risks. Nevertheless, artificial biomaterials are developed to imitate the myocardium to encourage cell growth and organ repair [29].

The nervous system is very essential to the normal function of human as it regulates and controls different body organ activities. Dysfunction of body organ and diseases can be caused if there are injuries to the nervous system [30]. Millions of people are suffering injuries in nervous system and the number are expected to be continue growing annually among the people ranges from 15 to 50 years of age [31, 32]. Nerves systems are composed of two major parts: peripheral nervous system (PNS) like ganglia that located external of the brain and spinal cord autonomic and spinal nerves while central nervous system (CNS) like the brain and spinal cord. PNS can perform self-repair and regeneration, however, such properties rarely occur on elderly people and these properties only exhibit in small injury; in large injuries, autograft is still needed for the treatment. While CNS on the other hand has no regenerative properties after disease or trauma due to lack of Schwann cells and compact glial scar tissue which sustain the growth of axon and inhibiting the neural regeneration, respectively. The only treatment for

CNS injury is reducing the secondary injury and physical therapy to restore the patient limited mobility [30, 32]. Yet, biomimetic materials with reasonable design can help in leading cell adhesion, proliferation, and growth and thus lead to neuroregeneration [30].

There are many nanomaterials, or their composites which have been fabricated and investigated due to the development in nanotechnology. Such nanoscale properties of those nanomaterials allow the manipulation on their behavior in cellular hierarchy level, such as cell adhesion, differentiation, gene expression, proliferation, migration, and signal transduction [20, 33]. Among those nanomaterials CNTs, graphite sheets in a cylindrical tubes conformation in nanoscale that are characterized into SWCNTs or MWCNTs, had been researched and achieved remarkable results as the tissue engineering and regenerative materials for bone, cardiac, nerves, and more organs. This is mainly due to its chemical and physical properties of CNTs, such as very high ratio of surface area, high thermal conductivity, high tensile strength, flexibility, and electrical conductivity [24, 34]. Based on those characteristics, many positive results had been achieved in bone, cardiac, and nerves regeneration, and tissue engineering (Table 14.1).

There are many methods used for tissue engineering and regeneration scaffold to produce scaffold organization with desired architectures to achieve the best outcome with their own pros and cons. The way of production including electrospinning, solvent casting, freeze drying, self-assembly, phase separation, and rapid prototyping technologies (3D bioprinting, laser-assisted bioprinting, fused deposition modeling, stereolithography, and digital light projection) [35]. Therefore, in this chapter, CNTs as scaffold application in bone, cardiac, and nerves will be focused with examples to provide a better and deeper understanding to the reader regarding to this field.

14.2.1 ADVANTAGES OF CNTS IN SCAFFOLD APPLICATION

CNTs are allotrope of carbon with carbon atom bonded with each other via sp^2 bonds. The structure of CNTs composed of one rolled hollow cylindrical nanostructure of graphene sheet. There are 2 subtypes of CNTs namely as SWCNTs, tubular graphene single-layer of graphene sheet and MWCNTs that formed via multiple graphene layers. Both CNTs can be a biomimetic nanocomposite as it had proven to have positive ability in stimulating cell adhesion due to excellent cell-binding proteins interaction. Moreover, due to cell binding of preferential affinity, it can help in cell morphology regulation and stem cell differentiation acceleration.

In terms of morphological features, the C–C bonds hybridization of CNTs with high stability and cylindrical shape provide special mechanical, chemical, thermal, and electrical properties to CNTs. Moreover, the nanoscale and rod-like morphology of CNTs allow the collagen fibers simulation in the ECM while the large surface-area-to-volume ratio of CNTs supplies more proteins adhesion sites for tissue engineering scaffold.

On the other hand, the mechanical properties of CNTs are among the most important properties in the scaffold production. CNTs are flexible, high strength and low density as compared to the other material like ceramic or conventional metals. The range of density and tensile strength, bending strength, and Young's modulus of CNTs are 1.3–2.0 g/cm^3, 11–52 GPa, 14.2 ± 8 GPa, and 32–1,470 GPa, respectively. Due to these significant mechanical properties, CNTs had been applied vastly with other polymers to improve the overall mechanical properties in composite forms.

For, chemical properties, CNTs have good adsorption capacity for organic compounds with chemical stability. The adsorption of proteins is mainly contributed by the high-delocalized π-bonds that located on the external surface of CNTs. Nonetheless, the disadvantages of CNTs in terms of chemical properties are mainly due to the hydrophobicity and low dissolution ability in solvent. Therefore, surfaces functionalized via functional groups, such as carboxyl and hydroxyl, are used to resolve the drawback of CNTs with increasing the ability of improving cellular interactions.

CNTs also acquired with electrical properties. The electronic conductivity of CNTs can be controlled depending on the diameter, alignment, chirality, and aspect ratio of CNTs. The conductivity of CNTs can promote cell proliferation and activity as it can improve the electron-conductive relativity and electrochemical of proteins as well as biomolecules that are related to cell or tissue engineering and regeneration. Apart from that, the conductivity also improves the function of calcium ion channels, allow the maintenance of cell membrane's electrical function with antibacterial activity [20, 35, 36]. Hence, owing to those unique properties, CNTs, and the composites of it have become the best material to be used in the tissue engineering and regeneration medical purpose.

14.2.2 BONE TISSUE ENGINEERING AND REGENERATION MEDICINE

The extracellular matrix (ECM) of bone tissue is built up via complex environment from nano- to macro-scale structure like osteoclasts, osteocytes, and osteoblasts surrounded with mineralized ECM entailing of collagen and other proteins [37–40]. This also allows the 3D architecture formation and causes synergy interaction of protein, cells, and other molecules to be possible [41]. Such complexity allows the bone to have regenerative when it comes to small defect. Nonetheless, when the defection is bigger than the critical-size defects that due to trauma, tumor, congenital etiology, surgery, and infection [19], the template of orchestrated regeneration will lost, thus limit the regeneration of bone and require clinical intervention [42].

Autologous and allogeneic bone are both the most widely used method for clinical intervention to treat patients with large bone defects. Autograft is limited by the availability of donor, and the mechanical stability will be effect with high chances of morbidity in the surgery area [43]. On the other hand, allografts might cause severe immune responses and infections [44]. Xenografts also had been chosen to use as a replacement of bone defects in patients, however it is rarely been used fur to strong host rejection [45–47]. Therefore, in this case the materials nanotechnology is involved to mimics the actual bone structure for replacement of the current treatment.

The treatment of the bone defects in humans, like autografts, allographs, and xenograft are mainly focusing on the replacement of the defected one, but no regenerate them [48, 49]. Recent years the artificial materials with nanostructure are being researched to create tissue replacement with the ability to culturing bone cells and tissue on nanocomposites and 3D scaffolds composites [36]. To achieve that there are some criteria that need to be achieved include:

1. **Good Biocompatibility:** Help in cell migration, differentiation, and safe implantation [50–52].
2. **Porosity, Roughness, Pore Size, and Interconnected Porosity:** For cell migration, nutrients exchange, affect cell behavior, angiogenesis, differentiation, proliferation, adhesion bone regeneration and good cell adhesion due to high surface area [53, 54].
3. **Good Mechanical Properties:** To support loading and hold the scaffold rigidity even with pores [53, 55].

For biocompatibility, from Table 14.1, it can be observed that most of the polymers, including both synthetic or natural substances, are incorporated into CNTs structure to improve its biocompatibility with some additional biological properties to enhance the overall suitability of the scaffold like improving cell adhesion, proliferation, growth, differentiation, and reduce possible toxicity that might cause by CNTs. While some of the materials are added for aiding the incorporation process to form CNTs nanocomposites or the production process like making the CNTs based scaffold can be more printable via electrospinning, three-dimensional (3D) printing or other method to produce the suitable structure [56].

The nanocomposite for scaffold also needs to be able to allow the colonization of cell and it can be achieved via the porosity and surface roughness [57, 58]. The surface roughness and the porosity are depended on the nanoscale morphology or surface of the composites. The porosity and surface roughness also important when it comes to bio-mimic the nanoarchitecture of the actual bone to allow cell colonization for example, From Table 14.1, it can be seen that the electrospinning and 3D structure formation technology had been used to create scaffold. 3D printing for the scaffold production is chosen is mainly due to the it promotes the proliferation, growth of human stem cells, more structural similar to actual bone, more applicable to *in vivo*, better bone regeneration and chondrogenic differentiation which is more suitable that 2D structure [59–61]. In 2D structure due to the structure and the ultra-small pores size, the penetration as well as the migration of cells on electrospun matrix restricted as the cell can only proliferate on the scaffold's top area and this block the cell colonization in depth. The combination of electrospinning and 3D structure allow to produce 3D electrospun scaffolds that acquired with larger pore sizes and better porosity with 3D structure that overcome the 2D structure's issues [56]. On the other hand, electrospinning can produce a scaffold with better cell attachment, growth, and differentiation as compared with another method. This is owing to the low-dimension fibrous structure provide large specific surface area for cell adhesion facilitation to the electrospun fibers [62].

In terms of mechanical properties, CNTs are added to improve the mechanical properties of scaffold as most of the polymer with good biocompatibility, moldability, elasticity, and other biological properties, such as PVA, BCP, HA, Cs, and more are having weak mechanical properties like tensile strength (Table 14.1). Such incorporations also allowed the scaffold to have good porosity, pore size, and interconnected porosity, while remaining mechanically robust. Combining with the lightweight properties of CNTs, this made CNTs the best candidate for scaffold materials [63].

Other characteristics, such as conductibility and hydrophilicity/hydrophobicity, are also preferable as according to Table 14.1. The conductivity that provided by the incorporation of CNTs can allow electrical stimulation to be given and help in cell/tissues regeneration in the scaffold like promoting cell growth, proliferation, and differentiation [64–67]. Even without the

TABLE 14.1 Applications of CNTs in Tissue Engineering and Regenerative Medicine for Bone, Nerve, and Cardiac

Structure of CNTs (MWCNTs/ SWCNTs)	Combination of Materials/ Substances	Functional Part		Function	Production Method	Remark	Reference
		Body Part	Specific Cells/Tissues/ Organism				
–	• Single-stranded deoxyribonucleic acid (ssDNA). • 3D-printed (poly(propylene fumarate) (PPF) scaffolds).	Bone	MC3T3 pre-osteoblast cells.	• Adhesion • Proliferation • Differentiation	1. Sonication is used for combining ssDNA and CNTs to get a negative charge. 2. Ammonolysis is performed on 3D-printed (PPF) scaffolds to produce a positive charge. 3. Combination of both product via electrostatic forces.	Biodegradable PPF provides rigidities that favor bone regeneration. ssDNA reduces cytotoxicity. Electrical stimulation is given through CNTs to modulate cell behavior.	[98]
–	• Polyvinyl alcohol (PVA). • Biphasic calcium phosphate (BCP).	Bone	MC3T3-E1 mouse calvaria-derived preosteoblast cell line.	• Cytocompatibility. • Cell proliferation. • Cell adhesion.	Freeze-thawing and freeze-drying method.	PVA and BCP have high biocompatibility but weak mechanical properties. CNTs are used to reinforce the mechanical properties.	[99]
MWCNTs	• Hydroxyapatite (HA). • Agarose gel (AG). • Collagens.	Bone	Mesenchymal stem cell lines and six eight-week-old female Sprague–Dawley (SD) rats.	• Proliferation. • Differentiation. • Thighbone's reparation *in vivo*.	1. CNTs–HA were produced via MWCNTs mineralization. 2. AG-CNTs-HA were produced by AG electrophoresis to achieved ordered CNT–HA array. 3. AG-CNTs-HA-collagen were produced by immersing the AG-CNTs-HA to collagen solution.	HA, a main inorganic component in bones with good biocompatibility osteogenic potential, tissue adhesion but weak in mechanical properties. • AG can help in cell growth, differentiation, proliferation, oxygen, and nutrients permeation for cell. • AG also help in forming ordered arrangement via electrophoresis. • But AG poorly adheres to cells. Collagen can promote cell adhesion and cell proliferation.	[98]

TABLE 14.1 *(Continued)*

Structure of CNTs (MWCNTs/SWCNTs)	Combination of Materials/Substances	Functional Part		Function	Production Method	Remark	Reference
		Body Part	Specific Cells/Tissues/Organism				
MWCNTs	• Montmorillonite (MMT). • Poly-l-lactic acid (PLLA).	Bone	MG-63	• Cell adhesion. • Growth. • Proliferation.	1. Chemical modification of CNTs via glacial acetic acid and aminopropyltriethoxysilane. 2. CNTs-MMT production through cation exchange. 3. Incorporated with PLLA via selected laser sintering (SLS).	CNT and MMT can enhance the mechanical properties of polymer, but aggregation will reduce their effect. The chemical modification and combining method provided well dispersion.	[100]
MWCNTs	–	Bone	Bone marrow derived mesenchymal stem cells (BMSCs).	• Biocompatible. • Osteogenic gene expression.	Unzipped CNTs produced via string acid treatment on MWCNTs.	The result indicated good osteogenic potential and biocompatibility for unzipped CNTs than pure CNTs.	[101]
MWCNTs	• Poly(ε-caprolactone) (PCL). • Keratin (Kr).	Bone	Mouse fibroblast cell line (3T3).	Cytocompatibility.	PCL/Kr/CNT was produced via electrospinning.	• KR have good hydrophilicity, biodegradability, biocompatibility, cell adhesion and proliferation supporting. • However, it has low mechanical strength and high swelling ratio.	[102]
			3T3 and human adipose-tissue-derived mesenchymal stem cells (hAD-MSCs).	Cell adhesion		PCL was introduced to maintain structural integrity and mechanical strength.	
			hAD-MSCs	Osteogenic differentiation. Cell proliferation.			

TABLE 14.1 *(Continued)*

Structure of CNTs (MWCNTs/SWCNTs)	Combination of Materials/Substances	Functional Part		Function	Production Method	Remark	Reference
		Body Part	Specific Cells/Tissues/Organism				
MWCNTs	• Poly[(alanine ethyl ester)-(glycine ethyl ester)] phosphazene (PAGP). • Dopamine hydrochloride solution (PDA).	Bone	BMSCs	• Proliferation. • Biocompatibility. • Osteogenic differentiation.	PAGP was blended with CNTs to produced PAGP/CNTs composite films with conductivity with PDA as surface modification.	PAGP is rich in phosphorus and nitrogen that can help in bone formation but with low cell attachment. PDA is added for providing the bio-adhesive feature. Electrical stimulation is applied to cell through PAGP/CNTs composite films to further. CNTs provided conductivity to the composites.	[103]
SWCNTs	• Poly(ε-caprolactone) (PCL). • Amine.	Bone	Rat bone marrow-derived mesenchymal stem cells (rMSCs).	• Cell adhesion. • Proliferation. • Differentiation.	Amine-CNTs are purchased while Amine-CNTs-PCL are produced via electrospinning.	PCL is biodegradable with good biocompatibility, but it is soft and lacks of functional groups for cellular responses. CNTs are used to increase the strength of the scaffold with PCL. Amine functionalized CNTs can improve osteogenesis, cellular responses and mechanical properties for PCL nanocomposite.	[104]
SWCNTs and MWCNTs	–	Bone	Canine mesenchymal stem cells (MSCs).	• Proliferation. • Differentiation. • Cytocompatibility.	CNTs with –OH functionalized was acquired.	MWCNTs with –OH functionalization osteogenic and chondrogenic differentiation.	[105]

TABLE 14.1 *(Continued)*

Structure of CNTs (MWCNTs/SWCNTs)	Combination of Materials/Substances	Functional Part		Function	Production Method	Remark	Reference
		Body Part	Specific Cells/Tissues/Organism				
MWCNTs	Polyion complex (PIC) hydrogels	Bone	rMSCs	• Biocompatibility. • Cell adhesion. • Proliferation. • Cell growth. • Osteogenic differentiation.	PIC/CNTs hydrogels were fabricated to interconnected porous scaffolds via extrusion-based 3D printing.	CNTs have good osteogenic effects while PIC hydrogels have good mechanical properties.	[74]
			Calvaria of sprague-Dawley (SD) rats (*in vivo*).	• Calvaria healing and regeneration.			
MWCNTs	Poly(lactic acid) (PLA). • Bioglass (BG).	Bone	rMSCs	• Biocompatible. • Cell activity. • Differentiation.	PLA/BG/CNT was produced via adding BG and CNTs into PLS membranes.	PLA has good mechanical features, flexibility, biocompatibility, and biodegradation. BG can help in osteoinduction and osteoconduction properties of nanocomposites. CNTs have good antimicrobial ability can block the proliferation of pathogens.	[106]

TABLE 14.1 *(Continued)*

Structure of CNTs (MWCNTs/ SWCNTs)	Combination of Materials/ Substances	Functional Part		Function	Production Method	Remark	Reference
		Body Part	Specific Cells/Tissues/ Organism				
MWCNTs	PCL	Bone	Human adipose-derived stem cells (hADSCs).	• Cell adhesion. • Proliferation.	• CNTs were produced by catalytic chemical vapor deposition technique. • PCL/CNTs was produced via melt blending method. • PCL/CNTs with 3D porous is produced via 3D printing through screw-assisted extrusion-based additive manufacturing.	3D printing is used to emulate the *in vivo* environment. PCL has good biocompatibility, can be processed easily, regulated degradation but low in cellular affinity, bioactivity, and poor mechanical properties with high hydrophobicity.	[75]
MWCNTs	• Polyurethane (PU). • Chitosan (Cs).	Cardiac	• Cardiac rat myoblast cells (H9C2). • Human umbilical vein endothelial cells (HUVEC).	• Cell adhesion. • Proliferation. • Biocompatibility.	• Electrospinning/spray process were utilized to produce Pu-Cs-CNTs composites.	Cs is biocompatible, with good wound healing property, antimicrobial activity and physicochemical properties but lack of mechanical properties. PU have good mechanical features and antimicrobial ability. CNTs were used to provide good conductive and mechanical properties.	[84]
MWCNTs	Silk fibroin	Cardiac	Neonatal rat cardiomyocytes.	• Biocompatibility. • Cell adhesion. • Guiding cell proliferating organization. • Expression of specific proteins for cardiac.	CNTs-silk fibroin composites are made by electrospinning procedure.	CNTs were used to provide good conductive and mechanical properties. Silk fibroin has good biodegradability, biocompatibility, with low immunogenicity.	[107]

TABLE 14.1 *(Continued)*

Structure of CNTs (MWCNTs/ SWCNTs)	Combination of Materials/ Substances	Functional Part		Function	Production Method	Remark	Reference
		Body Part	Specific Cells/Tissues/ Organism				
SWCNTs	• Polyvinyl alcohol (PVA). • Cs.	Cardiac	Rat mesenchymal stem cells (MSCs).	• Cell proliferation. • Cell adhesion. • Biocompatibility. • Cell differentiation.	Cs-PVA-CNT are produced mainly via electrospinning.	CNTs were used to provide good conductive, chemical stability, elastic, tensile strength, and crosslinking properties. Electrical stimulation is given from CNTs to cause differentiation. PVA is used to enhance the solubility of CNTs via forming hydrogen bonds. PVA also increase the interfacial strength and mechanical performance of the nanocomposites. CS are used as stabilizing agents in improving the solubility of CNTs and enhance the efficient fabrication of scaffolds	[108]
MWCNTs	Polyurethane	Cardiac	• H9c2 cells. • HUVECs.	• Cytocompatibility. • Cell adhesion. • Proliferation.	CNTs/PU nanocomposites are produced via electrospinning and electrospray.	CNTs were used to provide good conductive and mechanical properties and hydrophilicity. PU has good cytocompatibility, biodegradability.	[109]

TABLE 14.1 *(Continued)*

Structure of CNTs (MWCNTs/ SWCNTs)	Combination of Materials/ Substances	Functional Part		Function	Production Method	Remark	Reference
		Body Part	Specific Cells/Tissues/ Organism				
MWCNTs	• PCL. • Gelatine.	Cardiac-vascular	• Endothelial cells.	• Proliferation. • Biocompatibility. • Guiding cell proliferating organization.	PCL/Gelatin/CNT nanocomposites are produced via wet electrospinning.	CNTs were used to provide good conductive and mechanical properties but low in biocompatibility. • Using miscible solvents to mix CNTs and polymers shows high selectivity for polymers, while the usage of surface modified CNTs with high dispersal ability in the polymer matrix will alter the properties of materials and high method complexity required. • modified electrospinning are utilized to overcome those issues.	[110]
MWCNTs	Poly(octamethylene maleate (anhydride) 1,2,4-butanetricarboxylate) (124 polymer).	Cardiac	Neonatal rat heart tissue.	• Biocompatibility. • Cell maturation. • Tissue/cell function-beating.	• CNTs were dispersed into poly(ethylene glycol) dimethyl ether porogen with 124 polymer and crosslinking under ultraviolet light.	CNTs were used to provide good conductive and mechanical properties. 124 polymer allows the whole scaffolds to be high moldability and elasticity. The conductivity of CNTs caused the maturation of cell.	[111]

TABLE 14.1 *(Continued)*

Structure of CNTs (MWCNTs/ SWCNTs)	Combination of Materials/ Substances	Functional Part		Function	Production Method	Remark	Reference
		Body Part	Specific Cells/Tissues/ Organism				
MWCNTs	Polydimethylsiloxane (PDMS).	Cardiac	Neonatal rat ventricular myocytes (NRVMs).	• Biocompatibility. • Cell maturation. • Electrophysiological maturation. • Proliferation.	• MWCNTs were mixed with sugar to form sugar granules inside to create pores for spongy structure. • Then place on layers of PDMS and cured in oven. • The sugar was then be dissolved in distilled water.	PDMS has good biocompatibility with many applications in the medical sector with high stability that allow the incorporation of CNTs. CNTs were used to provide good conductive and mechanical properties, porosity to allow seeding integration, migration, and permeation of cardiomyocytes. The 3D structure of the scaffold provides the cardiac cells with good viability, maturation, and proliferation and reduced the proliferation of cardiac fibroblasts.	[82]
MWCNTs	–	Cardiac	Mouse embryoid bodies form by 129/ SVE-derived mouse stem cells.	• Cell differentiation. • Beating activity.	CNTs used in this procedure had been functionalized with carboxyl groups via an acid-treatment process.	The electrical stimulation given through the scaffold had caused cell differentiation and cause beating to the mouse embryoid bodies.	[112]

TABLE 14.1 *(Continued)*

Structure of CNTs (MWCNTs/SWCNTs)	Combination of Materials/Substances	Functional Part		Function	Production Method	Remark	Reference
		Body Part	Specific Cells/Tissues/Organism				
–	–	Cardiac	• Ovine (*in vivo*). • Rodent (*in vivo*).	• Toxicity. • Myocardial conduction and atrioventricular conduction. • Myocardial activation.	CNTs were treated with acid and spun under tension within acetone.	CNTs improved the conduction velocity (ovine study) with no toxicity and the conduction had lasted for 1 month (rodent study). CNTs with good mechanical properties and conductive properties help in myocardial conduction.	[85]
–	–	Cardiac	• Neonatal rat cardiomyocytes. • Mouse (*in vivo*).	• Cell morphology guided. • Electrical transmission.	• Super-aligned CNT (SA-CNTs) were produced by dry-spinning method. • CNT synthesized via chemical vapor deposition with no modification.	SA-CNTs were produced to mimic the structure with electrical-impulse transmission of myocardium.	[113]
MWCNTs	Poly(p-dioxanone) (PPDO)	Nerves (Peripheral nerve).	• Rabbit Schwann cells (rSCs). • Human adipose-derived mesenchymal stem cells (hADMSCs).	• Proliferation. • Growth. • Biocompatibility. • Differentiation. • Cell maturation.	PPDO/CNT nanoyarn nanocomposites is produced via electrospinning.	CNTs provided good mechanical properties and conductive properties to the composites. The electrical stimulation and chemical induction caused hADMSCs into SC-like cells (SCLCs) and further cell maturation, respectively. PPDO can help in host cells migration and axonal regeneration promotion.	[114]

TABLE 14.1 *(Continued)*

Structure of CNTs (MWCNTs/ SWCNTs)	Combination of Materials/ Substances	Functional Part		Function	Production Method	Remark	Reference
		Body Part	Specific Cells/Tissues/ Organism				
MWCNTs	• Cs. • Polyethylene glycol (PEG).	Nerves (Peripheral nerve).	• Culturing rat pheochromocytoma (PC12) cells.	• Cell adhesion. • Biocompatibility. • Proliferation. • Differentiation. • Neurite extension.	CS/PEG/CNTs scaffolds were produced by freeze-drying method.	• Conductivity and mechanical stability of CNTs can guide neuronal cell behavior, and induce axon regeneration. • CNTs provides roughness and hydrophobicity of scaffolds. PEG has adjustable biochemical and mechanical properties with hydrophilicity and biocompatibility. • CS has good biocompatibility and can promote differentiation and proliferation of nerve cells. • Cs also has less nerve inducibility, obvious nerve conductivity and is able to guide the differentiation as the neural networks.	[116]

TABLE 14.1 *(Continued)*

Structure of CNTs (MWCNTs/ SWCNTs)	Combination of Materials/ Substances	Functional Part		Function	Production Method	Remark	Reference
		Body Part	Specific Cells/Tissues/ Organism				
MWCNTs	PEG hydrogel	Nerves	• PC12 cells. • Adult neural stem cells (NSCs). • Primary hippocampal neurons.	• Differentiation. • Biocompatibility. • Neuronal network activity.	CNTs–PEG hydrogel composites are produced via *in situ* polymerization.	PC12 cells and adult NSCs were differentiated into astrocytes, neurons, and primary hippocampal neurons. Hydrogel has good biocompatibility to reduce the chances of fibroblast proliferation and abnormal immune cell activation caused by CNTs. CNTs give good conductivity to the nanocomposites.	[116]
MWCNTs	–	Nerves (Peripheral nerve).	Sprague Dawley rats (*in vivo*). • Gender: female. • Number:35. • Weight: 200–220 g. • Age: 8 weeks.	• Axons regeneration. • Repairing nerve defects.	1. The CNTs yarn was produced via dry drawing and spinning. 2. CNTs are produced via chemical vapor deposition.	Improvement in gait function observed at the 16th week according to sciatic nerve functional index (SFI). Electromyographical findings found axons regeneration 8 weeks after surgery.	[92]
MWCNTs	• Poly($_L$-lactide-*co*-D, $_L$-lactide) (PLDLLA). • 4-aminopyridine (4-AP)-loaded molecularly imprinted nanoparticles ($MIP_{4\text{-}AP}$).	Nerves (Peripheral nerve).	• PC12 cells. • Wistar rats. • (250 ± 25 g) Number=9	• Biocompatibility. • Proliferation. • Nerve generation.	PLDLLA/MWCNTs/$MIP_{4\text{-}AP}$ are produced via electrospinning.	Nerve generation is observed via histopathological images and SFI. PLDLLA is a polymer with electrospinable, biodegradable, and biocompatible properties. 4-aminopyridine (4-AP) are to use to multiple sclerosis and speed up the crashed sciatic nerve of rat recovery.	[117]

TABLE 14.1 *(Continued)*

Structure of CNTs (MWCNTs/SWCNTs)	Combination of Materials/Substances	Functional Part		Function	Production Method	Remark	Reference
		Body Part	Specific Cells/Tissues/Organism				
–	• Biodegradable poly(caprolactone fumarate) (PCLF). • Graphene. • [2-(methacryloyloxy) ethyl] trimethylammonium chloride (MTAC).	Nerves	PC12 cell	• Proliferation. • Differentiation. • Neurite extension. • Cellular migration.	PCLF-Graphene-CNT-MTAC composites are produced via ultraviolet (UV) photo-crosslinking.	CNTs and graphene had reduced electrochemical impedance and improved the surface roughness. When electric stimulation is applied, neurite protrusions increase. • PCLF have good non-immunogenicity and mechanical properties. • PCLF have better performance compared with PLGA and oligo [(polyethylene glycol) fumarate] (OPF). • PCLF provide nerve cell with good morphologic characteristics and electrophysiologic recovery. • PCLF will not produce harmful substances during degradation and can hold sutures. • But PCLF have low conductivity and smooth surface with is not favor to cell attachment and proliferation.	[94]

TABLE 14.1 *(Continued)*

Structure of CNTs (MWCNTs/ SWCNTs)	Combination of Materials/ Substances	Functional Part		Function	Production Method	Remark	Reference
		Body Part	Specific Cells/Tissues/ Organism				
MWCNTs	• Polycaprolactone (PCL). • Collagen.	Nerves (Peripheral nerve).	Human neuroblastoma cell line (IMR-32). • Adult Sprague-Dawley rats. • Gender: male. • Weight: 250–270 g.	• Biocompatibility. • Cell growth. • Proliferation. • Injured sciatic nerves healing. • Axonal regeneration.	• Electrospinning is used to produced PDMS/ PCL-collagen mixture and reinforced with CNTs coaxially.	CNTs in the scaffold had provided conductivity, tensile properties to the composite. The composite reached sciatic nerves healing within 30 days. Polydimethylsiloxane/ polycaprolactone and collagen have biodegradable ability.	[118]
MWCNTs	Sericin	Nerves	RSC96 Schwann cells.	• Biocompatibility. • Biodegradability. • Cell adhesion. • Cell growth.	–	CNTs improve the mechanical properties, contribute physical guidance for long nerve gap defect repair in the 12th week with electric conductive.	[119]
–	–	–	Sprague-Dawley rats Gander: Male Weight: 200–300 g.	• Sciatic nerve regeneration. • Structural repair. • Functional recovery.	–	Sericin have good biocompatibility, good biodegradability, low immunogenicity, allow neuron attachment, proliferation, axon extension, and prevent neuron apoptosis but sericin have weak mechanical properties.	–
MWCNTs	–	Kidney	Human embryonic kidney cell line (HEK293) cells.	• Cytotoxicity.	Two types of CNTs are produced via electric arc method with size of 90 to 150 nm and chemical vapor deposition method with size of 60 to 80 nm and test on HEK293 cells.	Both CNTs showed cytotoxicity.	[120]

TABLE 14.1 *(Continued)*

Structure of CNTs (MWCNTs/SWCNTs)	Combination of Materials/Substances	Functional Part		Function	Production Method	Remark	Reference
		Body Part	Specific Cells/Tissues/Organism				
MWCNTs	–	Liver	Primary rat hepatocytes	• Sustain liver-specific function. • Biocompatibility.	2D and 3D MWNTs scaffolds were produced.	Good biocompatibility and sustain liver-specific function was achieved.	[122]
MWCNTs	• N-carboxyethyl chitosan (CEC). • Benzaldehyde-terminated PF127 (PF127-CHO).	Skin	• Mouse fibroblast (L929) cells. • Kunming mice. ○ Weight: 30–35 g ○ Sex: female.	• Biocompatibility. • Antibacterial ability. • Healing effect.	CEC/PF/CNT hydrogels were prepared based on CEC and PF127-CHO/CNT dispersions.	–	[122]

electrical stimulation from the scaffold, the electroactive surfaces of it can also promote cell adhesion, maturation, proliferation, growth, and cellular functions [68–71]. This might be due to it helps the adsorption for adhesion-mediating proteins of cell and cellular processes of cell like activation of ion channels, allow easy movement of cell ions, enhanced proteosynthesis and up-regulated mitochondrial activity. Moreover, CNTs scaffold with conductivity also help in the chemical stability as it can block the ions or material particles move out from the scaffold [70]. While on the other hand, the hydrophilicity of the materials in the scaffold are mainly contributed by the addition of CNTs and the polymer (depending on the polymer type). The hydrophilic scaffolds are needed mainly because it can allow better cell adhesion and proliferation [72]. Nevertheless, hydrophobic surfaces are having better non-adhesive protein absorption like albumin for cell. Therefore, the best cell adhesion will only be achieved on moderately wettable surfaces [70]. Apart from that, the usage of the type of CNTs (MWCNTs and SWCNTs) is also very important in scaffold production. It can be observed that MWCNTs are the most used type CNTs in the research due to their relatively low toxicity.

From Table 14.1, the incorporation of CNTs-based nanocomposites had shown positive result in both *in vitro* and *in vivo* in various biological, regenerative, and tissue engineering properties via various cell and tissue, such as hAD-MSCs, Sprague–Dawley (SD) rats, MC3T3 pre-osteoblast cells, rMSCs, and more as shown in Figure 14.2 and Table 14.1. All of them had shown that CNTs are a good candidate for bones tissue engineering and regeneration medicine.

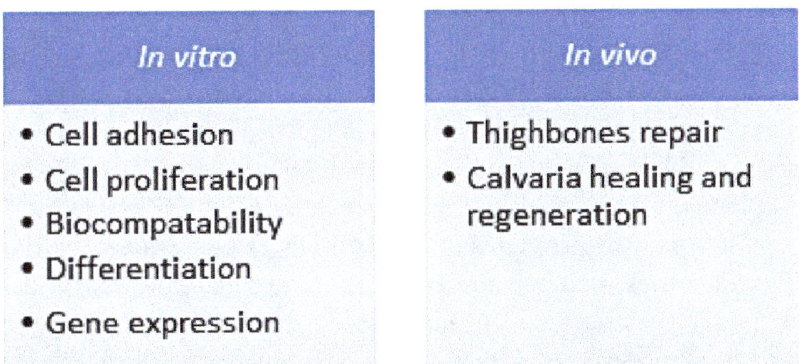

FIGURE 14.2 CNTs application for bone tissue engineering and regeneration on both *in vivo* and *in vitro*.

Xifeng et al. had produced CNTs scaffold combining with water-soluble single-stranded deoxyribonucleic acid (ssDNA) and poly(propylene fumarate) (PPF) scaffolds [73]. In this case, the material added is mainly to aid the scaffold production process. The production section is divided into 3 steps, the production of PPF 3D scaffold, a combination of ssDNA and CNTs and lastly the Combination of both PPF 3D structure and ssDNA-CNTs. Firstly, PPF was used to produce the 3D structure via 3D stereolithography with computer aiding. After that CNTs were incorporated with ssDNA via sonication to produce negative changed on ssDNA-CNTs. Before the final combination of both products, PPF 3D structure will be ammonolyzed and lead to the free amine groups with positive surface charge and the formation of PPF-ssDNA-CNTs composites scaffold product will be produced via electric-static force. The ssDNA had been found to decrease the cytotoxicity of the composites in both *in vivo* and *in vitro* study while PPF have mechanical strength for bone regeneration and can fabricate crosslinked scaffold. CNTs in this case had provided good conductivity which had also play a vital role in this experiment. For the result, the PPF-ssDNA-CNTs composites scaffold have positive result in MC3T3 pre-osteoblast cell adhesion, differentiation, and proliferation. Moreover, the scaffold can also modulate the cellular behavior like proliferation and gene expression via the application of electrical stimulation. On the other hand, Haomin et al. incorporated both CNTs (MWCNTs) and PIC to create PIC/CNTs hydrogels 3D scaffolds via extrusion-based 3D printing [74]. PIC's strong mechanical stiffness with pro-osteogenesis and -bone calcification of CNTs is combined and tested on rMSCs for *in vitro* and sprague-Dawley (SD) rats' calvaria (cranium) for *in vivo* test. For *in vitro* test, PIC/CNTs hydrogels 3D scaffolds show biocompatibility, cell growth, proliferation, adhesion, and promote better osteogenic differentiation as compared with PIC scaffolds alone. While on the other hand, Sprague-Dawley (SD) rats had shown regeneration on the cranium defect sites by using PIC/CNTs hydrogels 3D scaffolds as the template. The mechanism of the bone promotion via MWCNTs is due to it can induce alkaline phosphatase (ALP) releasing and recruit calcium for bone calcification. Moreover, it was also proven that the MWCNTs can lead to cell adhesion and angiogenesis, which are the best candidates in bone scaffold as bone tissue is highly vascularized. In this chapter, the researchers also found that there are blood vessels (new and mature) occupying the defects implanted with PIC/CNTs.

Huang et al. utilized PCL incorporated into MWCNTs to create composites scaffold by screw-assisted extrusion based additive manufacturing which is a

3D printing method to test on human adipose derived stem cells (hADSCs) [75]. PCL have good biocompatibility and good processibility that can allow to make CNTs more printable. Nonetheless, it is lack in cellular affinity, bioactivity, and mechanical strength with high hydrophobicity which could be fixed by the addition of CNTs. According to the result, the PIC/CNTs composite showed good hADSCs cell adhesion and proliferation with low cytotoxicity. By altering the concentration of CNTs within the scaffold, the mechanical properties of bone can also be produced. In this chapter, 3 wt.% of MWCNTs within the composite can give compressive modulus similar to cancellous bone.

In a nutshell, CNTs is a great bone scaffold candidate with its conductivity and mechanical properties. However, more *in vivo* and pre-clinical or clinical studies could be carried out to further ensure the applicability of this material in bone tissue engineering and regeneration.

14.2.3 CARDIAC TISSUE ENGINEERING AND REGENERATION MEDICINE

Heart function are to pump the oxygenated and deoxygenated blood throughout the body. Deoxygenated blood will be received from the body to the heart and later pumped into the lungs to oxygenate it while the oxygenated blood that come from lung will be distributed throughout the body to provide oxygen to the body. For the cardiac tissue, ECM with 3D environment that made up by network of fibrous structures is filled with cardiac cells [76]. The normal function and adaptation to workloads of the heart are sustained via the cellular properties of the heart. The cells within the heart can initiate electricity from one and propagate to another cardiac cell. Such properties allow the heart to contract synchronously and ensure the blood circulation to be run in the optimum level between lungs, heart, and the distal organs [77]. During puberty, human cardiomyocyte nuclei are polyploid and initiation of DNA synthesis with no nuclear division will happen when pathological workloads occur, and such DNA synthesis will increase cardiomyocyte nuclear ploidy but not cardiomyocyte proliferation. Therefore, if any injury occurs to the heart, repairing will be carried out instead of regeneration. Scar will be form by meshwork of extracellular matrix to replace the injured muscle tissue and decrease the contractility of the myocardium which might also lead to heart failure and even death [26, 27]. Currently, the only treatment is through transplantation, but it suffers with low donor availability and high surgery risk. However, through artificial cell-supportive materials, regeneration, and cardiac tissue engineering of diseased heart frameworks are doable via mimic the myocardium to encourage organ repair and cell growth.

Apart from the previous section about the CNTs properties that can aid in bone regeneration and tissue engineering, cardiac tissue engineering and regeneration can also be further improved through the conductivity provided by CNTs as it allows the fabrication of electroconductive material. Such materials can not only replace or regenerate the cardiac cell/tissue but functional regeneration which might be able to aid in CVD like congenital cardiovascular defects and myocardial infarction, valvular heart disease, coronary artery disease, etc. [78, 79]. The aims of the biomaterials are to fabricate composites that can give replacing some functions of the cardiac tissue while avoiding the dysfunction after myocardial infarction and cardiac remodeling [70]. The properties of the cardiovascular biomaterials are mainly focusing on the biodegradability and the conductivity [70, 80]. According to Table 14.1, the synthetic polymers like PU, PVA, 124 polymer, PDMS, PPDO, polyethylene glycol (PEG) hydrogel, and PLDLLA in the composites had provided with different mechanical and biological properties like antibacterial, cytocompatibility, biodegradability, solubility, interfacial strength, moldability, and elasticity while natural polymers such as Cs, silk fibroin, and collagen had provided mainly on biological properties like wound healing property, antimicrobial activity, biodegradability, biocompatibility, low immunogenicity and solubility with some minority of them contributing to the physicochemical properties. Some natural polymers also supplied with cell adhesion and proliferation properties [81]. However, they are lacking mechanical and conductivity properties. Therefore, CNTs is added to improve the mechanical and conductivity properties of the composites while the other polymer and substances are added to improve the biocompatibility.

Same as CNTs application on bone regeneration and tissue engineering research, 3D structures architectures in cardiac as transplantable devices with cell-enriched properties [70]. The 3D structure of the scaffold provides the cardiac cells with good viability, maturation, and proliferation and reduced the proliferation of cardiac fibroblasts and produce a favorable and stable ratio between cardiomyocyte/cardiac fibroblast [82]. Apart from that, electrospinning/spray are the most used method in producing cardiac tissue engineering and regeneration scaffold (Table 14.1). Moreover, CNTs application had also show positive result in cardiac tissue engineering and regeneration with some nanoscale applications in both in *vivo* and *in vitro* test on different cell/tissue and organism such as rat mesenchymal stem cells (MSCs), H9c2 cells, neonatal rat heart tissue, neonatal rat ventricular myocytes (NRVMs), ovine (*in vivo*), rodent (*in vivo*) and more via CNTs or CNTs-based composites as shown in Table 14.1 and Figure 14.3.

In vitro	*In vivo*
• Cell adhesion • Cell proliferation • Biocompatability • Differentiation • Gene expression • cell maturation • protein expression • guiding cell proliferating organization • electrophysiological maturation • Tissue functioning-beating • electrical transmission	• Cell differentiation • conduction • Cytotoxicity • Myocardial conduction and atrioventricular conduction • Myocardial activation

FIGURE 14.3 Applications of CNTs for cardiac tissue engineering and regeneration on both *in vivo* and *in vitro*.

One significant different in cardiac tissue engineering and regeneration is that the conductivity of the CNTs added allows the beating function, myocardial conduction, atrioventricular conduction and myocardial activation of cardiac tissue to be realized and improved in both *in vitro* and *in vivo* test, along with some other cellular function such as cell maturation, protein expression, guiding cell proliferating organization and electrical transmission (Table 14.1) [83].

Ahmadi et al. had used polyurethane (PU) and chitosan (Cs) to incorporate with CNTs (MWCNTs) [84]. Electrospinning/spray process are used to produce Pu-Cs-CNTs composites to test on cardiac rat myoblast cells (H9C2) and human umbilical vein endothelial cells (HUVEC). Cs is a natural polymer with good biocompatible and physicochemical properties for wound healing purposes. Nonetheless, Cs has low in mechanical properties, limiting its application as cardiac scaffold. Therefore, PU is added to give strong mechanical properties while maintaining the good biocompatible of Cs. MWCNTs are added to further enhance the mechanical and conductivity of the scaffold. Apart from that, MWCNTs are used as they have a large surface-to-volume ratio, which can promote electron transfer reactions and increase the surface roughness of composites which can lead to protein absorption and finally improve cell proliferation and adhesion. For the result, the researchers had found out that the cell adhesion, proliferation, and biocompatibility are observed on both cardiac rat myoblast cells (H9C2) and Human umbilical vein endothelial cells (HUVEC). The Alamar blue assay illustrated the HUVEC and H9C2 cells have more cell number than only bare PU scaffolds and control group in 1, 4, and 7 days.

In addition to that, Mertinelli et al. combined both polydimethylsiloxane (PDMS) and MWCNTs to be cardiac scaffold. In this case, the 3D structure is produced by dissolving MWCNTs with sugar to form granule [82]. The granule will cause connected pores to be form and produce a spongy structure. After that, the mixture is molded and dried. After dried, the mixture is sutured via the PDMS via vacuum and cured via oven. After that sugar was then be dissolved in distilled water. PDMS are used to give good biocompatibility and high stability to allow the incorporation of CNTs while CNTs improve the conductivity and mechanical properties of the composite scaffold. The composite produced have positive implications to the neonatal rat ventricular myocytes (NRVMs) in biocompatibility, cell maturation, proliferation, and electrophysiological maturation.

Mccauley et al. used CNTs on ovine and rodent for *in vivo* test [85]. In sheep, an acute open chest electrophysiology research was carried out and epicardial conduction delay was created via radiofrequency ablation after the application of CNTs while rodents' right atrioventricular junction was surgically sewn by CNTs with both acute and chronic electrophysiology studies were held. The addition of CNTs gives good mechanical, conductive, and biocompatibility properties that allow the restoration of electrical conduction of diseased myocardium. The result show improved conduction velocity in large animal studies with no significant toxicity observed. The conduction had maintained for 1 month in rats with no significant immunological and toxic response. Moreover, CNTs also proven to be able to reestablish the myocardial conduction in acute study and chronically allow atrioventricular conduction in the research. Moreover, CNTs can is also found out to enable the myocardial activation.

In conclusion, cardiac tissue engineering and regeneration had been successfully achieved via CNTs and CNTs based composites scaffold with satisfying mechanical strength and conductivity that allow functional improvement like cardiac beating. Moreover, multiple positive result also indicates that CNTs can be an excellent multifunctional cardiac scaffold.

14.2.4 NERVES TISSUE ENGINEERING AND REGENERATION MEDICINE

Nervous system is made up from a complex nerves network that regulate body organs to maintain body balance like breathing, digestion, sexual development during puberty and more [86–88]. The nervous system including two parts: CNS and PNS. CNS includes the brain and spinal cord while PNS is composed of nerves and ganglia at the external part of the brain and spinal cord. Neuroregeneration is the regeneration of nervous tissues, cells or cell products [30]. Yet, the regeneration and tissue engineering of the nerves tissue is challenging mainly due to the limitation of regenerative properties of both CNS and PNS. PNS have the ability for self-regeneration spontaneously after injury via disease or trauma. However, the self-generative properties only limited in small injuries and young people. Large injuries in PNS require clinical intervention, nevertheless, even if intervention is given, the functional recovery is inadequate. CNS on the other hand, have no generative properties at all after the disease or trauma. This is owing to there are not ample of Schwann cells to support axonal development and the glial scar tissue that form via astrocyte and meningeal cell activity is compact in CNS. This produces an unfavorable condition which restricts the neural regeneration. The current treatment for large PNS defect involves allografts and autografts as a connector to link the nerve stumps with the tubular prostheses such as cutaneous nerves or blood vessels. However, in most scenario, tubular implants are needed due to insufficiency of allografts and autografts. Moreover, many problems like immune response, inadequate functional recovery, rejection, and materials instability might occur after the clinical treatment which might further damage the nervous system. For CNS, especially for the spinal cord, the patient will only be subjected to physical therapy and minimizing the secondary injury. Yet, it does not ensure for fully recover but the limited mobility only [30, 32]. Therefore, a material that can fulfill the need of biocompatible, stable for both neural regeneration and total functional recovery is important. There are few criteria need to be met to be the competent material for neural regeneration and tissue engineering. Apart from preliminary standard like biocompatibility, mechanical, biological properties such as proliferation and differentiation promotion, functional restoration as well as nerve regeneration guidance or facilitation also very vital when it comes to materials for neural regeneration and tissue engineering as it can help blocking the outgrowth of the cell/tissue while reconnect other neurons and lead to functional restoration [89]. Nanostructured environment is more preferable for nerves cells interaction as the biological function like differentiation process are found out to be faster in nanoscale-fibrous as compare to microfibrous scaffolds [90]. Therefore, the nano-scale materials like nanotubes are used to imitate the tubular structures of the body.

CNTs are one of the best candidates for the nerves tissue regeneration and tissue engineering due to its nanoscale, flexibility, inertness, and mechanical strength of CNTs which allow to create an artificial ECM environment for nerve regeneration [31, 91, 92]. Moreover, it is found that the conductivity and the positive surface charge of functionalized CNTs is able to generate electrical conduction and promote nerves cell elongation, allow the communication between neuronal cells electrically, promote neural cell differentiation, adhesion, growth, maturation, and neurite outgrowth orientation [93–96]. With the combination of 2D and 3D scaffolds, this further enhance CNTs as the neural tissue engineering and regeneration medicine [97].

Same as bone and cardiac regeneration both natural and synthetic polymer had been incorporating into the CNTs scaffold such as poly(p-dioxanone) (PPDO), PEG, poly($_L$-lactide-*co*-D, $_L$-lactide) (PLDLLA), Poly-lactide-co-glycolide (PLGA), biodegradable poly(caprolactone fumarate) (PCLF), graphene, [2-(methacryloyloxy)ethyl] trimethylammonium chloride (MTAC), collagen, sericin, and polydimethylsiloxane/polycaprolactone (Table 14.1). Their purposes are to improve the biocompatibility as well as other biological function. While the incorporation of CNTs is to compensate or provide the poor mechanical strength and conductivity for the composite scaffold produced. Some other substances such as 4-aminopyridine (4-AP)-loaded molecularly imprinted nanoparticles (MIP4-AP) are also added to improve the neural recovery (Table 14.1). The most utilized method is electrospinning among all the method. Scaffold produced had applied in many types of cells *in vitro* including rabbit Schwann cells (rSCs), human adipose-derived mesenchymal stem cells (hADMSCs), culturing rat pheochromocytoma (PC12) cells, adult neural stem cells (NSCs), primary hippocampal neurons, human neuroblastoma cell line (IMR-32) cells and RSC96 while For *in vivo* test, Sprague Dawley rats and Wistar rats are used, and all the research had gotten satisfying result in various aspects (Table 14.1 and Figure 14.4).

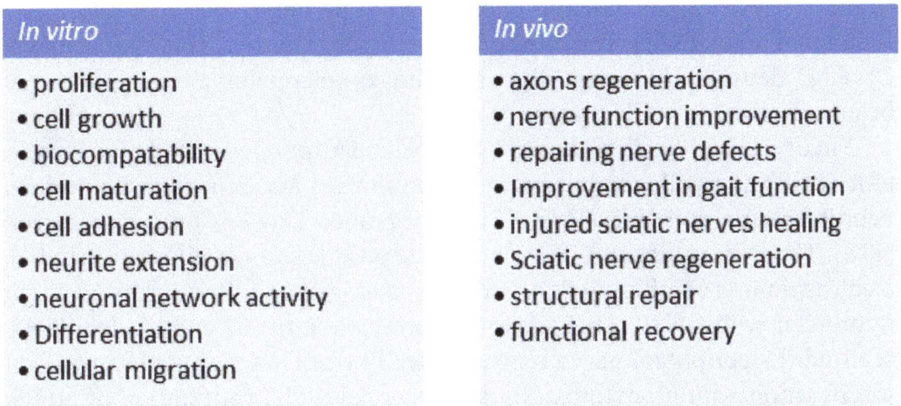

FIGURE 14.4 Applications of CNTs for nerves tissue engineering and regeneration on both in *vivo* and in *vitro*.

Ye et al. had combined both PEG hydrogel and MWCNTs and discovered cell differentiation and maintenance of neuronal network activity with good biocompatibility on pheochromocytoma 12 cells (PC12), adult neural stem cells (NSCs), and primary hippocampal neurons [116]. In this research, PEG is polymerized *in situ* around a CNT meshwork to produce CNTs-PEG hydrogel scaffold. PEG hydrogel had provided good biocompatibility that can reduce the chances of fibroblast proliferation and immunological response that might cause via insertion of CNTs while CNTs provided PEG hydrogel with good mechanical strength and conductivity that can promote neural regeneration. In the result, NSCs were differentiated astrocytes, neurons, and primary hippocampal neurons with improved synaptic connectivity via CNTs-PEG hydrogel composite. Moreover, neuronal network activity also found out to be maintained by CNTs-PEG hydrogel scaffold via spontaneous calcium oscillations. Therefore, the CNTs-PEG hydrogel scaffold can not only promote nerves cell differentiation but also maintaining neuronal homeostasis.

On the other hand, MWCNTs had been applied on Sprague Dawley rats for *in vivo* test by Kunisaki et al. [92]. Dry drawing and spinning method are used to produce CNT yarn. Acetylene and iron are both used as carbon source and catalyst, respectively, in vertically aligned MWCNTs production via chemical vapor deposition. CNTs yarns that were applied within the *in vivo* tests were 15 μm in diameter within the silicon tubes with a diameter of 15 mm. After 8 weeks, axons regeneration is found through electromyographical study with recovery on the muscle weight ratio at the lower leg.

In the 16th week, gait function is observed to be improved via sciatic nerve functional index (SFI). The most effective regeneration of nerves is achieved 2% CNT density. This result illustrated the peripheral nerve regeneration can be accomplished by CNT yarn.

Finally, Ghosh et al. had used MWCNTs incorporated with polycaprolactone (PCL) and collagen to apply on both *in vitro* and *in vivo* test on human neuroblastoma cell line (IMR-32) and Sprague-Dawley rats, respectively [118]. The PCL-collagen-CNTs composite production was first produced via electrospinning combining PCL and collagen together, following by coaxially reinforced with CNTs. This allows the production of 3D and biodegradable scaffold for peripheral nerve regeneration. For *in vitro* test, cell growth and proliferation with no cytotoxicity are observed with proliferation of around 184% (±8) at 72 h and around 240% (±9) at 120 h. For *in vivo* test, sciatic nerves injuries in rats were healed within 30 days. In addition to that, with the conductivity from CNTs, axonal regeneration was improved. Therefore, it can be concluded that PCL-collagen-CNTs composite is a very suitable in peripheral sciatic nerve regeneration.

To summarize, CNTs are applicable in neural regeneration and tissue engineering. With the application of electricity conduction properties of CNTs, the regeneration could be further improved according to both *in vitro* and *in vivo* research.

14.2.5 DIFFERENT BODY PART TISSUE ENGINEERING AND REGENERATION MEDICINE

It can be observed that in most of the tissue engineering and regeneration studies are mainly focusing on bone, cardiac, and neural related tissue and cell. However, there are some applications of CNTs on other cells and tissues. For example, Reddy et al. had utilized MWCNTs with 2 different synthesis method as electric arc method (size: 90–150 nm) and chemical vapor deposition method (size: 60–80 nm) to test on human embryonic kidney cell line (HEK293) cells via MTT assay, LDH assay with reduced glutathione (GSH), interleukin-8 (IL-8), as well as lipid peroxidation levels to be determined [120]. The results indicated that both CNTs showed severe cytotoxicity as increasing levels of LDH is observed which indicated the cell membrane damage with increasing production of IL-8 and lipid peroxidation. On the other hand, the intracellular glutathione levels had decreased, which can be linked to the oxidative stress provided via CNTs application. In short,

CNTs produced via both methods exhibit cytotoxicity in HEK293 cells, indicating that CNTs are not suitable for kidney cell and tissue engineering and regeneration.

Che Abdullah et al. also used 2D and 3D MWCNTs nano-scaffolds in liver tissue engineering on primary rat hepatocytes [121]. For the result, cell viability, hepatocyte specific marker albumin production, enzyme activity (CYP 1A2/3A4), and transporter activity are achieved and enhanced by MWCNTs. In addition to that, they also found out that MWCNTs yarns can induce high albumin secretion levels.

Apart from that, skin has also been treated with CNTs combined with N-carboxyethyl chitosan (CEC) and benzaldehyde-terminated PF127 via mixing CEC polymer and PF127-CHO/CNT dispersion at physiological conditions (PF127-CHO) [122]. The CNTs composites had been applied in both *in vivo* (Kunming mice) and *in vitro* test (mouse fibroblast (L929) cells). The produced composite had provided good mechanical properties, biodegradability, hemostatic properties, high water absorbency, and suitable gelation time. For the result, the CNTs composite with rapid photothermal properties improved the antibacterial activity in *in vitro* and *in vivo* studies. In addition to that, wound healing, angiogenesis, and collagen deposition were observed *in vivo* test while good biocompatibility was found in *in vitro* test with L929 cells. Apart from this study, other studies have tested CNTs-based nanocomposites application on skin tissue engineering and regeneration with good result in biocompatibility, bioactivity, antibacterial, and wound healing applications [123, 124].

14.3 BIOSENSING

Sensor is a device that detects and responds to the physical input and converts the measurement into output signals that are to be recorded. Temperature, pH, force, odor, and pressure, as well as the presence of particular chemicals, flow, position, and light intensity, are all detected and measured using sensors and their accompanying interfaces [125]. The output is a signal that can be translated to a human-readable display at the sensor location or sent over a network for additional processing. A biosensor is a device that combines a biological component that detects an analyte with a physicochemical component that generates a measurable signal. Sensitivity, selectivity, accuracy, signal stability, operating range, and regeneration time are all features of biosensors. The biosensor can be categorized into two components: (a) bioreceptor; and (b) transducer as shown in Figure 14.5. A bioreceptor is a biomolecule element that identifies the target analyte, such as an enzyme, DNA, antibody, entire cells, tissue, etc.

Then, the transducer converts a recognized event into a measurable signal that can be electrochemical, optical, thermal, or piezoelectric. According to IUPAC recommendations from 1999, a biosensor is defined as an autonomously integrated receptor transducer device, which is capable of giving selectable quantitative or semiquantitative analytical information utilizing a biological recognition element [126]. Biosensor development is a interdisciplinary field in which researchers use diverse molecular biology approaches, such as genetic engineering to identify or produce a variety of bioreceptors with better sensitivity and selectivity [127].

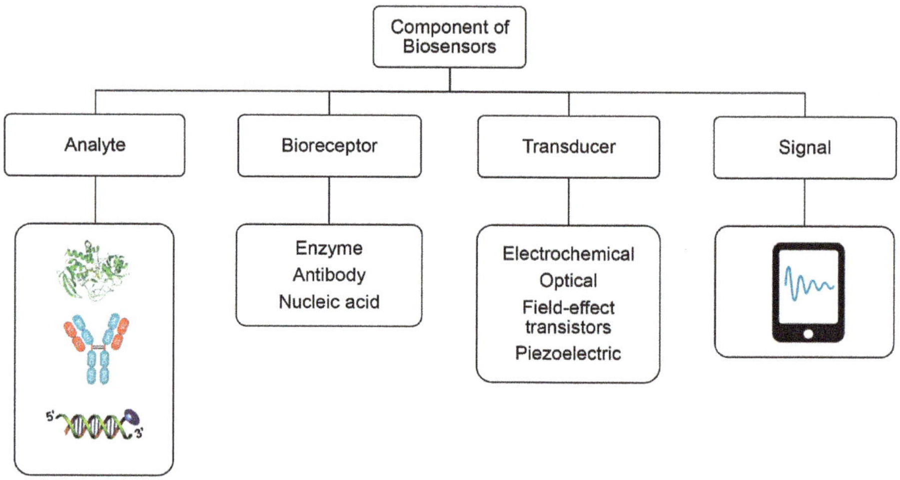

FIGURE 14.5 Schematic representation of biosensor operation principles.

Source: Kim et al. [128]; Nathani, Vishnu, & Sharma [129]; Grieshaber et al. [130]; Alfaleh et al. [131]; and Su et al. [132].

Biosensors have been widely employed in environmental, health, and food quality monitoring, as well as in evaluating and optimizing the optimum performance of any technique. The first biosensor demonstrated by Clark and Lyons in 1962 used an immobilized glucose oxidase electrode to quantify glucose in biological samples using an electrochemical detection technique for oxygen or hydrogen peroxide [133]. A biosensor is a small analytical instrument that includes a biological or biologically derived sensing element that is either integrated into or closely connected with a physicochemical transducer. A biosensor's goal is to deliver rapid, real-time, accurate, and dependable information about the interrogated analyte [134].

CNTs are a well-known and good contender for serving as a platform for the immobilization of biomolecules. CNTs possess various unique characteristics, such as high surface-to-volume ratio, radii comparable to the Debye length, and excellent electrical properties [135], making them a suitable material for signal transduction for the detection of analytes, metabolites, or disease biomarkers. Furthermore, CNTs possess a hollow core and large specific surface area (SSA), which allows for the immobilization of a large number of functional units, such as receptor moieties, on the CNT surface for the application of the biosensor [136, 137].

Nowadays, CNTs electrodes are being developed for the detection of biological agents, such as glucose, immunoglobulin G (IgG), immunoglobulin E (IgE), and other biomarkers in the medical field [138–140]. CNTs work as an amplifier, enhancing the detection signals and increasing the detection sensitivity [141]. CNTs paste enzyme electrodes, for example, are composite electrodes that combine CNTs's capacity to enhance electron-transfer processes with the appealing properties of paste electrode materials [142]. In this section, we will discuss the application of CNT-based biosensors for biomedical applications.

14.3.1 BIORECEPTORS

Bioreceptor is one of the most distinguishing features of biosensors, which is also known as biological recognition elements. The bioreceptor recognizes the target analyte, and then, the transducer turns this response into a different type of energy that is amplified, processed, and translated into the preferred signal format. CNTs-based biosensors can detect a variety of bioreceptors, including enzymes, antibodies, and nucleic acids.

14.3.1.1 CNTS-BASED ENZYME BIOSENSORS

Enzymes are typical biocatalysts that can speed up biological reactions. Enzymes are globular proteins made up primarily of the 20 amino acids found in nature that can catalyze biological reactions, as well as the well-known green catalysts with high selectivity [143]. An enzyme-based biosensor is a type of analytical instrument that combines an enzyme with a transducer to generate a signal which is proportional to the concentration of a target analyte. This signal can be caused by different mechanisms, such as change in proton concentration, release or uptake of gases (e.g., ammonia or oxygen), light emission (absorption or reflectance), heat emission, and so on, all of which are caused by the enzyme-catalyzed reaction [144]. CNTs-based enzyme biosensors are used for measuring various biomolecules. The benefit of these sensors is that electroactive materials are created by enzyme reactions, which may be detected with high sensitivity on CNT-modified electrodes. CNTs can react as the electrode surface functions for attaching biomolecules and a transducer for enhancing electrochemical response. Also, CNTs can promote electron-transfer reaction between the enzyme and the electrode [145].

Comba et al. [146] synthesized CNTs-mucin composite (CNTs-muc) for enzymatic matrix of a glucose biosensor for human blood samples. The amount of crosslinker used for the enzymatic matrix, as well as the ratio of CNTs-muc/alb, affects the analytical performance of the biosensor. The enzymatic matrix consists of 50% w/w CNTs-muc, 50% w/w albumin, 1.33 U glucose oxidase (GOx) per biosensor, and 5.0% v/v glutaraldehyde has the best relationship between sensitivity and response time among the different biosensors. The addition of CNTs to the enzymatic matrix reduces the viscosity of the matrix, resulting in higher diffusion coefficients for reagents and products of the enzymatic process than in an enzyme matrix without CNTs.

14.3.1.2 CNTs-BASED ANTIBODY BIOSENSORS

Antibodies are affinity biorecognition elements with a wide application range and strong antigen-antibody interactions that have been employed for over two decades. Antibodies have the structure of immunoglobulins (Ig), which are made up of two heavy and two light polypeptidic chains linked by disulfide bonds [147]. Biosensors using antibodies as ligands are called immunosensors. An immunosensor is a biosensor that combines a biological recognition mechanism with a transducer that provides a quantifiable signal in response to changes in a biomolecule's concentration [148].

CNTs can be employed as transduction materials in which enzymatic products and electroactive materials can be detected with high sensitivity at CNTs-modified electrodes. CNTs can be used as an immunoassay carrier and label to carry a significant amount of electroactive compounds [145]. Thus, a CNTs-based immunosensor might be used as a sensitive detector. Gulati et al. [149] demonstrated a flexible immunosensor for detecting multidrug-resistant myeloid leukemia cells at extremely low levels. The immunosensor was fabricated by VA-MWCNTs by using doxorubicin-treated leukemia K562 cells with different concentrations (1.5×10^2 cells mL^{-1} to 1.5×10^7 cells mL^{-1}), resulting detection limit of 10 cells mL^{-1}. Saify Nabiabad et al. fabricated immunosensor of tissue plasminogen activator (tPA) by immobilization of anti-tPA on SWCNTs/glassy carbon electrode (GCE) as a biomarker of myocardial infarction and breast cancer [150]. The biosensor was built with a linear response range of 0.1 to 1.0 ng mL^{-1} and a detection limit of 0.026 ng mL^{-1}.

14.3.1.3 CNTs-BASED NUCLEIC ACID BIOSENSORS

Aptamers are two-dimensional (2D) and three-dimensional (3D) synthetic single-stranded nucleic acids (DNA or RNA sequences) that attach to target molecules preferentially. Aptamers always deliver high selectivity and affinity to their targets [151]. Aptamer interactions between their molecular targets are precise that even minor changes in the target molecule can cause aptamer binding to be disrupted [152]. Besides, aptamer-based biosensor using CNTs-FET devices was also produced for disease diagnosis [153]. Applying monoclonal IgE antibody displayed very low sensitivity at ~50 ng/mL. CNTs-FET can block non-target proteins and selectively detect the target protein in an environment similar to human serum electrolytes. Park et al. [154] fabricated a polyaniline/CNTs (PANI/CNTs) electrode for aptamer biosensor designed for detecting vascular endothelial growth factor ($VEGF_{165}$) on a screen-printed carbon electrode (SPCE) used as a biomarker in tumor cells. PANI/CNTs exhibit high sensitivity for $VEGF_{165}$ sensing with a detection limit of 0.4 pg/mL.

14.3.2 TRANSDUCERS

The transducers' task is to transport the signal from the recognition system's output domain to the input domain. In CNTs based-biosensors, several transducer-based output signals have been used, such as electrochemical, optical, field-effect transistors (FET), and piezoelectric biosensors.

14.3.2.1 ELECTROCHEMICAL BIOSENSORS

An electrochemical biosensor is a self-contained and integrated device that employs a bioreceptor in direct spatial contact with an electrochemical transducer to generate quantitative or semiquantitative analytical data on a target analyte [125]. Electrochemical biosensors occur when a biomolecule interacts with the analyte, a chemical change occurs on the biosensor's surface, which is then transformed into an electric signal that changes in proportion to the quantity of the analyte [155]. Electrochemical biosensors can be classified into numerous categories based on the transduction principle, including amperometric, potentiometric, voltametric, and impedimetric. CNTs have been widely used in the development of electrochemical sensors. CNTs have a number of significant advantages in the fabrication of electrochemical sensors, including [156]:

i. Large SSA leading to high sensitivity;
ii. A tubular nanostructure and chemical stability that allows the fabrication of ultrasensitive sensors consisting of only one nanotube; and
iii. Good biocompatibility for electrochemical biosensors by enhancing the electron transfer of redox proteins and enzymes.

14.3.2.2 CNTS-BASED AMPEROMETRIC BIOSENSORS

Amperometric biosensors operate in a two or three-electrode systems by measuring the current created by from the oxidation or reduction of electroactive materials at the working electrode, when a potential is applied to the working electrode for the Ag/AgCl reference electrode [130, 157, 158]. The current generated on the working electrode's surface is proportional to the concentration of analyte in the solution. This approach offers a sensitive, rapid, precise, and linear response, which makes it more ideal for mass production than potentiometric biosensors [147]. CNTs are frequently used as working electrodes in sensing systems because of their extremely low detection limit. The hollow shape of CNTs is ideal for enzyme adsorption. In CNT-based amperometric biosensors, CNTs are frequently utilized to functionalize with enzymes to create enzyme/CNT electrodes or to change the electrode surface [159].

Shukla, Turner, & Tiwari [160] fabricated a cholesterol oxidase (ChOx) immobilized PANI/CNTs composite electrode for the amperometric detection of cholesterol. Blending with CNTs generates a network within the matrix, which strengthens the bioelectrode's mechanical properties. Thus, a linear current response to the cholesterol oleate was 30 to 280 μM with a response time of 10 s. Ramonas et al. [161] proposed an amperometric biosensor by immobilizing alcohol dehydrogenase on graphite electrode which was modified with CNTs and a redox mediator tetrathiafulvalene for the detection of glycerol concentration in human urine. Wang & Musameh [162] reported CNTs-based amperometric biosensors made up of polypyrrole/CNTs-glucose oxidase (PPy/CNT-GOx). When entrapped within the PPy network, the CNTs dopant preserves its electrocatalytic activity toward hydrogen peroxide, resulting in high sensitivity where linearity prevails up to ca. 50 mM glucose.

14.3.2.3 CNTS-BASED POTENTIOMETRIC BIOSENSORS

Potentiometric biosensors measure the accumulation of charge potential at the working electrode compared to the reference electrode [130]. Potentiometric biosensors can detect pH, H^+, NH_4^+, and other ions, as well as biomolecules, including glucose, urea, and penicillin, among other things. The potentiometric biosensor can be divided into several types such as ion-selective electrodes, ion-sensitive field-effect transistors, screen-printed electrodes, solid-state devices, and chemically modified electrodes [163, 164]. Although potentiometric biosensors have lower sensitivity and slower response times than amperometric biosensors they have very high detection limits [155]. Ahuja et al. [165] analyzed ureases/MWCNTs/silica/indium tin oxide electrode for potentiometric biosensor applications. The electrode demonstrates an excellent performance with a wide linear range from 2.18×10^{-5} to 1.07×10^{-3} M urea and high sensitivity of 23 mV/decade/cm^2 in the shortest response time of 10–25 s.

14.3.2.4 CNTS-BASED VOLTAMETRIC BIOSENSORS

Voltammetric biosensors measure current during a controlled fluctuation of the applied voltage to detect the analyte. The current peak size is related to the electroactive materials, and the potential where the redox peaks arise is distinct for the tested electroactive materials. There are several types of voltammetric methods, for example cyclic voltammetry (CV), linear sweep voltammetry (LSV), square wave voltammetry (SWV), differential pulse voltammetry (DPV), stripping voltammetry, AC voltammetry, polarography, etc. [166]. The advantages of voltammetric biosensors are high sensitivity readings and simultaneous detection of numerous analytes [147]. Goyal, Gupta, & Chatterjee [167] applied SWV method for SWCNTs modified edge plane pyrolytic graphite electrode (EPPGE) to detect paracetamol. For SWCNTs modified EPPGE, the sensitive oxidation peak of paracetamol was observed at ~187 mV with pH 7.2 ($\mu = 0.5$ M) and was used to quantitate the drug between 5 and 1,000 nM with the lowest detection limit of 2.9×10^{-9} M.

14.3.2.5 CNTS-BASED IMPEDIMETRIC BIOSENSORS

Impedimetric biosensors measure the electrical impedance spectroscopy generated on the electrode/electrolytes interface, which characterizes the response of an electrochemical cell to a small amplitude sinusoidal voltage signal, as a function of frequency. In a usual alternate current (AC) circuit for impedance analysis, several activities for example kinetics of antigen-antibody interactions, redox reactions, and other molecular interactions at the electrode's surface can be measured to impede the flow of electrons [158]. Liu et al. [168] demonstrated impedimetric biosensor usage for the detection of cancer cells at low concentrations. The electrode sensor was constructed by MWCNTs/PEI electrodes and epithelial cell adhesion molecule (EpCAM) over-expressed on the surface of liver cancer cell line ($HepG_2$) cells. The detection limit of the cancer cells is a minimum concentration of 10 cells per mL in whole blood samples. Palomar et al. [169] conducted an impedimetric immunosensor for the detection of dengue virus antibodies. For consistent highly sensitive monitoring of the Dengue Virus 2 NS1 antibody in a complicated environment, controlled CNTs layers were produced and functionalized with the Dengue virus 2 NS1 glycoprotein. This immunosensor has good linearity in the 10^{-13}–10^{-5} g mL^{-1} range and low sensitivity of 39.5 ± 3.8 Ω per order of magnitude.

14.3.3 OPTICAL BIOSENSORS

Optical biosensors are analytical devices consisting of a biorecognition element integrated into an optical transducer system. Optical biosensors are made up of a light source and a variety of optical components that work together to generate a light beam with specified properties and direct it toward a modulating agent, a modified sensing head, and a photodetector [170]. As biorecognition elements, the optical biosensor can use a variety of biological components such as nucleic acids, enzymes, antibodies, entire cells, and tissues. The transduction process in optical biosensors causes a change in light absorption, transmission, reflection, refraction, phase, amplitude, frequency, or polarization in response to the physical/chemical change caused by biorecognition events.

They may be classified into two modes based on the optical biosensor's principle, i.e., label-free and label-based. In label-free mode, the interaction between the examined material and the transducer, and in label-based mode the optical signal is generated by colorimetric, fluorescence, or luminescent methods [171]. Surface plasmon resonance (SPR), evanescent wave (EW) fluorescence, optical waveguide interferometry, chemiluminescence, fluorescence, refractive index, and surfaced-enhanced Raman scattering (SERS) are some of the optical concepts that can be used to create optical biosensors. The most often used optical-based biosensors are fluorescence-based optical biosensors, chemiluminescence-based biosensors, SPR-based biosensors, and fiber-based biosensors [147]. Detection of biomolecules employing near-infrared light between 0.9 and 1.3 eV has crucial biomedical applications because of improved tissue penetration and lower auto-fluorescent background in thick tissue or whole-blood medium. CNTs offer outstanding luminescence qualities, high luminous intensity, and a good wavelength conversion function, particularly for tunable near-infrared emission that responds to changes in the local dielectric function while remaining stable against photobleaching [172]. From these excellent advantages, CNTs can be applied in optical biosensors.

14.3.3.1 CNTS-BASED FLUORESCENCE BIOSENSORS

The fluorescence-based biosensors are based on the measurement of fluorescence intensity which is proportional to the concentration of the target analyte [164]. Because of its excellent selectivity, sensitivity, and fast reaction time, this type of biosensor is the most studied for medical diagnosis, environmental, and food quality monitoring applications. There are three types of fluorescence-based biosensors: (a) fluorescent quenching (turning off); (b) fluorescent amplification (turning on); and (c) fluorescence resonance energy transfer (FRET) [147].

CNTs have been widely used in fluorescence sensors and biosensors because their fluorescent characteristics are greatly reliant on their physical structure [173]. Wojtera et al. [174] investigated the feasibility of attaching structurally diverse fluorophores to the surface of CNTs to create fluorescent biosensors that can be used in medical diagnostics to identify disease early. Fluorescent acidic, base, and neutral dyes were successfully connected to the surface of CNTs, and the fluorescent markers were successfully linked to their surface.

14.3.3.2 CNTS-BASED SPR BIOSENSORS

SPR-based biosensors measure the changes in the refractive index produced by molecule interactions at a metal surface through surface plasmon waves [147]. Surface plasma oscillations, also known as surface plasmons, are coherent fluctuations induced by electron charges at a metal-dielectric contact. The plasmons can produce an electric field up to ~100 nm. When monochromatic, polarized light strikes an interface between a prism and a buffer solution with the highest RI, the light can be partially reflected and refracted toward the interface plane [158, 171]. SPR sensors may be a good option for detecting tiny compounds that interact with biomolecules. Lee et al. [175] developed a CNTs-based signal amplification approach for SPR immunoassays that can be used to monitor pharmaceutical processes. This method improves detection sensitivity and widens the dynamic range, which is over four orders of magnitude for human erythropoietin (EPO) and human granulocyte macrophage colony-stimulating factor (GM-CSF).

14.3.4 FIELD-EFFECT TRANSISTORS BIOSENSORS

Field-effect transistors (FET) biosensors are three-terminal devices that use an electric field to regulate the current flowing through them. FET devices consist of a source, a drain, and a gate terminal, with the electric field created by the voltage at the gate (V_G) and the voltage supplied between the source and drain (V_{SD}) terminals causing modulation of the current (I_D) in the semi-conducting channel [176]. There have two types of transistor-based sensing platforms ion-sensitive field-effect transistors (ISFETs) and metal-oxide-semiconductor field-effect transistors (MOSFETs) [147].

For the detection of biological species, CNTs-based FETs have several advantages, i.e., biocompatibility, size compatibility, and sensitivity to minute electrical disturbances. CNTs-FET can be used to detect protein, glucose, enzyme, antigen, and antibody molecules, DNA, bacteria, and hormones [172]. Bobba, Carrara, & Micheli [177] proposed an array of CNTs-FETs to improve specificity and sensitivity by using a multi-gate controller at the nano-scale. By multiplexing distinct P450 probes, this research will be applied to the detection of drugs in multi-component samples. Thanihaichelvan et al. [178] reported a CNTs-based FET biosensor for rapid detection of severe acute respiratory syndrome coronavirus 2 (SARS-CoV-2) responded selectively to the positive target sequence, with a detection limit of 10 fM.

14.4 DRUG DELIVERY

CNTs have been a great interest for researcher to use as biological delivery carrier due to the possibility of various modifications and adsorption capabilities of the nanotubes to load small molecules, such as drug, gene, vaccine, etc. In general, the CNTs will first undergo modifications to make it biocompatible and then drug molecules can be adsorbed or chemically bonded on the surface of CNTs, lastly the drug loaded CNTs nanocomposites can be delivered to the targeted cell to release the drug molecules in the intracellular space. The modifications of CNTs, drug loading mechanism and drug delivery mechanism will be discussed in subsections.

14.4.1 MODIFICATION OF CNTS

Although CNTs are fascinating material to use as biological delivery carrier, its hydrophobicity characteristic makes them hard to be dispersed in water. Due to the lack of solubility of CNTs in aqueous media, modifications of CNTs are needed to improve the compatibility of CNT in biological systems [179]. Various studies reported oxidation of CNTs to yield functional groups (carboxylic acid (-COOH), aldehyde (-HC=O), and alcohol (-OH)) on the CNTs. The presence of these functional groups not only allow the CNTs become more soluble and easily disperse in water, but it also provides active sites for chemical reaction to take place [1, 2]. There are two types of modifications of CNTs which are covalent functionalization via chemically modified and non-covalent functionalization via van der Waals, π-π stacking, ionic bond, hydrogen bonding, and hydrophobic interactions [180]. These modifications include processes, such as oxidation, esterification, and amidation on the oxidized CNTs, functionalizing them with polar organic molecules, polymer grafting, and dispersion with polymer or amphiphilic surfactants [181–183]. Researchers had utilized these active sites for further chemical reactions, including esterification, amidation, etherification, etc., to form covalent bond with other compounds, such as polymers (PEG, PEI), organic molecules (folate, cyclodextrin), drugs, etc. [181–186]. Yu et al. [184] had prepared PEG-modified CNTs to load lobaplatin (chemotherapy drug) as pH-controlled release carrier on HepG2 cells [184]. The CNTs underwent oxidation process to obtained COOH-containing CNTs. Then, the COOH-modified CNTs was undergo acyl chlorination to enable the grafting of hydrophilic PEG on the CNTs. After that, the PEG-modified CNTs can be used to load the lobaplatin. Das et al. [185] had prepared a cancer cell-selective PEG-linked 17β-Estradiol grafted on MWCNTs for intranuclear drug delivery to breast cancer cell [185]. Firstly, the PEG was linked with Estradiol 17 β-hemisuccinate and the CNTs was undergo oxidation process to obtain COOH modified MWCNT, Then, the MWCNTs functionalized with 7β-estradiol-hemisuccinyl-poly(ethylene glycol)-amine to obtain the drug delivery carrier. Then, the doxorubicin can be loaded into the MWCNTs via π-π stacking interaction.

Besides, modifications can also be done through non-covalent functionalization via physical interactions between on the CNTs' surface in the form of hydrogel, microgel, nanofibers, and nanocomposites [186–189]. With these chemical and physical modifications, various molecules can be attached on the surface of the CNTs, which is useful for drug delivery system, as shown in Figure 14.6. Moreover, it can enhance the uptake into biological cells and also reduce the cytotoxicity and oxidative stress towards cells [179].

14.4.2 DRUG LOADING MECHANISMS

Physical loading of drug compounds on CNTs by adsorption of active drug compounds on the surface of CNTs via interactions, such as electrostatic, hydrophobic, hydrogen bonding, covalent bonding, π-π stacking, etc. [190]. Furthermore, some studies had also loaded the drug via formation chemical bond on the surface of CNTs and then controlled release of the drug compound either through cleavable disulfide bond or hydrolytic cleavage [190]. Besides, researchers had also utilized the hollow internal cavities of the nanotubes (both single- and multi-wall) to carry small drug molecules, peptides, DNA, and RNA [191]. Tsai et al. [192] had studied the drug loading capacity of doxorubicin onto anionic amphiphilic polymer-grafted MWCNTs with carboxylic acid, heparin, and polyglycolic acid [192]. The polyglycolic acid-modified MWCNTs exhibit excellent loading capacity as compared with carboxylic acid and heparin-modified MWCNT due to via hydrophobic

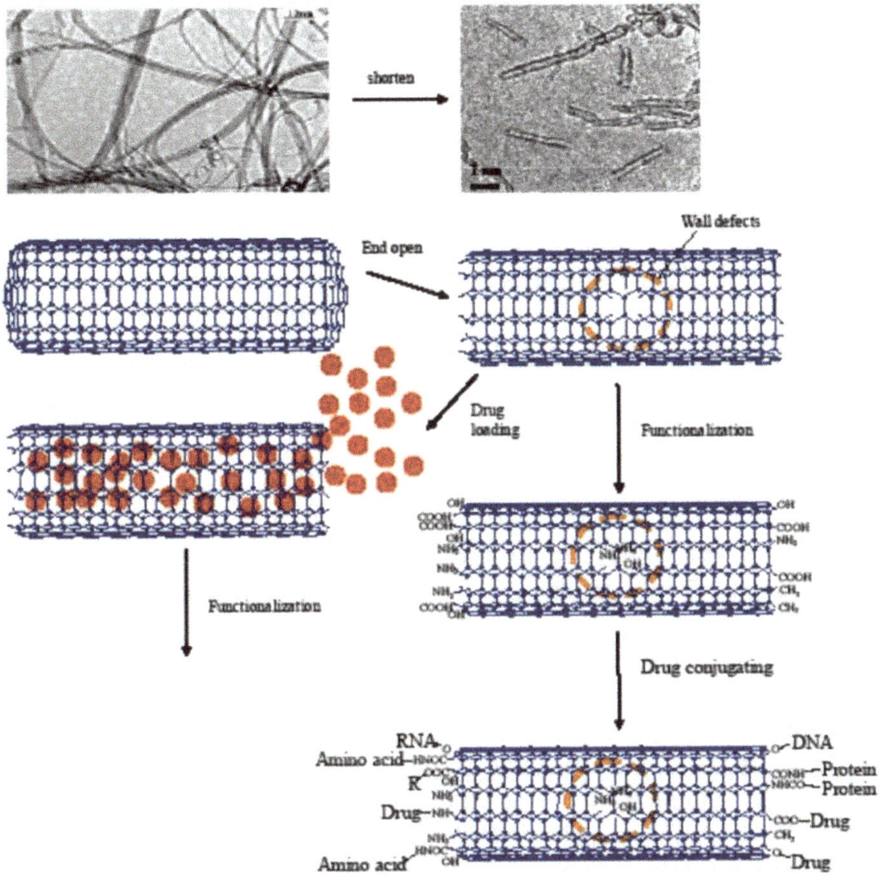

FIGURE 14.6 The TEM images and an illustration of the possible modifications of CNTs via functionalization and drug conjugating for drug delivery systems.

Source: Adapted with revisions from: Liu [180].

interactions and π-π stacking with the loaded drug. Recent years, many studies reported in using computational studies via molecular dynamics simulation to investigate the adsorption capacity of the active drug onto the CNTs' surface [193–197]. Contreras et al. [195] had studied the intermolecular interactions of PEG-functionalized SWCNTs and doxorubicin [195]. The molecular dynamics simulation shows that the adsorption of doxorubicin occurred on the surface and internal cavity of the CNTs via π-π stacking and N-H…π electrostatic interactions with equilibrium distances of 3.1–3.9 Å. Nikfar & Shariatinia [198] had investigated the phosphate-functionalized

SWCNT adsorbed with risedronate and zolendronate using the density functional theory computations [198]. The presence of phosphate on the surface of CNTs introduced dipole moment in the molecule which can carry the adsorbed drug passing through the lipophilic phospholipid cellular membranes. Karimzadeh et al. [194] had studied the adsorption mechanism of doxorubicin on hydroxyl- and carboxyl-functionalized SWCNTs [194]. The functionalized SWCNTs shows improvement in adsorption of doxorubicin in aqueous and gas phases compared with the pristine SWCNTs due to the formation of hydrogen bonding between active sites of doxorubicin molecules and the oxygen containing functional groups of CNTs via physisorption process (exothermic and thermodynamically favorable).

14.4.3 DRUG DELIVERY MECHANISM

The modifications on the CNTs which makes it water dispersible had improve its workability in biological medium. Typically, the drug delivery mechanism of CNTs (Figure 14.7) from the extracellular environment into biological cell undergo processes via direct diffusion and endocytosis processes (mediated and non-mediated). Mediated endocytosis processes are the approach of targeted delivery via specific receptor protein binding on cellular membrane. These type of specific binding targeted delivery can be achieved with approaches such as encapsulation of the drug loaded CNTs with ligand functionalized biopolymers and covalently conjugation of specific binding protein on the surface of CNTs [199, 200]. Studies show that the polymer modifications on CNTs can also makes possibility for a slower drug release rate due to the secondary physical interaction of the drug molecules with the extended polymers that prolong the desorption process in the nanocarrier. These slower release rate favors biomedical applications because it can prolong drug activity in the biological system extend the therapeutic time and reduce the cytotoxicity of the drug delivery system. An illustration of pathways for the delivery of CNTs into the biological cell is shown in Figure 14.7.

Huang et al. [199] had prepared CNTs encapsulated with folic acid-conjugated chitosan to load doxorubicin via π-π stacking interaction onto the CNTs surface [199]. The hydrophilicity of the nanocarrier had been improved with functionalization of cationic charge of chitosan enhances the stability of CNTs in the aqueous medium. *In vitro* test had been conducted to study the drug release response of CNTs at a temperature of 37°C in the

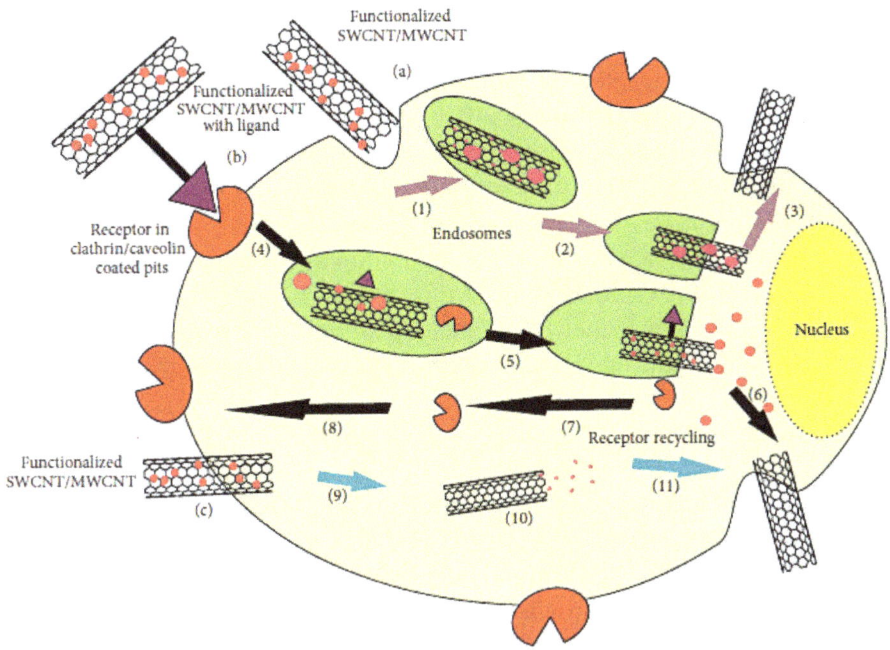

FIGURE 14.7 Penetration pathway of CNTs into the cell—(a) nonreceptor mediated endocytosis: (1) membrane that surrounds the drug loaded functionalized CNTs; (2) internalization of drug loaded CNTs; and (3) release of drug; (b) receptor mediated endocytosis: (4) membrane surrounds the CNT-receptor conjugate by forming endosomes followed by internalization; (5) release of drug; and (6–8) regeneration of receptor; and (c) endocytosis diffusion pathway: (9) direct penetration of drug loaded functionalized CNT; and (10, 11) release of the drug.

Source: Reprinted from Ref. [201]. https://creativecommons.org/licenses/by/4.0/

phosphate buffer solution. When the phosphate buffer solution was adjusted to pH 5.3 from pH 7.4, the rate of doxorubicin release increased by 25% for CNTs loaded doxorubicin samples. With the CNTs encapsulated with folic acid-conjugated chitosan, the encapsulation allows controlled release of doxorubicin at a lower rate at both pHs after 72 h. The slower release rate of doxorubicin may be due to the hydrogen bonding interaction between doxorubicin and folic acid in the encapsulated CNTs.

Taghavi et al. [200] had prepared a targeted delivery system using carboxylated SWCNT grafted with modified branched polyethylenimine using PEG linker [200]. The AS1411 aptamer as the nucleolin ligand was covalently attached on the nanocarrier to target deliver the doxorubicin and Bcl-xL-specific shRNA into nucleolin-abundant gastric cancer cell. The nanocarrier exhibit excellent tumoricidal efficacy and strong cell selectivity The combination of these two chemotherapeutic drug and gene-silencing shRNA can provide a safer approach for antitumor activity.

Wu et al. [202] had prepared PEI grafted MWCNTs covalently bonded with prostate stem cell antigen monoclonal antibody and fluorescein isothiocyanate for targeted drug delivery [202]. They had conducted *in vivo* study using PC-3 tumor-bearing mice as animal model which successful target deliver the nanocarrier to the tumor and suppress the tumor growth. The nanocarrier carrying doxorubicin was able to slowdown the tumor growth by 1.58-fold due to the presence of monoclonal antibody on the nanocarrier can specifically bind with the prostate stem cell antigen receptor on the tumor cell.

Cifuentes-Riu et al. [203] had prepared flexible and rigid CNTs coated with positively charged polyallylamine by plasma enhanced chemical vapor deposition and electrostatically bind GFP plasmid reporter on its surface for gene delivery application [203]. The rigid CNTs showed a lower amount of GFP plasmid loaded on CNTs, but it can have better release of DNA into the cell and tissue accumulation when investigated *in vivo* studies on rat.

14.5 BIOIMAGING

In this section, we will review studies on the application of CNTs in biomedical imaging (biomedical imaging). Bioimaging plays a significant role especially in clinical practice, especially in identifying the abnormal processes related to diseases and understanding of the operating mechanism of cells, tissues, and organs [204]. CNTs possess many unique properties, especially in terms of the unique physical properties, such as their compelling size, shape, and structure, which have motivated the development of biological applications. CNTs are potentially used in various bioimaging applications, including near-infrared (NIR) photoluminescence imaging [205], Raman imaging [206], magnetic resonance imaging (MRI) [207] and photoacoustic (PA) imaging [208].

14.5.1 FLUORESCENCE BIOIMAGING

Besides the application in fluorescence biosensing, CNTs can also be used for fluorescence bioimaging because living systems are transparent and Near-Infrared radiation (NIR) is not harmful. Hence, fluorescence imaging is particularly important in scientific research and medical diagnosis. In 2002, the near infrared photoluminescence in individual semiconducting SWCNTs was discovered [209]. CNTs as fluorescent imaging agents *in vitro* and *in vivo* imaging agents has been studied widely [210, 211]. CNTs were used as the Near-Infrared (NIR) label for the immunoassay (*in vitro* assay) where the intrinsic photoluminescence of SWNTs in the NIR above 1,000 nm could be a potential candidate for biological probes with low scattering by bio-organic molecules and deep tissue penetration [212]. Besides, MWCNTs have also been modified into a nanocomposite by covalently decorating the surface of the MWCNTs using magnetite nanoparticles (Fe_3O_4), poly(ethylene glycol) (PEG), and fluorophore fluorescein isothiocyanate (FITC). The CNTs nanocomposite can respond to an external magnetic field while maintaining strong fluorescence characteristic [211]. It was found that the nanocomposite can deliver a greater amount of FITC into the cytoplasm of the cells than the extracellular exposure of free FITC with MCF7 cells. This finding further confirmed that the produced fluorescent nanocomposite can serve as a versatile probe and could be a promising candidate for bioimaging.

Meanwhile, for *in-vivo* fluorescence imaging, CNTs could generally improve tissue penetration with better spatial resolutions [213, 214]. Welsher et al. prepared SWCNTs coated with phospholipid-PEG which were then injected into athymic nude mice's tail vein. The SWCNTs are useful fluorophores in the low albedo NIR II region in which the *in vivo* distributions of the SWCNTs were tracked by recording the fluorescence images using NIR light [215]. Huang et al. demonstrated an approach by utilizing the fluorescent bioimaging to trace the location of *in-vivo* implanted biomaterials [216]. The MWCNTs were prepared by electrospun with poly(lactide-co-glycolide) (PLGA), followed by further shaping into multichannel nerve guide conduits (NGCs) to repair the injured rat sciatic nerve. The distribution of the MWCNTs could be detected via bioimaging. On the other hand, Yin et al. had developed a nanoplatform of chlorin e6-manganese dioxide/CNTs (Ce6-MnO_2/CNTs) for *in vivo* imaging. The Ce6-MnO_2/CNTs were injected intravenously into tumor-bearing mouse where the fluorescence was mainly observed in the kidney [217]. However, after 12 hours of post-injection, the fluorescence moved to the tumor sides by showing the strongest fluorescence intensity. After 36 hours, the intensity of fluorescence started to decrease due to the metabolized of Ce6-MnO_2/CNTs. This could be a great potential in fluorescence imaging for tumor imaging.

14.5.2 RAMAN IMAGING

The intrinsic spectroscopic properties of CNTs are not restricted in the application of NIR fluorescence bioimaging. CNTs could also be potentially used as Raman probes for bioimaging [124, 218]. Zavaleta et al. has demonstrated an optimized non-invasive Raman microscope to evaluate the tumor targeting and localization of SWCNTs in mice [219]. Raman imagings were obtained in two groups of tumors bearing mice that received the SWCNTs intravenously (Control group: plain SWCNTs, experimental group: arginine-glycine-asparatic acid (RGD) peptide with single-walled CNTs (RGD-SWCNTS)). It was found that after 72 h, an increased accumulation of RGD-SWCNTs in tumor was observed as compared to plain-SWCNTs. This work has led to the further development of highly sensitive non-invasive Raman imaging tool for diagnostic strategies and therapies in small animal models and eventually to the care of cancer patients. Bajaj et al. has reported an immunoassay that used biotinylated SWCNTs as a Raman label [220], in which they used avidin-biotin chemistry to link targeting ligands in order to image the whole cells by using a breast tumor cell model.

Raman spectroscopy has been studied widely and is a well-established bioanalytical tool [221]. However, the main drawback is the weak Raman intensity which has resulted in low sensitivity. Hence, surface-enhanced Raman scattering (SERS) has been studied widely because it can increase the Raman signal effectively [222, 223]. A ratiometric SERS nanoprobe for imaging hypoxic living cells or tissues has been reported [224]. The SERS nanoprobe was synthesized using azo-alkynes assembled on SWCNTs and surface-functionalized with Ag/Au alloy nanoparticles (SWCNTs/Ag/AuNPs). The hypoxia level (in different cell lines and rat tissue samples derived from hepatic ischemia surgery) was determined based on the peak intensities (I_{2578}/I_{2207}) where the alkyne Raman band (2,207 cm^{-1}) as target-dependent, and the 2D-band of SWCNTs (2,578 cm^{-1}) is used as an internal standard. As a result, the ratiometric SERS probe could be an assuring tool for both *in vitro* and *in vivo* imaging of hypoxia.

14.5.3 MAGNETIC RESONANCE IMAGING

Magnetic resonance imaging (MRI) is one of the most powerful and non-invasive methods of imaging [225, 226]. CNTs are widely used as contrast agent in MRI. Kakavand et al. has reported the use of CNTs as an MRI contrast agent *in vitro* [227]. They managed to synthesize a superparamagnetic gadolinium (Gd) nanoparticle-catalyzed SWCNTs (Gd-CNT) and reduced the toxicity and solubility of CNTs by coated with polyethylene glycol (PEG). The *in vitro* MRI studies showed that the produced Gd-CNTs-PEG displayed an enhanced signal intensity in T1-W images. Choi et al. reported the use of SWCNTs as T2 contrast agent for T2 weighted MRI [228]. Iron oxide nanoparticles were attached at the end of SWCNTs without the need of additional labeling. A recent study produced oxidized MWCNTs via the [2+1] cycloaddition of nitrenes, particularly salicylic acid nitrene generated by the thermal decomposition of 4-azidosalicylic acid [229]. The oxygen functional groups on the MWCNTs' surface have a great effect on the T2 relaxometric properties, leading to a high contrast enhancement.

Meanwhile, CNTs could also be used as the carbon nanotube electrode for MRI. Test disk electrodes were fabricated from CNTs using the CNTs-templated microfabrication technique (CNT-M) [230]. The produced CNTs electrodes demonstrated a closely matched magnetic susceptibility (–5.9 to –8.1 ppm) with tissue. In phantom MR imaging experiments, there was almost no distortion caused by these electrodes as compared to reference electrodes (Cu and Pt-Ir). This has shown great potential for significant improvement in accurate tip visualization. Zheng et al. studied and produced an intramuscular electrode made from a soft and elastomeric conducting polymer composite (consisting of polyethylene glycol (PEG) end-capped poly(3,4-ethylene-dioxythiophene (PEDOT-PEG) copolymer, silicone, and CNTs with fluorosilicone insulation) [231]. The produced electrodes have a mechanical modulus much closer to the muscle tissue than metal wires, which is stable *in vivo for* up to 4 weeks. This intramuscular electrode can be CT and MRI imaged without undesired metal artifacts.

14.5.4 PHOTOACOUSTIC IMAGING

Photoacoustic (PA) imaging is an imaging modality that has been widely used in the biological field [232, 233]. Both SWCNTs and MWCNTs have been used as a photothermal agent due to its strong NIR absorbance [234]. Thus, CNTs can be served as an ideal contrast agent for PA imaging. Commonly, a thin layer of gold or some organic molecules with NIR absorbance were coupled with SWCNTs or MWCNTs. Kim et al. synthesized golden carbon nanotube (GNTs) by coating the SWCNTs with a thin layer of gold [235]. The GNTs were conjugated with antibodies to target lymphatic vessels in mice with low laser fluence levels of a few $mJcm^{-2}$. The antibody conjugated GNTs were used to map the lymphatic endothelial receptor. The obtained results show that the produced nanomaterials could be a promising alternative for fluorescent labels and non-invasive targeted imaging of molecular structures *in-vivo*. Later, Cui et al. reported the preparation of ultrathin gold nanowires-incorporated MWCNTs (GNW-MWCNTs) hybrid as NIR PA imaging [236]. The produced GNW-MWCNTs show an extraordinary optical absorption, thermal, and electric conductivity. A detection limit of 0.01 ng/mL for the alpha-fetoprotein (AFP) antigen with high selectivity.

On the other hand, CNTs composite film can be used as laser ultrasonic transducer that could enhance the PA signal. Mosse et al. fabricated an ultrasound transducer which consist of CNTs and polydimethylsiloxane (PDMS) [237]. The produced composite was dip coated onto the end faces of optical fibers. An optical fiber hydrophone positioned adjacent to the coated 200 μm core optical fiber. Ultrasound reflectance measurements were obtained from the outer surface of a sheep heart ventricle. In their study, an ultrasound transducer consists of optical fibers with CNT-PDMS composite coatings showing a promising result that may be suitable for miniature medical imaging probes. Meanwhile, Choi et al. reported a dual-mode imaging system that utilizes optical ultrasound without a transmission circuit [238]. The ultrasonic pulse-echo system can generate high-power PA signal, whereas a thin CNTs-polydimethylsiloxane (PDMS) composite as semi-absorption of the laser. A single-shot imaging system was then developed. A single-shot dual-mode imaging experiment on point and line phantoms, as well as the particle spread in the soft tissue was performed and successfully obtained volumetric image results.

14.6 TOXICITY

Carbon-based nanomaterials (CBNs) have become one of the most appealing nanomaterials due to their many forms, including fullerenes, single- and multiple-walled CNTs, carbon nanoparticles, and nanofibers, etc. Biological applications that use CBNs for DNA, proteins, and pharmaceutical delivery, in particular, have received much interest. Nevertheless, the literature on the possible dangers of CBN exposure is few and still being debated. Because of their structural similarity to asbestos, the scientific community is mainly worried about CNT toxicity [239, 240]. Seo et al. [241] investigated the shape effect of CBNs on cell toxicity by exposing cells *in vitro* to CBNs with various aspect ratios, including multi-walled CNTs, and carbon nanofibers (CNFs), and lastly, flakelike-shaped carbon nanoparticles (carbon black) [241]. All CBNs were suspended in a very diluted gelatin solution. Nanotechnology and nanomedicines have been discovered to be an emerging prospective sector with increased characteristics attracting numerous investigators. Nanomaterials have been made commercially and are widely employed in various sectors [242]. Recent research has shown that exposure to ultrafine particles, such as air pollution, welding fumes, and silica dust, has a deleterious influence [243]. The chemical reactivity and biological activity of nanoparticles are much higher than large particles [244]. The principal reason for CNTs' toxicity is related to reactive oxygen species (ROS) and free radical generation, which causes oxidative stress, inflammation, and protein and DNA damage (apoptosis, impairment of genetic material, oxidation of amino acid, and enzymes inactivation) [245]. Impurities, shape, length, chemical composition, surface charge, surface structure, aggregation, solubility [246], route of exposure such as dermal, intravenous injection, inhalation, and action mechanisms such as oxidative stress, DNA damage, and interstitial fibrosis all influence toxicity [247]. Metal-oxides generated by CNTs have been reported to enter the blood and harm the lungs [248]. Toxicity studies for CNTs in biomedical applications must encompass implant toxicity, cytotoxicity, carcinogenicity, and genotoxicity. These toxicity studies must establish the safety problems before being employed as biomaterials [249]. Figure 14.8 summarizes the mechanisms, classifications, and variables influencing toxicity. A few *in vitro* cytotoxicity assessments of water-dispersible single-walled carbon nanotubes nano-tubes (SWCNT) on A549 cells, a human lung cell line, confirmed that SWCNT had no intracellular localization in A549 cells and demonstrated that SWCNT could induce indirect cytotoxicity through cell culture medium modification, resulting in a false-positive toxic effect [250, 251]. Dumortier et al. discovered that fluorescein-labeled water-soluble SWCNTs were harmless to mouse B- and T-lymphocytes and macrophages and kept their function [252]. Other research sought to assess the possible toxicity and general mechanism of two diameter types of water soluble multiwalled carbon nanotubes (MWCNT)-induced cytotoxicity in the C6 rat glioma cell line [253].

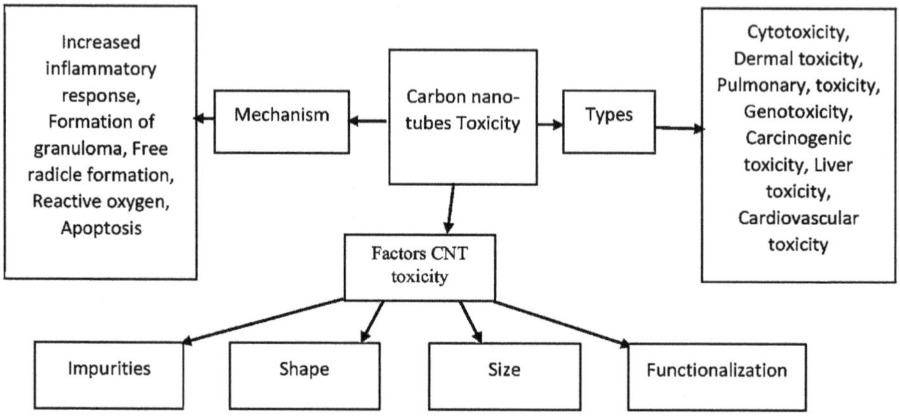

FIGURE 14.8 Summary of the factor's affection CNT toxicity.
Source: Adapted with revisions from: Prajapati et al. [254].

The results showed that smaller MWCNTs seemed more harmful than bigger ones—the enhanced oxidative stress caused by MWCNT-induced cytotoxicity in C6 rat glioma cells. However, pure, water-insoluble CNTs have been shown *in vitro* to be highly hazardous to various cell types, including human keratinocytes, rat brain neuronal cells, human embryonic kidney cells, and human lung cancer cells [255–257]. It is said that these insoluble pure CNTs cannot be exploited as carriers for medication and gene delivery in therapies and can only be discovered in CNT manufacturing facilities. According to Yang et al.'s intriguing comprehensive article on CNT toxicity, several *in vivo* toxicological evaluations have been undertaken in different species using IV or S.C. injections and gastrointestinal exposure with functionalized or dispersed SWCNTs or/and MWCNTs (rats, mice) [255]. The existing safety studies suggest that carbon nanotubes have low toxicity through numerous exposure paths for biological purposes. CNTs generated significant toxicity in mice only at very high doses (60 mg/kg) in the form of Polyethylene-Glycol-MWCNTs (PEG-MWCNTs) [255, 258]. Regardless of the delivery method, the toxicity of SWCNTs is tightly connected to oxidative stress.

CNTs, on the other hand, displayed extremely strong biocompatibility and did not cause any significant toxicity, save for minimal inflammation, when employed as tissue engineering materials for cell development by implanting subcutaneously [259]. Folkmann et al. discovered that SWCNTs might cause oxidative damage to DNA in mice following oral gavage [260], while Fraczek et al. discovered that implanted SWCNTs and MWCNTs cause inflammation. Other research on the toxicity of CNTs to the skin, on the other hand, revealed that CNTs were biocompatible to skin with high biocompatibility following subcutaneous planting [259]. Takanashi et al. discovered that MWCNTs injected into the subcutaneous tissue of rasH2 mice did not cause neoplasms when tested for carcinogenicity [261]. Other researchers discovered that CNTs put into the abdomen cavity of mice exhibited asbestos-like pathogenicity. Various factors influence CNT toxicity *in vivo*. Metal impurities may add to oxidative stress. Hence rigorous purification of CNTs is required. Chemically functionalized carbon nanotubes are more biocompatible than pure carbon nanotubes. As a result, Yang et al. found that functionalized carbon nanotubes are typically biocompatible and low toxic for biological applications. More toxicity studies are recommended to determine the safety threshold value of various CNTs and understand the toxicological mechanism [255]. CNTs are insoluble in water and accumulate in sediment, where they are hazardous to benthic organisms in rivers and disrupt the transit of other contaminants [262]. Zhu et al. discovered that SWCNTs had a significant impact on the growth of artemia salina in saltwater, with the higher the concentration of SWCNTs, the greater the larval mortality [262]. Da Rocha et al. [263] investigated the toxicity of carbon nanotubes to zebrafish [263]. It was discovered that CNTs accessing the lungs would cause severe toxicity, that the damage caused by CNTs would worsen with time, and that long-term inhalation of CNTs would be exceedingly hazardous to health. Russ et al. discovered that inhaling MWCNTs may cause an inflammatory reaction in the lungs, causing disruptions in pulmonary mechanics and airway epithelial function, eventually leading to alterations in lung function [264]. It has been shown that the smaller the CNTs, the more difficult it is for macrophages to remove them fast. The size and quantity of CNTs are linked to lung injury. The greater the interaction between CNTs and alveolar epithelial cells and macrophages, the greater the likelihood of inflammatory cell bursts. The placental barrier is an organ that exchanges nutrients and metabolites between the mother and the fetus, preventing dangerous chemicals from entering the fetus. The placental barrier serves as an important protective barrier to safeguard the baby during maternal pregnancy. Nanoparticles smaller than 100 nm have been found in studies on the embryotoxicity of nanomaterials to enter fetal blood through the placenta and alter fetal growth and development [265]. Despite their enormous potential therapeutic advantages, CNTs' toxicity is a key worry that has to be better researched and understood. Understanding the molecular pathways behind CNT-induced toxicity and disease is essential for elucidating and preventing the negative impacts of employing CNT as novel materials in human life. Furthermore, the findings of the CNT toxicity study will bring fresh insights into the development, production, and use of innovative nanomaterials that are safe for people and the environment. We predict a flurry of new discoveries and vigorous study in the area of nanotoxicology in the future years.

14.7 CONCLUSION

Emerging and rapid development of nanotechnology have offered unprecedented opportunity for CNTs to be used in biomedical applications. In this chapter, the biomedical application of CNTs in tissue engineering, biosensing, drug delivery, and bioimaging had been covered. We have highlighted the potential of CNTs and summarized many efforts in optimizing the use of CNTs as potential nanomaterial for different applications in the biomedical field.

KEYWORDS

- **carbon**
- **cytotoxicity**
- **functionalization**
- **modification**

REFERENCES

1. Iijima, S., (1991). Helical microtubules of graphitic carbon. *Nature, 354*, 56–58.
2. Ajayan, P. M., (1999). Nanotubes from carbon. *Chemical Reviews, 99*(7), 1787–1799. https://doi.org/10.1021/cr970102g.
3. Karousis, N., Nikos, T., & Dimitrios, T., (2010). Current progress on the chemical modification of carbon nanotubes. *Chemical Reviews, 110*(9), 5366–5397. https://doi.org/10.1021/cr100018g.
4. Zhang, R., Yingying, Z., Qiang, Z., Huanhuan, X., Weizhong, Q., & Fei, W., (2013). Growth of half-meter long carbon nanotubes based on Schulz–Flory distribution. *ACS Nano, 7*(7), 6156–6161. https://doi.org/10.1021/nn401995z.

5. Martin, C., & Punit, K., (2008). Smart nanotubes for biotechnology and biocatalysis. *Dekker Encyclopedia of Nanoscience and Nanotechnology – Set (Print Version)* (2nd edn., Vol. 6, pp. 4147–4157). https://doi.org/10.1201/noe0849396397.ch358.
6. Tasis, D., Nikos, T., Alberto, B., & Maurizio, P., (2006). Chemistry of carbon nanotubes. *Chemical Reviews, 106*(3), 1105–1136. https://doi.org/10.1021/cr050569o.
7. Mestre, R., Tania, P., & Samuel, S., (2021). Biohybrid robotics: From the nanoscale to the macroscale. *WIREs Nanomedicine and Nanobiotechnology, 13*(5), e1703. https://doi.org/10.1002/wnan.1703.
8. Huang, Shao-Ling, & David, D. M., (2014). Ultrasound for drug/gene delivery. In: *Cancer Theranostics* (pp. 269–283). Elsevier. https://doi.org/10.1016/B978-0-12-407722-5.00016-5.
9. Shoulders, M. D., & Ronald, T. R., (2009). Collagen structure and stability. *Annual Review of Biochemistry, 78*(1), 929–958. https://doi.org/10.1146/annurev.biochem.77.032207.120833.
10. Makareeva, E., & Sergey, L., (2014). Collagen structure, folding and function. In: *Osteogenesis Imperfecta* (pp. 71–84). Elsevier. https://doi.org/10.1016/B978-0-12-397165-4.00007-1.
11. Wieland, A., Pamela, L. S., Hannah, S., Ezgi, B., Dieter, J., Matthias, W. B., Markus, E., et al., (2021). Brain and breast cancer cells with PTEN loss of function reveal enhanced durotaxis and RHOB Dependent amoeboid migration utilizing 3D scaffolds and aligned microfiber tracts. *Cancers, 13*(20), 5144. https://doi.org/10.3390/cancers13205144.
12. Vonsattel, J. P. G., Christian, K., & Etty, P. C. R., (2011). *Huntington's Disease – Neuropathology* (pp. 83–100). In. https://doi.org/10.1016/B978-0-444-52014-2.00004-5.
13. Skoog, S. A., Girish, K., Roger, J. N., & Peter, L. G., (2018). Biological responses to immobilized microscale and nanoscale surface topographies. *Pharmacology & Therapeutics, 182*, 33–55. https://doi.org/10.1016/j.pharmthera.2017.07.009.
14. Dawson, K. A., & Yan, Y., (2021). Current understanding of biological identity at the nanoscale and future prospects. *Nature Nanotechnology, 16*(3), 229–242. https://doi.org/10.1038/s41565-021-00860-0.
15. Shi, J., & Bing, X., (2015). Nanoscale assemblies of small molecules control the fate of cells. *Nano Today, 10*(5), 615–630. https://doi.org/10.1016/j.nantod.2015.09.001.
16. Cavallaro, S., Federico, P., Fredrik, S., André, G., Carolina, P., Siddharth, S. S., Doste, R. M., et al., (2021). Multiparametric profiling of single nanoscale extracellular vesicles by combined atomic force and fluorescence microscopy: Correlation and heterogeneity in their molecular and biophysical features. *Small, 17*(14), 2008155. https://doi.org/10.1002/smll.202008155.
17. Boskey, A. L., (2013). Bone composition: Relationship to bone fragility and anti-osteoporotic drug effects. *Bonekey Reports, 2*, 447. https://doi.org/10.1038/bonekey.2013.181.
18. Ruppel, M. E., Miller, L. M., & Burr, D. B., (2008). The effect of the microscopic and nanoscale structure on bone fragility. *Osteoporosis International, 19*(9), 1251–1265. https://doi.org/10.1007/s00198-008–0579-1.
19. Fernandez De, G., Gabriel, L. K., Idoux-Gillet, Q. W. Y., Anne-Marie, M., Benkirane-Jessel, N., Fabien, B., & Damien, O., (2018). Bone substitutes: A review of their characteristics, clinical use, and perspectives for large bone defects management. *Journal of Tissue Engineering, 9*, 204173141877681. https://doi.org/10.1177/2041731418776819.

20. Pei, B., Wei, W., Nicholas, D., & Xiaoming, L., (2019). Applications of carbon nanotubes in bone tissue regeneration and engineering: Superiority, concerns, current advancements, and prospects. *Nanomaterials, 9*(10), 1501. https://doi.org/10.3390/nano9101501.
21. Li, D., Zhouyuan, Y., Xin, Z., Yue, L., Yi, O., Pengde, K., & Meng, T., (2021). A bone regeneration strategy via dual delivery of demineralized bone matrix powder and hypoxia-pretreated bone marrow stromal cells using an injectable self-healing hydrogel. *Journal of Materials Chemistry B, 9*(2), 479–493. https://doi.org/10.1039/D0TB01924K.
22. Bai, X., Mingzhu, G., Sahla, S., Jerry, Z., Xiaoyang, X., & Xue-Qing, Z., (2018). Bioactive hydrogels for bone regeneration. *Bioactive Materials, 3*(4), 401–417. https://doi.org/10.1016/j.bioactmat.2018.05.006.
23. Cheng, X., Qianbing, W., & Xibo, P., (2018). Graphene family materials in bone tissue regeneration: Perspectives and challenges. *Nanoscale Research Letters, 13*(1), 289. https://doi.org/10.1186/s11671-018-2694-z.
24. Martins-Júnior, P. A., Alcântara, C. E., Resende, R. R., & Ferreira, A. J., (2013). Carbon nanotubes: Directions and perspectives in oral regenerative medicine. *Journal of Dental Research, 92*(7), 575–583. https://doi.org/10.1177/0022034513490957.
25. Chandika, P., Seong-Yeong, H., Tae-Hee, K., Gun-Woo, O., Geun-Hyeong, K., Min-Sung, K., & Won-Kyo, J., (2020). Recent advances in biological macromolecule-based tissue-engineered composite scaffolds for cardiac tissue regeneration applications. *International Journal of Biological Macromolecules, 164*, 2329–2357. https://doi.org/10.1016/j.ijbiomac.2020.08.054.
26. Vujic, A., Niranjana, N., & Richard, T. L., (2020). Molecular mechanisms of heart regeneration. *Seminars in Cell & Developmental Biology, 100*, 20–28. https://doi.org/10.1016/j.semcdb.2019.09.003.
27. Laflamme, M. A., & Charles, E. M., (2011). Heart regeneration. *Nature, 473*(7347), 326–335. https://doi.org/10.1038/nature10147.
28. Karperien, L., Ali, N., Brent, G., Dolatshahi-Pirouz, A., Mohsen, A., & Mehdi, N., (2019). Nanoengineered biomaterials for cardiac regeneration. In: *Nanoengineered Biomaterials for Regenerative Medicine* (pp. 95–124). Elsevier. https://doi.org/10.1016/B978-0-12-813355-2.00005-3.
29. Barrejón, M., Silvia, M., Nuria, A., & Maurizio, P., (2021). Carbon nanotubes for cardiac tissue regeneration: State of the art and perspectives. *Carbon 184*, 641–650. https://doi.org/10.1016/j.carbon.2021.08.059.
30. Reddy, S., Xiaoting, X., Ting, G., Rong, Z., Liumin, H., & Seeram, R., (2018). Allotropic carbon (graphene oxide and reduced graphene oxide) based biomaterials for neural regeneration. *Current Opinion in Biomedical Engineering, 6*, 120–129. https://doi.org/10.1016/j.cobme.2018.05.001.
31. Qian, Y., Han, L., Zhiwen, Y., Jianlin, S., & Cunyi, F., (2021). Functional nanomaterials in peripheral nerve regeneration: Scaffold design, chemical principles and microenvironmental remodeling. *Materials Today, 51*, 165–187. https://doi.org/10.1016/j.mattod.2021.09.014.
32. Fraczek-Szczypta, A., (2014). Carbon nanomaterials for nerve tissue stimulation and regeneration. *Materials Science and Engineering: C, 34*, 35–49. https://doi.org/10.1016/j.msec.2013.09.038.

33. Tay, C. Y., Scott, A. I., Freddy, Y. C. B., Lay, P. T., & Subbu, V., (2011). Micro-/nano-engineered cellular responses for soft tissue engineering and biomedical applications. *Small, 7*(10), 1361–1378. https://doi.org/10.1002/smll.201100046.
34. Veetil, J. V., & Kaiming, Y., (2009). Tailored carbon nanotubes for tissue engineering applications. *Biotechnology Progress, 25*(3), 709–721. https://doi.org/10.1002/btpr.165.
35. Szymański, T., Adam, A. M., Magdalena, R., Tomasz, T., Ewa, F., Jakub, D. R., & Michael, G., (2020). Utilization of carbon nanotubes in manufacturing of 3d cartilage and bone scaffolds. *Materials, 13*(18), 4039. https://doi.org/10.3390/ma13184039.
36. Tanaka, M., Kaoru, A., Hisao, H., Takayuki, K., Takashi, T., Atsushi, S., Kazushige, Y., et al., (2020). Applications of carbon nanotubes in bone regenerative medicine. *Nanomaterials, 10*(4), 659. https://doi.org/10.3390/nano10040659.
37. Lemos, R., Raquel, M. F., Rui, L. R., & Joaquim, M. O., (2022). Engineering of extracellular matrix-like biomaterials at nano- and macroscale toward fabrication of hierarchical scaffolds for bone tissue engineering. *Advanced NanoBiomed Research, 2*(2), 2100116. https://doi.org/10.1002/anbr.202100116.
38. McKee, M. D., Betty, H., William, N. A., Nilana, M. T. B., José, L. M., & Catherine, C., (2013). Extracellular matrix mineralization in periodontal tissues: Noncollagenous matrix proteins, enzymes, and relationship to hypophosphatasia and x-linked hypophosphatemia. *Periodontology, 63*(1), 102–122. https://doi.org/10.1111/prd.12029.
39. Pham, Q. P., Kurtis, K. F., Scott, B. L., Robert, M. R., John, A. J., & Antonios, G. M., (2008). The influence of an *in vitro* generated bone-like extracellular matrix on osteoblastic gene expression of marrow stromal cells. *Biomaterials, 29*(18), 2729–2739. https://doi.org/10.1016/j.biomaterials.2008.02.025.
40. Wen, L., Jiepeng, C., Lili, D., & Shuzhuang, L., (2018). Vitamin K-dependent proteins involved in bone and cardiovascular health (review). *Molecular Medicine Reports, 18*, 3–15. https://doi.org/10.3892/mmr.2018.8940.
41. Urbanczyk, M., Shannon, L. L., & Schenke-Layland, K., (2020). The role of extracellular matrix in biomechanics and its impact on bioengineering of cells and 3D tissues. *Matrix Biology, 85, 86*, 1–14. https://doi.org/10.1016/j.matbio.2019.11.005.
42. Dantas, P. C. De. L., Martins-Júnior, P. A., Danielle, C. O. C., Vanessa, B. A., Thalita, M. V., Erick De, S. Á., Tatiane, C. S. A., et al., (2021). Nanohybrid composed of graphene oxide functionalized with sodium hyaluronate accelerates bone healing in the tibia of rats. *Materials Science and Engineering: C, 123*, 111961. https://doi.org/10.1016/j.msec.2021.111961.
43. Sohn, Hoon-Sang, & Jong-Keon, O., (2019). Review of bone graft and bone substitutes with an emphasis on fracture surgeries. *Biomaterials Research, 23*(1), 9. https://doi.org/10.1186/s40824-019-0157-y.
44. Moraschini, V., Daniel, C. F. A., Calasans-Maia, M. D., Ingrid, C. C. K., Rafael, S. L., & José, M. G., (2020). Immunological response of allogeneic bone grafting: A systematic review of prospective studies. *Journal of Oral Pathology & Medicine, 49*(5), 395–403. https://doi.org/10.1111/jop.12998.
45. Vidal, L., Carina, K., Meadhbh, Á. B., Alain, H., & Pierre, L., (2020). Reconstruction of large skeletal defects: Current clinical therapeutic strategies and future directions using 3D printing. *Frontiers in Bioengineering and Biotechnology, 8*, 61. https://doi.org/10.3389/fbioe.2020.00061.
46. Gashtasbi, F., Shahriar, H., Sadegh, H., Mohammad, M. D., Farzin, S., & Abbas, S., (2020). Comparative study of impact of animal source on physical, structural, and

biological properties of bone xenograft. *Xenotransplantation, 27*(6), e12628. https://doi.org/10.1111/xen.12628.

47. Bracey, D. N., Natalie, E. C., Alexander, H. J., Austin, V. S., Bettina, M. G., Patrick, W. W., & Aaron, T. S., (2020). Bone xenotransplantation: A review of the history, orthopedic clinical literature, and a single-center case series. *Xenotransplantation, 27*(5), e12600. https://doi.org/10.1111/xen.12600.
48. Sheikh, Z., Nader, H., Mohamed-Nur, A., Michael, G., & Marc, G., (2019). Natural and synthetic bone replacement graft materials for dental and maxillofacial applications. In: *Advanced Dental Biomaterials* (pp. 347–376). Elsevier. https://doi.org/10.1016/B978-0-08-102476-8.00015-3.
49. Balaji, V. R., Manikandan, D., & Ramsundar, A., (2020). Bone grafts in periodontics. *Matrix Science Medica, 4*(3), 57. https://doi.org/10.4103/MTSM.MTSM_2_19.
50. Eivazzadeh-Keihan, R., Ali, M., Miguel De La, G., Milad, S. B., Karim, K. C., Pashazadeh-Panahi, P., Behzad, B., Ahad, M., & Michael, R. H., (2019). Carbon based nanomaterials for tissue engineering of bone: Building new bone on small black scaffolds: A review. *Journal of Advanced Research, 18*, 185–201. https://doi.org/10.1016/j.jare.2019.03.011.
51. Xue, J., Dario, P., & Younan, X., (2020). Maneuvering the migration and differentiation of stem cells with electrospun nanofibers. *Advanced Science, 7*(15), 2000735. https://doi.org/10.1002/advs.202000735.
52. Lotfi, M., Nejib, M., & Naceur, M., (2013). Cell adhesion to biomaterials: Concept of biocompatibility. In: *Advances in Biomaterials Science and Biomedical Applications*. Intech. https://doi.org/10.5772/53542.
53. Resende-Gonçalves, C. I., Nuno, S., Joaquim, M., Oscar, C., João, C., Manzanares-Céspedes, M. C., Filipe, S., Bruno, H., & Júlio, S., (2022). Porous zirconia blocks for bone repair: An integrative review on biological and mechanical outcomes. *Ceramics, 5*(1), 161–172. https://doi.org/10.3390/ceramics5010014.
54. Wang, Ya-Wu, Qiong, W., & Guo-Qiang, C., (2004). Attachment, proliferation and differentiation of osteoblasts on random biopolyester poly(3-hydroxybutyrate-Co-3-hydroxyhexanoate) scaffolds. *Biomaterials, 25*(4), 669–675. https://doi.org/10.1016/S0142-9612(03)00561-1.
55. Sakr, M. A., Kabilan, S., Towsif, H., Su Ryon, S., Sumi, S., Jaehwan, K., & Keekyoung, K., (2022). Recent trends in gelatin methacryloyl nanocomposite hydrogels for tissue engineering. *Journal of Biomedical Materials Research Part A, 110*(3), 708–724. https://doi.org/10.1002/jbm.a.37310.
56. Lin, W., Miao, C., Tao, Q., Jidong, L., & Yi, M., (2020). Three-dimensional electrospun nanofibrous scaffolds for bone tissue engineering. *Journal of Biomedical Materials Research Part B: Applied Biomaterials, 108*(4), 1311–1321. https://doi.org/10.1002/jbm.b.34479.
57. Campodoni, E., Ellinor, B. H., Ahmad, R., Ramírez-Rodríguez, G. B., Kamal, M., Kristin, S., Anna, T., & Monica, S., (2019). Polymeric 3D scaffolds for tissue regeneration: Evaluation of biopolymer nanocomposite reinforced with cellulose nanofibrils. *Materials Science and Engineering: C, 94*, 867–878. https://doi.org/10.1016/j.msec.2018.10.026.
58. Dwivedi, R., Sumit, K., Rahul, P., Aman, M., Deepti, N., Dhirendra, S. K., & Divya, M., (2020). Polycaprolactone as biomaterial for bone scaffolds: Review of literature. *Journal of Oral Biology and Craniofacial Research, 10*(1), 381–388. https://doi.org/10.1016/j.jobcr.2019.10.003.

59. Su, X., Ting, W., & Shu, G., (2021). Applications of 3D printed bone tissue engineering scaffolds in the stem cell field. *Regenerative Therapy, 16*, 63–72. https://doi.org/10.1016/j.reth.2021.01.007.
60. Zhang, M., Rongcai, L., Xin, W., Jianmin, X., Cuijun, D., Chun, F., Hui, Z., et al., (2020). 3D Printing of haversian bone–mimicking scaffolds for multicellular delivery in bone regeneration. *Science Advances, 6*(12), eaaz6725. https://doi.org/10.1126/sciadv.aaz6725.
61. Lee, Se-Hwan, Kang-Gon, L., Jong-Hyun, H., Yong, S. C., Kang-Sik, L., Hun-Jin, J., Sang-Hyug, P., et al., (2019). Evaluation of mechanical strength and bone regeneration ability of 3D printed Kagome-structure scaffold using rabbit calvarial defect model. *Materials Science and Engineering: C, 98*, 949–959. https://doi.org/10.1016/j.msec.2019.01.050.
62. Pramanik, S., Pingguan-Murphy, B., & Noor, A. A. O., (2012). Progress of key strategies in development of electrospun scaffolds: Bone tissue. *Science and Technology of Advanced Materials, 13*(4), 043002. https://doi.org/10.1088/1468-6996/13/4/043002.
63. Sun, Z., Song, J., Hongchang, J., Zhenzhen, D., Yanwu, Z., Anyuan, C., Hengxing, J., & Li-Jun, W., (2018). Robust expandable carbon nanotube scaffold for ultrahigh-capacity lithium-metal anodes. *Advanced Materials, 30*(32), 1800884. https://doi.org/10.1002/adma.201800884.
64. Chen, C., Xue, B., Yahui, D., & In-Seop, L., (2019). Electrical stimulation as a novel tool for regulating cell behavior in tissue engineering. *Biomaterials Research, 23*(1), 25. https://doi.org/10.1186/s40824-019-0176-8.
65. Yao, Q., Haixiao, L., Xin, L., Liwei, M., Xiao, Z., Yu, L., Pingping, H., et al., (2019). 3D interpenetrated graphene foam/58S bioactive glass scaffolds for electrical-stimulation-assisted differentiation of rabbit mesenchymal stem cells to enhance bone regeneration. *Journal of Biomedical Nanotechnology, 15*(3), 602–611. https://doi.org/10.1166/jbn.2019.2703.
66. Li, Y., Lu, Y., Yue, H., Zhenzhen, Z., Miao, C., Maoxia, W., Jin, L., et al., (2022). Polydopamine-mediated graphene oxide and nanohydroxyapatite-incorporated conductive scaffold with an immunomodulatory ability accelerates periodontal bone regeneration in diabetes. *Bioactive Materials, 18*, 213–227. https://doi.org/10.1016/j.bioactmat.2022.03.021.
67. Dixon, D. T., & Cheryl, T. G., (2021). Conductive scaffolds for bone tissue engineering: Current state and future outlook. *Journal of Functional Biomaterials, 13*(1), 1. https://doi.org/10.3390/jfb13010001.
68. Ning, C., Zhengnan, Z., Guoxin, T., Ye, Z., & Chuanbin, M., (2018). Electroactive polymers for tissue regeneration: Developments and perspectives. *Progress in Polymer Science, 81*, 144–162. https://doi.org/10.1016/j.progpolymsci.2018.01.001.
69. Huang, J., Xueyu, H., Lei, L., Zhengxu, Y., Quanyu, Z., & Zhuojing, L., (2010). Electrical regulation of Schwann cells using conductive polypyrrole/chitosan polymers. *Journal of Biomedical Materials Research Part A, 93*, 164–174. https://doi.org/10.1002/jbm.a.32511.
70. Bosi, S., Laura, B., & Maurizio, P., (2013). Carbon nanotubes in tissue engineering. In: *Peptide-Based Materials* (Vol. 310, pp. 181–204). https://doi.org/10.1007/128_2013_474.
71. Yang, K., Seung, J. Y., Jong, S. L., Hak-Rae, L., Gyeong-Eon, C., Jungmok, S., Taeyoon, L., et al., (2017). Electroconductive nanoscale topography for enhanced

neuronal differentiation and electrophysiological maturation of human neural stem cells. *Nanoscale, 9*(47), 18737–18752. https://doi.org/10.1039/C7NR05446G.

72. Ju, Y. M., Kwideok, P., Jun, S. S., Jae-Jin, K., Jong-Won, R., & Dong, K. H., (2008). Beneficial effect of hydrophilized porous polymer scaffolds in tissue-engineered cartilage formation. *Journal of Biomedical Materials Research Part B: Applied Biomaterials, 85B*(1), 252–260. https://doi.org/10.1002/jbm.b.30943.
73. Liu, L., Bo, Y., Lan, Q. W., Jin, P. H., Wu, Y. C., Qing, B., Yi, Z., Rong, Y., Liang, Y., & Yan, Q. G., (2020). Biomimetic bone tissue engineering hydrogel scaffolds constructed using ordered CNTs and HA induce the proliferation and differentiation of BMSCs. *Journal of Materials Chemistry B, 8*(3), 558–567. https://doi.org/10.1039/c9tb01804b.
74. Cui, H., Yaling, Y., Xiaokeng, L., Ziyang, S., Jihao, R., Ziliang, W., Jin, Q., & Jun, Y., (2019). Direct 3D printing of a tough hydrogel incorporated with carbon nanotubes for bone regeneration. *Journal of Materials Chemistry B, 7*(45), 7207–7217. https://doi.org/10.1039/c9tb01494b.
75. Huang, B., Cian, V., Iwan, R., Quentin, A. P., Wei, H. C., Jonny, J. B., Zhucheng, H., & Paulo, B., (2019). Fabrication and characterization of 3D printed MWCNT composite porous scaffolds for bone regeneration. *Materials Science and Engineering C, 98*, 266–278. https://doi.org/10.1016/j.msec.2018.12.100.
76. Capulli, A. K., MacQueen, L. A., Sean, P. S., & Parker, K. K., (2016). Fibrous scaffolds for building hearts and heart parts. *Advanced Drug Delivery Reviews, 96*, 83–102. https://doi.org/10.1016/j.addr.2015.11.020.
77. Arackal, A., & Khalid, A., (2022). Histology, heart. *StatPearls*. May, 8, 2022; https://www.ncbi.nlm.nih.gov/books/NBK545143/.
78. Lui, G. K., Susan, F., & Doff, B. M., (2014). Management of cardiovascular risk factors in adults with congenital heart disease. *Journal of the American Heart Association, 3*(6), e001076. https://doi.org/10.1161/JAHA.114.001076.
79. Lockhart, P. B., & Yee-Ping, S., (2021). Diseases of the cardiovascular system. In: *Burket's Oral Medicine* (pp. 505–552). Wiley. https://doi.org/10.1002/9781119597797.ch14.
80. Ghanbari, H., Brian, G. C., & Alexander, M. S., (2011). A nanocage for nanomedicine: Polyhedral oligomeric silsesquioxane (POSS). *Macromolecular Rapid Communications, 32*(14), 1032–1046. https://doi.org/10.1002/marc.201100126.
81. Joyce, K., Georgina, T. F., Yagmur, B., & Abhay, P., (2021). Bioactive potential of natural biomaterials: Identification, retention and assessment of biological properties. *Signal Transduction and Targeted Therapy, 6*(1), 122. https://doi.org/10.1038/s41392-021-00512-8.
82. Martinelli, V., Susanna, B., Brisa, P., Gabriele, B., Carlin, S. L., Orfeo, S., Mauro, G., Maurizio, P., & Luisa, M., (2018). 3D carbon-nanotube-based composites for cardiac tissue engineering. *ACS Applied Bio Materials, 1*(5), 1530–1537. https://doi.org/10.1021/acsabm.8b00440.
83. Gorain, B., Hira, C., Manisha, P., Prashant, K., Muhammad, M. A., Rakesh, K. T., & Zahid, H., (2018). Carbon nanotube scaffolds as emerging nanoplatform for myocardial tissue regeneration: A review of recent developments and therapeutic implications. *Biomedicine & Pharmacotherapy, 104*, 496–508. https://doi.org/10.1016/j.biopha.2018.05.066.
84. Ahmadi, P., Niloofar, N., Mohammad, A. D., & Hossein, G., (2021). Preparation and characterization of polyurethane/chitosan/CNT nanofibrous scaffold for cardiac tissue

engineering. *International Journal of Biological Macromolecules, 180*, 590–598. https://doi.org/10.1016/j.ijbiomac.2021.03.001.
85. Mccauley, M. D., Flavia, V., Stephen, Y. J., Colin, C. Y., Brian, G., Marco, O., Srikanth, P., et al., (2019). *In vivo* restoration of myocardial conduction with carbon nanotube fibers. *Circulation: Arrhythmia and Electrophysiology, 12*(8), 1–15. https://doi.org/10.1161/CIRCEP.119.007256.
86. Urfy, M. Z., & Jose, I. S., (2014). *Breathing and the Nervous System* (pp. 241–250). In. https://doi.org/10.1016/B978-0-7020-4086-3.00017-5.
87. Styne, D. M., (1994). Physiology of puberty. *Hormone Research, 41*(2), 3–6. https://doi.org/10.1159/000183949.
88. Furness, J. B., (2012). The enteric nervous system and neurogastroenterology. *Nature Reviews Gastroenterology & Hepatology, 9*(5), 286–294. https://doi.org/10.1038/nrgastro.2012.32.
89. Kehoe, S., Zhang, X. F., & Boyd, D., (2012). FDA approved guidance conduits and wraps for peripheral nerve injury: A review of materials and efficacy. *Injury, 43*(5), 553–572. https://doi.org/10.1016/j.injury.2010.12.030.
90. Yang, Y., Aditya, C., Jin, Z., Adam, E., Hae, L. J., & Ali, K., (2019). Applications of nanotechnology for regenerative medicine; healing tissues at the nanoscale. In: *Principles of Regenerative Medicine* (pp. 485–504). Elsevier. https://doi.org/10.1016/B978-0-12-809880-6.00029-1.
91. Mathur, V., Saikat, T., Swastik, K., & Zachariah, H., (2021). *In vivo* partial restoration of neural activity across severed mouse spinal cord bridged with ultralong carbon nanotubes. *ACS Applied Bio Materials, 4*(5), 4071–4078. https://doi.org/10.1021/acsabm.1c00248.
92. Kunisaki, A., Akira, K., Masakazu, I., Takahiro, U., Marcio, D. L., Takeshi, K., & Nobuo, A., (2021). Carbon-nanotube yarns induce axonal regeneration in peripheral nerve defect. *Scientific Reports, 11*(1), 1–10. https://doi.org/10.1038/s41598-021-98603-7.
93. Sun, Y., Qi, Q., Haoye, M., Yudong, Z., Jiang, P., Yaxin, H., Zhaoxuan, F., et al., (2019). Enhanced neurite outgrowth on a multiblock conductive nerve scaffold with self-powered electrical stimulation. *Advanced Healthcare Materials, 8*(10), 1900127. https://doi.org/10.1002/adhm.201900127.
94. Sun, Y., Xifeng, L., Matthew, N. G., Sungjo, P., Bipin, G., Andre, T., & Lichun, L., (2021). Enhanced nerve cell proliferation and differentiation on electrically conductive scaffolds embedded with graphene and carbon nanotubes. *Journal of Biomedical Materials Research – Part A, 109*(2), 193–206. https://doi.org/10.1002/jbm.a.37016.
95. Chowdhry, A., Jasreen, K., Madhu, K., Veena, P., Rakesh, T., & Sanjeev, P., (2019). Characterization of functionalized multiwalled carbon nanotubes and comparison of their cellular toxicity between HEK 293 cells and zebra fish *in vivo*. *Heliyon, 5*(10), e02605. https://doi.org/10.1016/j.heliyon.2019.e02605.
96. Kam, N. W. S., Edward, J., & Nicholas, A. K., (2009). Electrical stimulation of neural stem cells mediated by humanized carbon nanotube composite made with extracellular matrix protein. *Nano Letters, 9*(1), 273–278. https://doi.org/10.1021/nl802859a.
97. Oprych, K. M., Raymond, L. D. W., Sergey, V. M., Paul, T., & Jimi, A., (2016). Repairing peripheral nerves: Is there a role for carbon nanotubes? *Advanced Healthcare Materials, 5*(11), 1253–1271. https://doi.org/10.1002/adhm.201500864.
98. Liu, X., Matthew, N. G., Sungjo, P., Lee, M. II. A., Bipin, G., Linli, L., Brian, E. W., et al., (2020). 3D-printed scaffolds with carbon nanotubes for bone tissue engineering:

Fast and homogeneous one-step functionalization. *Acta Biomaterialia, 111*, 129–140. https://doi.org/10.1016/j.actbio.2020.04.047.

99. Lan, W., Xiumei, Z., Mengjie, X., Liqin, Z., Di, H., Xiaochun, W., & Weiyi, C., (2019). Carbon nanotube reinforced polyvinyl alcohol/biphasic calcium phosphate scaffold for bone tissue engineering. *RSC Advances, 9*(67), 38998–38910. https://doi.org/10.1039/c9ra08569f.
100. Shuai, C., Peng, B., Liu, M., Peng, S., & Feng, P., (2021). A self-assembled montmorillonite-carbon nanotube hybrid nanoreinforcement for poly-L-lactic acid bone scaffold. *Materials Today Advances, 11*, 100158. https://doi.org/10.1016/j.mtadv.2021.100158.
101. Patel, D. K., Sayan, D. D., Keya, G., Jin, W. K., & Ki Taek, L., (2021). Enhanced osteogenic potential of unzipped carbon nanotubes for tissue engineering. *Journal of Biomedical Materials Research – Part A, 109*(10), 1869–1880. https://doi.org/10.1002/jbm.a.37179.
102. Mahmoodi, M., Vida, H., Marjan, M., Maryam, T., Fatemeh, S., & Ali, D., (2021). Highly osteogenic and mechanically strong nanofibrous scaffolds based on functionalized multi-walled carbon nanotubes-reinforced electrospun keratin/poly(ε-caprolactone). *Materials Today Communications, 27*, 102401. https://doi.org/10.1016/j.mtcomm.2021.102401.
103. Huang, Y., Wei, J., Yechen, L., Qing, C., & Xiaoping, Y., (2021). Composites made of polyorganophosphazene and carbon nanotube up-regulating osteogenic activity of BMSCS under electrical stimulation. *Colloids and Surfaces B: Biointerfaces 204*, 111785. https://doi.org/10.1016/j.colsurfb.2021.111785.
104. Tohidlou, H., Seyedeh, S. S., Shahsanam, A., Asadi-Eydivand, M., & Fathi-Roudsari, M., (2019). Amine-functionalized single-walled carbon nanotube/polycaprolactone electrospun scaffold for bone tissue engineering: *In vitro* study. *Fibers and Polymers, 20*(9), 1869–1882. https://doi.org/10.1007/s12221-019-1262-1.
105. Madhusoodan, A. P., Kinsuk, D., Bhabesh, M., Kuldeep, K., Ajay, K., Saxena, A. C., Praveen, S., et al., (2019). *In vitro* proliferation and differentiation of canine bone marrow derived mesenchymal stem cells over hydroxyl functionalized CNT substrates. *Biotechnology Reports 24*, e00387. https://doi.org/10.1016/j.btre.2019.e00387.
106. Moura De, N. K., Eduardo, F. M., Rodrigo, L. M. S. O., Idália, A. W. De. B. S., João, P. B. M., Elisa, E., Suelen, S. A., et al., (2020). Synergistic effect of adding bioglass and carbon nanotubes on poly (lactic acid) porous membranes for guided bone regeneration. *Materials Science and Engineering C, 117*, 111327. https://doi.org/10.1016/j.msec.2020.111327.
107. Zhao, G., Xu, Z., Bingcheng, L., Guoyou, H., Feng, X., & Xiaohui, Z., (2020). Solvent-free fabrication of carbon nanotube/silk fibroin electrospun matrices for enhancing cardiomyocyte functionalities. *ACS Biomaterials Science and Engineering, 6*(3), 1630–1640. https://doi.org/10.1021/acsbiomaterials.9b01682.
108. Mombini, S., Javad, M., Behnaz, B., Asghar, N., Jhamak, N., Sadaf, V., & Shahrzad, Z., (2019). Chitosan-PVA-CNT nanofibers as electrically conductive scaffolds for cardiovascular tissue engineering. *International Journal of Biological Macromolecules, 140*, 278–287. https://doi.org/10.1016/j.ijbiomac.2019.08.046.
109. Shokraei, N., Shiva, A., Shabnam, S., Mehrdad, N. S., Faridi-Majidi, R., & Hossein, G., (2019). Development of electrically conductive hybrid nanofibers based on CNT-polyurethane nanocomposite for cardiac tissue engineering. *Microscopy Research and Technique, 82*(8), 1316–1325. https://doi.org/10.1002/jemt.23282.

110. Jiang, C., Kan, W., Yi, L., Chuck, Z., & Ben, W., (2021). Using wet electrospun PCL/gelatin/CNT yarns to fabricate textile-based scaffolds for vascular tissue engineering. *ACS Biomaterials Science and Engineering, 7*(6), 2627–2637. https://doi.org/10.1021/acsbiomaterials.1c00097.
111. Ahadian, S., Locke, D. H., Mehdi, E., Bess, Y., Nathaniel, S., Zhensong, X., Yu, S., & Milica, R., (2017). Moldable elastomeric polyester-carbon nanotube scaffolds for cardiac tissue engineering. *Acta Biomaterialia, 52*, 81–91. https://doi.org/10.1016/j.actbio.2016.12.009.
112. Ahadian, S., Shukuyo, Y., Mehdi, E., Xiaobin, L., Ramin, B. S., Ken, N., Hitoshi, S., Tomokazu, M., & Ali, K., (2017). Carbon nanotubes embedded in embryoid bodies direct cardiac differentiation. *Biomedical Microdevices, 19*(3), 57. https://doi.org/10.1007/s10544-017-0184-1.
113. Ren, J., Quanfu, X., Xiaomeng, C., Wei, L., Kai, G., Yang, Z., Qian, W., et al., (2017). Super aligned carbon nanotubes guide oriented cell growth and promote electrophysiological homogeneity for synthetic cardiac tissues. *Advanced Materials, 29*(44), 1–8. https://doi.org/10.1002/adma.201702713.
114. Wu, S., Ye, Q., Wen, S., Mitchell, K., Shaojuan, C., & Bin, D., (2022). Electrospun conductive nanofiber yarns for accelerating mesenchymal stem cells differentiation and maturation into Schwann cell-like cells under a combination of electrical stimulation and chemical induction. *Acta Biomaterialia, 139*, 91–104. https://doi.org/10.1016/j.actbio.2020.11.042.
115. Sang, S., Rong, C., Yanyan, C., Yayun, Y., Zhizhong, S., Yajing, Z., & Yanqing, H., (2022). Biocompatible chitosan/polyethylene glycol/multi-walled carbon nanotube composite scaffolds for neural tissue engineering. *Journal of Zhejiang University: Science B, 23*(1), 58–73. https://doi.org/10.1631/jzus.B2100155.
116. Ye, L., Haichao, J., Jie, L., Chien-Hua, T., Michael, K., Kaloian, K., Johannes, V., & Hans-Jürgen, B., (2021). Carbon nanotube–hydrogel composites facilitate neuronal differentiation while maintaining homeostasis of network activity. *Advanced Materials, 33*(41), 2102981. https://doi.org/10.1002/adma.202102981.
117. Fallah-Darrehchi, M., Payam, Z., Shahrokh, S., Ghaffari-Bohlouli, P., & Robabeh, A., (2021). Conductive conduit based on electrospun poly (L-lactide-Co-D, L-lactide) nanofibers containing 4-aminopyridine-loaded molecularly imprinted poly (methacrylic acid) nanoparticles used for peripheral nerve regeneration. *International Journal of Biological Macromolecules, 190*, 499–507. https://doi.org/10.1016/j.ijbiomac.2021.09.009.
118. Ghosh, S., Swati, H., Sumeet, G., Ankita, B., Samrat, C., Viney, K., Partha, R., & Debrupa, L., (2020). Anisotropically conductive biodegradable scaffold with coaxially aligned carbon nanotubes for directional regeneration of peripheral nerves. *ACS Applied Bio Materials, 3*(9), 5796–5812. https://doi.org/10.1021/acsabm.0c00534.
119. Li, X., Wen, Y., Hongjian, X., Jian, W., Lei, Z., Zheng, W., & Lin, W., (2020). CNT/sericin conductive nerve guidance conduit promotes functional recovery of transected peripheral nerve injury in a rat model. *ACS Applied Materials and Interfaces, 12*(33), 36860–36872. https://doi.org/10.1021/acsami.0c08457.
120. Reddy, A. R. N., Yellu, N. R., Devarakonda, R. K., & Vurimindi, H., (2010). Multi wall carbon nanotubes induce oxidative stress and cytotoxicity in human embryonic kidney (HEK293) cells. *Toxicology, 272*(1–3), 11–16. https://doi.org/10.1016/j.tox.2010.03.017.

121. Che, A., Che, A., Chihye, L. A., Ovalle-Robles, R., Shaoli, F., Marcio, D. L., Xavier, L., Steve, C., et al., (2014). Primary liver cells cultured on carbon nanotube substrates for liver tissue engineering and drug discovery applications. *ACS Applied Materials & Interfaces, 6*(13), 10373–10380. https://doi.org/10.1021/am5018489.
122. He, J., Mengting, S., Yongping, L., & Baolin, G., (2020). Conductive adhesive self-healing nanocomposite hydrogel wound dressing for photothermal therapy of infected full-Thickness skin wounds. *Chemical Engineering Journal, 394*, 124888. https://doi.org/10.1016/j.cej.2020.124888.
123. Santos, J. C. C., Alexandra, A. P. M., Virginia, S. T. C., & Herman, S. M., (2014). Nanocomposites of poly(vinyl alcohol)/functionalized-multiwall carbon nanotubes conjugated with glucose oxidase for potential application as scaffolds in skin wound healing. *International Journal of Polymeric Materials and Polymeric Biomaterials, 63*(4), 185–196. https://doi.org/10.1080/00914037.2013.812090.
124. Liang, F., & Chen, B., (2009). A review on biomedical applications of single-walled carbon nanotubes. *Current Medicinal Chemistry, 17*(1), 10–24. https://doi.org/10.2174/092986710789957742.
125. Ensafi, A. A., (2019). An introduction to sensors and biosensors. In: *Electrochemical Biosensors* (pp. 1–10). Elsevier Inc. https://doi.org/10.1016/B978-0-12-816491-4.00001-2.
126. Thevenot, D. R., Klara, T., Richard, A. D., & George, S. W., (1999). Electrochemical biosensors: Recommended definitions and classification. *Electroanalytical Chemistry, 71*(12), 2333–2348.
127. Sawant, S. N., (2017). Development of biosensors from biopolymer composites. In: *Biopolymer Composites in Electronics* (pp. 353–383). Elsevier Inc. https://doi.org/10.1016/B978-0-12-809261-3.00013-9.
128. Kim, J., Alan, S. C., Berta, E. F. De. Á., & Joseph, W., (2019). Wearable biosensors for healthcare monitoring. *Nature Biotechnology, 37*(4), 389–406. https://doi.org/10.1038/s41587-019-0045-y.
129. Nathani, A., Nandimalla, V., & Chandra, S. S., (2020). Review—Pencil graphite electrodes as platform for enzyme and enzyme-like protein immobilization for electrochemical detection. *Journal of The Electrochemical Society, 167*(3), 37520–37531. https://doi.org/10.1149/2.0202003jes.
130. Grieshaber, D., MacKenzie, R., Janos, V., & Erik, R., (2008). Electrochemical biosensors – sensor principles and architectures. *Sensors, 8*(3), 1400–1458. https://doi.org/10.3390/s8031400.
131. Alfaleh, M., A., Hashem, O. A., Ahmad, B. M., Almohanad, A. A., Martina, L. J., Stephen, M. M., & Anwar, M. H., (2020). Phage display derived monoclonal antibodies: From bench to bedside. *Frontiers in Immunology, 11*, 1–37. https://doi.org/10.3389/fimmu.2020.01986.
132. Su, Y., Shitou, X., Ruozhong, W., & Langtao, X., (2017). Phytohormonal quantification based on biological principles. In: *Hormone Metabolism and Signaling in Plants* (pp. 431–470). https://doi.org/10.1016/B978-0-12-811562-6.00013-X.
133. Vigneshvar, S., Sudhakumari, C. C., Balasubramanian, S., & Hridayesh, P., (2016). Recent advances in biosensor technology for potential applications – an overview. *Frontiers in Bioengineering and Biotechnology, 4*, 1–9. https://doi.org/10.3389/fbioe.2016.00011.

134. Karunakaran, C., Raju, R., & Kalpana, B., (2015). Introduction to biosensors. In: *Biosensors and Bioelectronics* (pp. 1–68). Elsevier Inc. https://doi.org/10.1016/B978-0-12-803100-1.00001-3.
135. Oh, J., Seunghwan, Y., Young, W. C., Kookjin, L., & Kyung, H. Y., (2009). Carbon nanotube-based biosensor for detection hepatitis B. *Current Applied Physics, 9*, e229–231. https://doi.org/10.1016/j.cap.2009.06.045.
136. Tîlmaciu, C. M., & May, C. M., (2015). Carbon nanotube biosensors. *Frontiers in Chemistry, 3*, 1–21. https://doi.org/10.3389/fchem.2015.00059.
137. Hwang, H. S., Jae, W. J., Yoong, A. K., & Mincheol, C., (2020). Carbon nanomaterials as versatile platforms for biosensing applications. *Micromachines, 11*(9), 1–27. https://doi.org/10.3390/MI11090814.
138. Sun, T. P., Hsiu, L. S., Congo, T. S. C., Yan, D. Y., Su, H. H., Chia, M. L., Wei, H. L., & Chung, Y. C., (2010). Carbon nanotube composites for glucose biosensor incorporated with reverse iontophoresis function for noninvasive glucose monitoring. *International Journal of Nanomedicine, 5*(1), 343–349. https://doi.org/10.2147/ijn.s10247.
139. Shen, G., & Youming, S., (2019). Covalent functionalized carbon nanotube with ionic liquid and its application for human immunoglobulin G immunosensor. *International Journal of Electrochemical Science, 14*, 7560–7569. https://doi.org/10.20964/2019.08.77.
140. Kase, H., Ryota, N., Michiharu, A., Noriko, K., & Yoshihiro, K., (2018). Biosensor response from target molecules with inhomogeneous charge localization. *Journal of Applied Physics, 124*(6), 064502. https://doi.org/10.1063/1.5036538.
141. Xu, T., Zhihong, W., & Jianmin, M., (2009). Fabrication of carbon-nanotube enhanced piezoelectric membrane for biosensor application. *International Journal of Nanotechnology, 6*(7, 8), 762–771. https://doi.org/10.1504/IJNT.2009.025314.
142. Madhurantakam, S., Jayanth, B. K., John, B. B. R., & Uma, M. K., (2017). Enzyme-free monitoring of glucose utilization in stimulated macrophages using carbon nanotube-decorated electrochemical sensor. *Applied Nanoscience, 7*(8), 773–780. https://doi.org/10.1007/s13204-017-0617-4.
143. Zhu, Y. C., Li, P. M., Yi, F. R., Nan, Z., Wei, W. Z., Jing, J. X., & Hong, Y., C., (2019). Enzyme-based biosensors and their applications. In: *Biomass, Biofuels, Biochemicals: Advances in Enzyme Technology* (pp. 201–223). Elsevier B.V. https://doi.org/10.1016/B978-0-444-64114-4.00008-X.
144. Mulchandani, A., (1998). Principles of enzyme biosensors. In: *Methods in Biotechnology* (Vol. 6, pp. 3–14).
145. Wang, J., & Yuehe, L., (2008). Functionalized carbon nanotubes and nanofibers for biosensing applications. *TrAC – Trends in Analytical Chemistry, 27*(7), 619–626. https://doi.org/10.1016/j.trac.2008.05.009.
146. Comba, F., N., Marcelo, R. R., Fernando, S. G., & Ana, M. B., (2018). Mucin and carbon nanotube-based biosensor for detection of glucose in human plasma. *Analytical Biochemistry, 550*, 34–40. https://doi.org/10.1016/j.ab.2018.04.006.
147. Naresh, V., & Nohyun, L., (2021). A review on biosensors and recent development of nanostructured materials-enabled biosensors. *Sensors, 21*(4), 1109–1143. https://doi.org/10.3390/s21041109.
148. Emon, J. M. V., (2011). Immunoassays in biotechnology. In: *Comprehensive Biotechnology* (2nd edn., Vol. 1, pp. 659–667). Elsevier B.V. https://doi.org/10.1016/B978-0-08-088504-9.00076-3.

149. Gulati, P., Prabhjot, K., Rajam, M. V., Tapasya, S., Prabhash, M., & Islam, S. S., (2019). Vertically aligned multi-walled carbon nanotubes based flexible immunosensor for extreme low-level detection of multidrug resistant leukemia cells. *Sensors and Actuators, B: Chemical, 301*, 127047–127058. https://doi.org/10.1016/j.snb.2019.127047.
150. Saify, N. H., Khosro, P., Fatemeh, K., Abbas, A., & Tayyebeh, M., (2018). Fabrication of an immunosensor for early and ultrasensitive determination of human tissue plasminogen activator (TPA) in myocardial infarction and breast cancer patients. *Analytical and Bioanalytical Chemistry, 410*(16), 3683–3691. https://doi.org/10.1007/s00216-018-1005-y.
151. Mehlhorn, A., Parvaneh, R., & Yvonne, J., (2018). Aptamer-based biosensors for antibiotic detection: A review. *Biosensors, 8*(2), 54–116. https://doi.org/10.3390/bios8020054.
152. Song, B., Piao, X., Guangming, Z., Jilai, G., Peng, Z., Haopeng, F., Yang, L., & Xiaoya, R., (2018). Carbon nanotube-based environmental technologies: The adopted properties, primary mechanisms, and challenges. *Reviews in Environmental Science and Biotechnology, 17*(3), 571–590. https://doi.org/10.1007/s11157-018-9468-z.
153. Kim, J. P., Seunghun, H., & Sang, J. S., (2011). Apta-biosensors for nonlabelled real time detection of human IgE based on carbon nanotube field effect transistors. *Journal of Nanoscience and Nanotechnology, 11*(5), 4182–4187. https://doi.org/10.1166/jnn.2011.3692.
154. Park, Y., Min, S. H., Woo, H. L., Jung, G. K., & Kyunghoon, K., (2021). Highly sensitive electrochemical aptasensor for detecting the VEGF165 tumor marker with PANI/CNT nanocomposites. *Biosensors, 11*(4), 114–124. https://doi.org/10.3390/bios11040114.
155. Bhardwaj, T., (2015). Review on biosensor technologies. *International Journal of Advanced Research in Engineering and Technology, 6*(2), 36–62.
156. Hu, C., & Shengshui, H., (2009). Carbon nanotube-based electrochemical sensors: Principles and applications in biomedical systems. *Journal of Sensors, 2009*, 1–40. https://doi.org/10.1155/2009/187615.
157. Maehashi, K., & Kazuhiko, M., (2009). Label-free electrical detection using carbon nanotube-based biosensors. *Sensors, 9*(7), 5368–5378. https://doi.org/10.3390/s90705368.
158. Malhotra, B. D., & Md Azahar, A., (2018). Nanomaterials in biosensors. In: *Nanomaterials for Biosensors*, 1–74. https://doi.org/10.1016/b978-0-323-44923-6.00001-7.
159. Sireesha, M., Veluru, J. B., Sandeep, K. K. A., & Seeram, R., (2018). A review on carbon nanotubes in biosensor devices and their applications in medicine. *Nanocomposites, 4*(2), 36–57. https://doi.org/10.1080/20550324.2018.1478765.
160. Shukla, S. K., Anthony, P. F. T., & Ashutosh, T., (2015). Cholesterol oxidase functionalized polyaniline/carbon nanotube hybrids for an amperometric biosensor. *Journal of Nanoscience and Nanotechnology, 15*(5), 3373–3377. https://doi.org/10.1166/jnn.2015.10209.
161. Ramonas, E., Dalius, R., Marius, D., Rolandas, M., & Juozas, K., (2019). Highly sensitive amperometric biosensor based on alcohol dehydrogenase for determination of glycerol in human urine. *Talanta, 200*, 333–339. https://doi.org/10.1016/j.talanta.2019.03.063.
162. Wang, J., & Mustafa, M., (2005). Carbon-nanotubes doped polypyrrole glucose biosensor. *Analytica Chimica Acta, 539*(1, 2), 209–213. https://doi.org/10.1016/j.aca.2005.02.059.

163. Yin, T., & Wei, Q., (2013). Applications of nanomaterials in potentiometric sensors. *TrAC – Trends in Analytical Chemistry, 51*, 79–86. https://doi.org/10.1016/j.trac.2013.06.009.
164. Salouti, M., & Fateme, K. D., (2020). Biosensors and nanobiosensors in environmental applications. In: *Biogenic Nano-Particles and Their Use in Agro-Ecosystems* (pp. 515–591). https://doi.org/10.1007/978-981-15-2985-6.
165. Ahuja, T., Kumar, D., Nahar, S., Biradar, A. M., & Rajesh, (2011). Potentiometric urea biosensor based on multi-walled carbon nanotubes (MWCNTs)/silica composite material. *Materials Science and Engineering C, 31*(2), 90–94. https://doi.org/10.1016/j.msec.2010.08.001.
166. Dziąbowska, K., Elżbieta, C., & Dawid, N., (2018). Application of electrochemical methods in biosensing technologies. In: *Biosensing Technologies for the Detection of Pathogens – A Prospective Way for Rapid Analysis* (pp. 151–71). https://doi.org/10.5772/intechopen.72175.
167. Goyal, R. N., Vinod, K. G., & Sanghamitra, C., (2010). Voltammetric biosensors for the determination of paracetamol at carbon nanotube modified pyrolytic graphite electrode. *Sensors and Actuators, B: Chemical, 149*(1), 252–258. https://doi.org/10.1016/j.snb.2010.05.019.
168. Liu, Y., Zhu, F., Dan, W., Fu, Y., & Liu, S., (2014). Construction of carbon nanotube based nanoarchitectures for selective impedimetric detection of cancer cells in whole blood. *Analyst 139*(20), 5086–5092. https://doi.org/10.1039/c4an00758a.
169. Palomar, Q., Chantal, G., Robert, M., Serge, C., & Michael, H., (2018). Impedimetric quantification of anti-dengue antibodies using functional carbon nanotube deposits validated with blood plasma assays. *Electrochimica Acta, 274*, 84–90. https://doi.org/10.1016/j.electacta.2018.04.099.
170. Mehrotra, P., (2016). Biosensors and their applications – A review. *Journal of Oral Biology and Craniofacial Research, 6*(2), 153–159. https://doi.org/10.1016/j.jobcr.2015.12.002.
171. Pisoschi, A. M., (2013). Biosensors as bio-based materials in chemical analysis: A review. *Journal of Biobased Materials and Bioenergy, 7*(1), 19–38. https://doi.org/10.1166/jbmb.2013.1274.
172. Yang, N., Xianping, C., Tianling, R., Ping, Z., & Daoguo, Y., (2015). Carbon nanotube-based biosensors. *Sensors and Actuators, B: Chemical, 207*, 690–715. https://doi.org/10.1016/j.snb.2014.10.040.
173. Ferrier, D. C., & Kevin, C. H., (2021). Carbon nanotube (CNT)-based biosensors. *Biosensors, 11*, 486–518.
174. Wojtera, K., Malgorzata, W., Lukasz, P., Justyna, F., Lukasz, S., & Sobczyk-Guzenda, A., (2020). Synthesis of functionalized carbon nanotubes for fluorescent biosensors. *Nanotechnology Reviews, 9*(1), 1237–1244. https://doi.org/10.1515/ntrev-2020–0096.
175. Lee, E. G., Kyung, M. P., Jin, Y. J., Seung, H. L., Jung, E. B., Hong, W. L., Joon, K. J., & Bong, H. C., (2011). Carbon nanotube-assisted enhancement of surface plasmon resonance signal. *Analytical Biochemistry, 408*(2), 206–211. https://doi.org/10.1016/j.ab.2010.09.026.
176. Alabsi, S. S., Abdelaziz, Y. A., Dennis, J. O., Md Khir, M. H., & Algamili, A. S., (2020). A Review of carbon nanotubes field effect-based biosensors. *IEEE Access, 8*, 69509–69521. https://doi.org/10.1109/ACCESS.2020.2987204.
177. Bobba, S., Sandro, C., & Giovanni De, M., (2010). Design of a CNFET array for sensing and control in P450 based biochips for multiple drug detection. *ISCAS 2010 – 2010*

IEEE International Symposium on Circuits and Systems: Nano-Bio Circuit Fabrics and Systems, 1711–1714.

178. Thanihaichelvan, M., Surendran, S. N., Kumanan, T., Sutharsini, U., Ravirajan, P., Valluvan, R., & Tharsika, T., (2022). Selective and electronic detection of COVID-19(coronavirus) using carbon nanotube field effect transistor-based biosensor: A proof-of-concept study. *Materials Today: Proceedings, 49*, 2546–2549. https://doi.org/10.1016/j.matpr.2021.05.011.
179. Tan, J. M., Saifullah, B., Sharida, F., & Mohd, Z. H., (2020). Preparation, characterization and biological evaluation of biopolymer-coated multi-walled carbon nanotubes for sustained-delivery of silibinin. *Scientific Reports, 10*(1), 16941. https://doi.org/10.1038/s41598-020-73963-8.
180. Liu, P., (2013). Modification strategies for carbon nanotubes as a drug delivery system. *Industrial and Engineering Chemistry Research, 52*(38), 13517–13527. https://doi.org/10.1021/ie402360f.
181. Al-Qattan, M., N., Pran, K. D., & Rakesh, K. T., (2018). Molecular dynamics simulation strategies for designing carbon-nanotube-based targeted drug delivery. *Drug Discovery Today, 23*(2), 235–250. https://doi.org/10.1016/j.drudis.2017.10.002.
182. Mahajan, S., Abhimanyu, P., Kaushik, K., Rahul, M., Pran, K. D., Kiran, K., & Rakesh, K. T., (2018). Functionalized carbon nanotubes as an emerging delivery system for the treatment of cancer. *International Journal of Pharmaceutics, 548*(1), 540–558. https://doi.org/10.1016/j.ijpharm.2018.07.027.
183. Li, Z., Andre, L. B. D. B., Daniel, C. F. S., Sara, N. M., & Laleh, A., (2017). Functionalized single-walled carbon nanotubes: Cellular uptake, biodistribution and applications in drug delivery. *International Journal of Pharmaceutics, 524*(1, 2), 41–54. https://doi.org/10.1016/j.ijpharm.2017.03.017.
184. Yu, S., Qiang, L., Junli, W., Jinglei, D., Yuduan, G., Li, Z., Lin, C., et al., (2018). A targeted drug delivery system based on carbon nanotubes loaded with lobaplatin toward liver cancer cells. *Journal of Materials Research, 33*(17), 2565–2575. https://doi.org/10.1557/jmr.2018.197.
185. Das, M., Raman, P. S., Satyajit, R. D., & Sanyog, J., (2013). Intranuclear drug delivery and effective *in vivo* cancer therapy via estradiol-peg-appended multiwalled carbon nanotubes. *Molecular Pharmaceutics, 10*(9), 3404–3416. https://doi.org/10.1021/mp4002409.
186. Yun, J., Ji, S. I., Young, S. L., & Hyung, I. K., (2011). Electro-responsive transdermal drug delivery behavior of PVA/PAA/MWCNT nanofibers. *European Polymer Journal, 47*(10), 1893–1902. https://doi.org/10.1016/j.eurpolymj.2011.07.024.
187. Spizzirri, U. G., Silke, H., Giuseppe, C., Fiore, P. N., Abdelwahab, H., Orazio, V., Nevio, P., & Francesca, I., (2013). Spherical gelatin/CNTs hybrid microgels as electro-responsive drug delivery systems. *International Journal of Pharmaceutics, 448*(1), 115–122. https://doi.org/10.1016/j.ijpharm.2013.03.013.
188. Tamahkar, I. E., (2017). Carbon nanotube based polyvinylalcohol-polyvinylpyrolidone nanocomposite hydrogels for controlled drug delivery applications. *Anadolu University Journal of Science and Technology A – Applied Sciences and Engineering, 18*(2), 543–553. https://doi.org/10.18038/aubtda.322138.
189. Niezabitowska, E., Jessica, S., Mark, R. P., Riaz, A., Felix, W. V. A., Yan, L., Ali-Boucetta, H., & Tom, O. M., (2018). Facile production of nanocomposites of carbon

nanotubes and polycaprolactone with high aspect ratios with potential applications in drug delivery. *RSC Advances, 8*(30), 16444–16454. https://doi.org/10.1039/c7ra13553j.
190. Mehra, N. K., & Srinath, P., (2016). Interactions between carbon nanotubes and bioactives: A drug delivery perspective. *Drug Discovery Today, 21*(4), 585–597. https://doi.org/10.1016/j.drudis.2015.11.011.
191. Martincic, M., & Gerard, T., (2015). Filled carbon nanotubes in biomedical imaging and drug delivery. *Expert Opinion on Drug Delivery, 12*(4), 563–581. https://doi.org/10.1517/17425247.2015.971751.
192. Tsai, H. C., Jeng, Y. L., Faiza, M., Chun, C. H., & Toyoko, I., (2013). Drug-loading capacity and nuclear targeting of multiwalled carbon nanotubes grafted with anionic amphiphilic copolymers. *International Journal of Nanomedicine, 8*, 4427–4440. https://doi.org/10.2147/IJN.S53636.
193. Maleki, R., Hamid, H. A., Mirollah, H., Davood, T., & Sara, R., (2020). Molecular dynamics simulation of doxorubicin loading with N-isopropyl acrylamide carbon nanotube in a drug delivery system. *Computer Methods and Programs in Biomedicine, 184*, 10503. https://doi.org/10.1016/j.cmpb.2019.105303.
194. Karimzadeh, S., Babak, S., & Tien, C. J., (2021). Theorical investigation of adsorption mechanism of doxorubicin anticancer drug on the pristine and functionalized single-walled carbon nanotube surface as a drug delivery vehicle: A DFT study. *Journal of Molecular Liquids, 322*, 114890. https://doi.org/10.1016/j.molliq.2020.114890.
195. Contreras, M. L., Camila, T., Ignacio, V., & Roberto, R., (2019). Molecular dynamics assessment of doxorubicin–carbon nanotubes molecular interactions for the design of drug delivery systems. *Structural Chemistry, 30*(1), 369–384. https://doi.org/10.1007/s11224-018-1210-5.
196. Mazumdar, P., Diganta, C., & Gargi, B., (2021). A DFT and molecular dynamics simulation study of single-walled carbon nanotube as a drug delivery system for few model nitrogen mustard drugs. *Journal of Molecular Structure, 1243*, 130877. https://doi.org/10.1016/j.molstruc.2021.130877.
197. Tohidifar, L., & Birgit, S., (2021). Molecular dynamics studies for enhancing the anticancer drug efficacy: Toward designing a new carbon nanotube-based paclitaxel delivery system. *Journal of Molecular Liquids, 323*, 114638. https://doi.org/10.1016/j.molliq.2020.114638.
198. Nikfar, Z., & Zahra, S., (2017). DFT computational study on the phosphate functionalized SWCNTs as efficient drug delivery systems for anti-osteoporosis zolendronate and risedronate drugs. *Physica E: Low-Dimensional Systems and Nanostructures, 91*, 41–59. https://doi.org/10.1016/j.physe.2017.04.011.
199. Huang, H., Yuan, Q., Shah, J. S., & Misra, R. D. K., (2011). A new family of folate-decorated and carbon nanotube-mediated drug delivery system: Synthesis and drug delivery response. *Advanced Drug Delivery Reviews, 63*(14, 15), 1332–1339. https://doi.org/10.1016/j.addr.2011.04.001.
200. Taghavi, S., Azadeh, H. N., Khalil, A., & Mohammad, R., (2017). Polyethylenimine-functionalized carbon nanotubes tagged with AS1411 aptamer for combination gene and drug delivery into human gastric cancer cells. *International Journal of Pharmaceutics, 516*(1, 2), 301–312. https://doi.org/10.1016/j.ijpharm.2016.11.027.
201. Rastogi, V., Pragya, Y., Shiv, S. B., Arun, K. M., Navneet, V., Anurag, V., & Jayanta, K. P., (2014). Carbon nanotubes: An emerging drug carrier for targeting cancer cells. *Journal of Drug Delivery, 2014*, 1–23. https://doi.org/10.1155/2014/670815.

202. Wu, H., Haili, S., Hao, Z., Xue, W., Yan, Y., Chao, Y., Caiqin, H., et al., (2014). Prostate stem cell antigen antibody-conjugated multiwalled carbon nanotubes for targeted ultrasound imaging and drug delivery. *Biomaterials, 35*(20), 5369–5380. https://doi.org/10.1016/j.biomaterials.2014.03.038.
203. Cifuentes-Rius, A., Nathan, R. B. B., Ines, F., Nuria, C., Ramos-Perez, V., Kristofer, J. T., & Salvador, B., (2017). *In vivo* fate of carbon nanotubes with different physicochemical properties for gene delivery applications. *ACS Applied Materials and Interfaces, 9*(13), 11461–11471. https://doi.org/10.1021/acsami.7b00677.
204. Li, J., Huamin, Z., Zhaowu, Z., Yiying, Z., & Tian, X., (2021). Promising graphene-based nanomaterials and their biomedical applications and potential risks: A comprehensive review. *ACS Biomaterials Science and Engineering, 7*(12), 5363–5396. https://doi.org/10.1021/acsbiomaterials.1c00875.
205. Lefebvre, J., David, G. A., Jeffery, B., & Paul, F., (2006). Photoluminescence imaging of suspended single-walled carbon nanotubes. *Nano Letters, 6*(8), 1603–1608. https://doi.org/10.1021/nl060530e.
206. Doorn, S. K., Lianxi, Z., Michael, J. O., Yuntian, Z., Shaoming, H., & Jie, L., (2005). Raman spectroscopy and imaging of ultralong carbon nanotubes. *Journal of Physical Chemistry B, 109*(9), 3751–3758. https://doi.org/10.1021/jp0463159.
207. Wu, H., Gang, L., Xue, W., Jiamin, Z., Yu, C., Jianlin, S., Hong, Y., He, H., & Shiping, Y., (2011). Solvothermal synthesis of cobalt ferrite nanoparticles loaded on multiwalled carbon nanotubes for magnetic resonance imaging and drug delivery. *Acta Biomaterialia, 7*(9), 3496–3504. https://doi.org/10.1016/j.actbio.2011.05.031.
208. Hoelen, C. G. A., De Mul, F. F. M., Pongers, R., & Dekker, A., (1998). Three-dimensional photoacoustic imaging of blood vessels in tissue. *Opt. Lett., 23*(8), 648–650. https://doi.org/10.1364/OL.23.000648.
209. Connell, M. J. O., Sergei, M. B., Chad, B. H., Valerie, C. M., Michael, S. S., Erik, H. H., Kristy, L. R., et al., (2002). Band gap fluorescence from individual single-walled carbon nanotubes. *Science, 297*(5581), 593–596.
210. Gong, H., Rui, P., & Zhuang, L., (2013). Carbon nanotubes for biomedical imaging: The recent advances. *Advanced Drug Delivery Reviews, 65*(15), 1951–1963. https://doi.org/10.1016/j.addr.2013.10.002.
211. Khandare, J. J., Jalota-Badhwar, A., Sneha, D. S., Sujit, G. B., Naval, D. A., Firuza, K., & Shashwat, S. B., (2012). PEG-conjugated highly dispersive multifunctional magnetic multi-walled carbon nanotubes for cellular imaging. *Nanoscale, 4*(3), 837–844. https://doi.org/10.1039/c1nr11540e.
212. Iizumi, Y., Toshiya, O., Yuzuru, I., Mutsuo, O., Shinsuke, F., & Masako, Y., (2013). Immunoassay with single-walled carbon nanotubes as near-infrared fluorescent labels. *ACS Applied Materials and Interfaces, 5*(16), 7665–7670. https://doi.org/10.1021/am401702q.
213. Shi, D., Hoon, S. C., Chris, H., Feng, W., Zhongyun, D., Giovanni, M. P., Jie, L., et al., (2009). Conjugation of quantum dots and Fe_3O_4 on carbon nanotubes for medical diagnosis and treatment. *Applied Physics Letters, 95*(22), 223702. https://doi.org/10.1063/1.3268469.
214. Guo, Y., Donglu, S., Hoonsung, C., Zhongyun, D., Amit, K., Giovanni, M. P., Wei, W., et al., (2008). *In vivo* imaging and drug storage by quantum-dot-conjugated carbon nanotubes. *Advanced Functional Materials, 18*(17), 2489–2497. https://doi.org/10.1002/adfm.200800406.

215. Welsher, K., Sarah, P. S., & Hongjie, D., (2011). Deep-tissue anatomical imaging of mice using carbon nanotube fluorophores in the second near-infrared window. *Proceedings of the National Academy of Sciences of the United States of America, 108*(22), 8943–8948. https://doi.org/10.1073/pnas.1014501108.
216. Huang, Z., Yizhan, M., Wei, J., Yanling, Z., Xiaolong, J., Qing, C., Qiang, A., & Xiaoping, Y., (2020). Tracing carbon nanotubes (CNTs) in rat peripheral nerve regenerated with conductive conduits composed of poly(lactide-co-glycolide) and fluorescent CNTs. *ACS Biomaterials Science and Engineering, 6*(11), 6344–6355. https://doi.org/10.1021/acsbiomaterials.0c01065.
217. Yin, Z., Dapeng, C., Jianhua, Z., Jinjun, S., Hao, T., Hong, X., Weili, S., & Xiaochen, D., (2018). Tumor microenvironment responsive oxygen-self-generating nanoplatform for dual-imaging guided photodynamic and photothermal therapy. *Chemistry Select., 3*(16), 4366–4373. https://doi.org/10.1002/slct.201800498.
218. Kostarelos, K., Bianco, A., & Prato, M., (2009). Promises, facts and challenges for carbon nanotubes in imaging and therapeutics. *Nature Nanotechnology, 4*(10), 627–633. https://doi.org/10.1038/nnano.2009.241.
219. Zavaleta, C., De, A. L. Z., Liu, Z., Keren, S., Cheng, Z., Schipper, M., Chen, X., et al., (2008). Noninvasive Raman spectroscopy in living mice for evaluation of tumor targeting with carbon nanotubes. *Nano Letters, 8*(9), 2800–2805. https://doi.org/10.1021/nl801362a.
220. Bajaj, P., Carole, M., Ruhung, W., David, K. B., Pauras, M., Rockford, K. D., Gregg, R. D., Paul, P., & Inga, H. M., (2014). A carbon nanotube-based Raman-imaging immunoassay for evaluating tumor targeting ligands. *Analyst, 139*(12), 3069–3076. https://doi.org/10.1039/c4an00258j.
221. Cialla-May, D., Zheng, X. S., Weber, K., & Popp, J., (2017). Recent progress in surface-enhanced Raman spectroscopy for biological and biomedical applications: From cells to clinics. *Chemical Society Reviews, 46*(13), 3945–3961. https://doi.org/10.1039/C7CS00172J.
222. Li, Y., Qiaolin, W., Fei, M., Xin, L., Fengyong, L., & Min, Z., (2018). Surface-enhanced Raman nanoparticles for tumor theranostics applications. *Acta Pharmaceutica Sinica B, 8*(3), 349–359. https://doi.org/https://doi.org/10.1016/j.apsb.2018.03.007.
223. Zhang, Y., Xue, M., Xiaoyue, T., & Rong, X., (2019). Recent progress on liquid biopsy analysis using surface-enhanced Raman spectroscopy. *Theranostics, 9*(2), 491–525. https://doi.org/10.7150/thno.29875.
224. Qin, X., Yanmei, S., Dawei, W., Zhaoyang, W., Jishan, L., & Yadong, Y., (2019). Nanoconjugates of Ag/Au/carbon nanotube for alkyne-meditated ratiometric SERS imaging of hypoxia in hepatic ischemia. *Analytical Chemistry, 91*(7), 4529–4536. https://doi.org/10.1021/acs.analchem.8b05487.
225. Sitharaman, B., Kissell, K. R., Hartman, K. B., Tran, L. A., Baikalov, A., Rusakova, I., Sun, Y., et al., (2005). Superparamagnetic gadonanotubes are high-performance MRI contrast agents. *Chemical Communications (Cambridge, England), 31*, 3915–3917. https://doi.org/10.1039/b504435a.
226. Tweedle, M. F., (2002). The chemistry of contrast agents in medical magnetic resonance imaging edited by André E. Merbach and Éva Tóth (University of Lausanne). J. Wiley & Sons: Chichester, New York, Weinheim, Brisbane, Singapore, Toronto. Xii + 472 pp. ISBN: 978-1-119-99176-2.

227. Mehri-Kakavand, G., Hadi, H., Rouzbeh, J., Maryam, A., Reza, N., Bitarafan-Rajabi, M. J. A., Darbandi-Azar, A., & Alireza, E., (2019). Gdn^{3+}@cnts-Peg versus Gadovist®: *In vitro* assay. *Oman Medical Journal, 34*(2), 147–155. https://doi.org/10.5001/OMJ.2019.27.
228. Choi, J. H., Freddy, T. N., Paul, W. B., Daniel, A. H., Anthonie, E. M., Dhaval, P., Stephen, A. B., & Michael, S. S., (2007). Multimodal biomedical imaging with asymmetric single-walled carbon nanotube/iron oxide nanoparticle complexes. *Nano Letters, 7*(4), 861–867. https://doi.org/10.1021/nl062306v.
229. Tomczyk, M. M., Sławomir, B., Artur, H., Tomasz, K., Jakóbik-Kolon, A., Mirosława, P., Maciej, K., et al., (2020). Oxygen functional groups on MWCNT surface as critical factor boosting T2 relaxation rate of water protons: Towards improved CNT-based contrast agents. *International Journal of Nanomedicine, 15*, 7433–7450. https://doi.org/10.2147/IJN.S257230.
230. Chen, G., Berg, D., Francis, J., Ileana, H., Eric, F., Wanming, Z., Craig, G., et al., (2018). Tissue-susceptibility matched carbon nanotube electrodes for magnetic resonance imaging. *Journal of Magnetic Resonance, 295*, 72–79. https://doi.org/10.1016/j.jmr.2018.08.003.
231. Zheng, X. S., Azante, Y. G., Emily, C., Michael, J. L., Lee, E. F., Brady, C., & Tracy, X. C., (2020). Evaluation of a conducting elastomeric composite material for intramuscular electrode application. *Acta Biomaterialia, 103*, 81–91. https://doi.org/10.1016/j.actbio.2019.12.021.
232. Ku, G., & Lihong, V. W., (2005). Deeply penetrating photoacoustic tomography in biological tissues enhanced with an optical contrast agent. *Optics Letters, 30*(5), 507. https://doi.org/10.1364/ol.30.000507.
233. Wang, X., Yongjiang, P., Geng, K., Xueyi, X., George, S., & Lihong, V. W., (2003). Noninvasive laser-induced photoacoustic tomography for structural and functional *in vivo* imaging of the brain. *Nature Biotechnology, 21*(7), 803–806. https://doi.org/10.1038/nbt839.
234. Liu, X., Huiquan, T., Kai, Y., Shuai, Z., Shuit-Tong, L., & Zhuang, L., (2011). Optimization of surface chemistry on single-walled carbon nanotubes for *in vivo* photothermal ablation of tumors. *Biomaterials, 32*(1), 144–151. https://doi.org/10.1016/j.biomaterials.2010.08.096.
235. Kim, J. W., Ekaterina, I. G., Evgeny, V. S., Hyung, M. M., & Vladimir, P. Z., (2009). Golden carbon nanotubes as multimodal photoacoustic and photothermal high-contrast molecular agents. *Nature Nanotechnology, 4*(10), 688–694. https://doi.org/10.1038/nnano.2009.231.
236. Cui, H., Chenglin, H., Andrew, Y., Xinmai, Y., & Shenqiang, R., (2013). Ultrathin gold nanowire-functionalized carbon nanotubes for hybrid molecular sensing. *ACS Nano, 7*(9), 7805–7811. https://doi.org/10.1021/nn4027323.
237. Mosse, C. A., Richard, J. C., Davinder, S. B., Edward, Z. Z., Ioannis, P., & Adrien, E. D., (2014). Fiber optic ultrasound transducers with carbon/PDMS composite coatings. *Photons Plus Ultrasound: Imaging and Sensing – 2014, 8943*, 89430P. https://doi.org/10.1117/12.2037283.
238. Choi, W. Y., Kwon, S. W., Kim, Y. H., Kang, K. C., & Park, K. K., (2020). Single-shot near-field volumetric imaging system for optical ultrasound and photoacoustics using capacitive micromachined ultrasonic transducer without transmission mode. *IEEE*

Transactions on Ultrasonics, Ferroelectrics, and Frequency Control, 67(6), 1151–1158. https://doi.org/10.1109/TUFFC.2020.2965600.

239. Chen, X., Un Chong, T., Jennifer, L. C., Goo, S. L., David, R., Alex, Z., & Carolyn, R. B., (2006). Interfacing carbon nanotubes with living cells. *Journal of the American Chemical Society, 128*(19), 6292–6293. https://doi.org/10.1021/ja060276s.
240. Singh, R., Davide, P., Lara, L., Giorgia, P., Cédric, K., Maurizio, P., Alberto, B., & Kostas, K., (2006). Tissue biodistribution and blood clearance rates of intravenously administered carbon nanotube radiotracers. *Proceedings of the National Academy of Sciences of the United States of America, 103*(9), 3357–3362. https://doi.org/10.1073/pnas.0509009103.
241. Seo, J. W., Magrez, A., Milas, M., Lee, K., Lukovac, V., & Forró, L., (2007). Catalytically grown carbon nanotubes: From synthesis to toxicity. *Journal of Physics D: Applied Physics, 40*(6), R109. https://doi.org/10.1088/0022-3727/40/6/R01.
242. Malik, M. A., Mohmmad, Y. W., Mohd, A. H., & Firdosa, N., (2011). Nanotoxicity: Dimensional and morphological concerns. *Advances in Physical Chemistry, 2011*, 1–15. https://doi.org/10.1155/2011/450912.
243. Zheng, W., Walter, M., Michael, L. K., Daniel, P., Vincent, C., & Hong, K., (2018). The effects of inhaled multi-walled carbon nanotubes on blood pressure and cardiac function. *Nanoscale Research Letters, 13*, 189. https://doi.org/10.1186/s11671-018-2603-5.
244. Duffin, R., Nicholas, L. M., & Ken, D., (2007). Nanoparticles – a thoracic toxicology perspective. *Yonsei Medical Journal*. https://doi.org/10.3349/ymj.2007.48.4.561.
245. Mohanta, D., Soma, P., Sanchit, S., & Nilanjan, D., (2019). Carbon nanotubes: Evaluation of toxicity at biointerfaces. *Journal of Pharmaceutical Analysis, 9*(5), 293–300. https://doi.org/10.1016/j.jpha.2019.04.003.
246. Holsapple, M. P., William, H. F., Timothy, D. L., Monteiro-Riviere, N. A., Janet, M. C., Nigel, J. W., & Karluss, V. T., (2005). Research strategies for safety evaluation of nanomaterials, part II: Toxicological and safety evaluation of nanomaterials, current challenges and data needs. *Toxicological Sciences, 88*(1), 12–17. https://doi.org/10.1093/toxsci/kfi293.
247. Song, B., Piao, X., Guangming, Z., Jilai, G., Xiaoxiao, W., Jin, Y., Shengfan, W., Peng, Z., et al., (2018). Modeling the transport of sodium dodecyl benzene sulfonate in riverine sediment in the presence of multi-walled carbon nanotubes. *Water Research, 129*, 20–28. https://doi.org/10.1016/j.watres.2017.11.003.
248. Kushwaha, S. K. S., Saurav, G., Awani, K. R., & Satyawan, S., (2013). Carbon nanotubes as a novel drug delivery system for anticancer therapy: A review. *Brazilian Journal of Pharmaceutical Sciences, 49*(4), 629–643. https://doi.org/10.1590/S1984-82502013000400002.
249. Saito, N., Hisao, H., Yuki, U., Kaoru, A., Kazuo, H., Seiji, T., Masayuki, S., et al., (2014). Safe clinical use of carbon nanotubes as innovative biomaterials. *Chemical Reviews, 114*(11), 6040–6079. https://doi.org/10.1021/cr400341h.
250. Chang, Y., Sheng, T. Y., Jia, H. L., Erya, D., Yanwen, W., Aoneng, C., Yuanfang, L., & Haifang, W., (2011). *In vitro* toxicity evaluation of graphene oxide on A549 cells. *Toxicology Letters, 200*(3), 201–210. https://doi.org/10.1016/j.toxlet.2010.11.016.
251. Firme, C. P., & Prabhakar, R. B., (2010). Toxicity issues in the application of carbon nanotubes to biological systems. *Nanomedicine: Nanotechnology, Biology, and Medicine, 6*(2), 245–256. https://doi.org/10.1016/j.nano.2009.07.003.

252. Dumortier, H., Stéphanie, L., Giorgia, P., Riccardo, M., Wei, W., Davide, B., Jean, P. B., et al., (2006). Functionalized carbon nanotubes are non-cytotoxic and preserve the functionality of primary immune cells. *Nano Letters, 6*(7), 1522–1528. https://doi.org/10.1021/nl061160x.
253. Han, Y. G., Jing, X., Zhi, G. L., Guo, G. R., & Zhuo, Y., (2012). *In vitro* toxicity of multi-walled carbon nanotubes in C6 rat glioma cells. *Neuro Toxicology, 33*(5), 1128–1134. https://doi.org/10.1016/j.neuro.2012.06.004.
254. Prajapati, S. K., Akanksha, M., Payal, K., Deeksha, S., & Aakanchha, J., (2022). Biomedical applications and toxicities of carbon nanotubes. *Drug and Chemical Toxicology, 45*(1), 435–450. https://doi.org/10.1080/01480545.2019.1709492.
255. Yang, S. T., Jianbin, L., Qinghan, Z., & Haifang, W., (2012). Pharmacokinetics, metabolism and toxicity of carbon nanotubes for bio-medical purposes. *Theranostics, 2*(3), 271–282. https://doi.org/10.7150/thno.3618.
256. Fisher, C., Amanda, E. R., Zhao, J. H., Shailesh, K., Igor, L., & Kostya, O., (2012). Applications and nanotoxicity of carbon nanotubes and graphene in biomedicine. *Journal of Nanomaterials 2012*, 1–19. https://doi.org/10.1155/2012/315185.
257. Ursini, C. L., Delia, C., Anna, M. F., Aureliano, C., Raffaele, M., Stefano, C., Francesca, T., et al., (2012). Study of cytotoxic and genotoxic effects of hydroxyl-functionalized multiwalled carbon nanotubes on human pulmonary cells. *Journal of Nanomaterials, 2012*, 1–9. https://doi.org/10.1155/2012/815979.
258. Zhang, D., Xiaoyong, D., Zongfei, J., Xizhong, S., Ling, D., Minghong, W., Taoying, G., & Yuanfang, L., (2010). Long-term hepatotoxicity of polyethylene-glycol functionalized multi-walled carbon nanotubes in mice. *Nanotechnology, 21*(17). https://doi.org/10.1088/0957-4484/21/17/175101.
259. Fraczek, A., Elzbieta, M., Czeslawa, P., & Marta, B., (2008). Comparative *in vivo* biocompatibility study of single- and multi-wall carbon nanotubes. *Acta Biomaterialia, 4*(6), 1593–1602. https://doi.org/10.1016/j.actbio.2008.05.018.
260. Folkmann, J. K., Lotte, R., Nicklas, R. J., Håkan, W., Steffen, L., & Peter, M., (2009). Oxidatively damaged DNA in rats exposed by oral gavage to C60 fullerenes and single-walled carbon nanotubes. *Environmental Health Perspectives, 117*(5), 703–708. https://doi.org/10.1289/ehp.11922.
261. Takanashi, S., Kazuo, H., Kaoru, A., Yuki, U., Masayuki, S., Hisao, H., Nobuhide, O., et al., (2012). Carcinogenicity evaluation for the application of carbon nanotubes as biomaterials in rasH2 mice. *Scientific Reports, 2*, 1–7. https://doi.org/10.1038/srep00498.
262. Zhu, B., Song, Z., Jian, L., Xin, H., & Gao, X. W., (2018). The developmental toxicity, bioaccumulation and distribution of oxidized single walled carbon nanotubes in: Artemia salina. *Toxicology Research, 7*(5), 897–906. https://doi.org/10.1039/c8tx00084k.
263. Rocha, A. M. D., Kist, L. W., Almeida, E. A., Silva, D. G. H., Bonan, C. D., Altenhofen, S., Kaufmann, C. G., et al., (2019). Neurotoxicity in zebrafish exposed to carbon nanotubes: Effects on neurotransmitters levels and antioxidant system. *Comparative Biochemistry and Physiology Part – C: Toxicology and Pharmacology 218*, 30–35. https://doi.org/10.1016/j.cbpc.2018.12.008.
264. Russ, K. A., Janet, A. T., Michael, K., Dale, W. P., Sherri, A. F., McKinney, W., & Jeffrey, S. F., (2019). Comparison of multi-wall carbon nanotube and nitrogen-doped multi-wall carbon nanotube effects on lung function and airway reactivity in rats. *Toxicology and Applied Pharmacology, 364*, 153–163. https://doi.org/10.1016/j.taap.2018.11.004.

265. Dong, J., & Qiang, M., (2015). Advances in mechanisms and signaling pathways of carbon nanotube toxicity. *Nanotoxicology, 9*(5), 658–676. https://doi.org/10.3109/17435390.2015.1009187.
266. Liang, Y., Xin, Z., Tianli, H., Yong, H., & Baolin, G., (2019). Mussel-inspired, antibacterial, conductive, antioxidant, injectable composite hydrogel wound dressing to promote the regeneration of infected skin. *Journal of Colloid and Interface Science, 556*, 514–528. https://doi.org/10.1016/j.jcis.2019.08.083.
267. Song, S., Lihua, W., Jiang, L., Chunhai, F., & Jianlong, Z., (2008). Aptamer-based biosensors. *TrAC – Trends in Analytical Chemistry, 27*(2), 108–117. https://doi.org/10.1016/j.trac.2007.12.004.
268. Khan, Waseem, Rahul Sharma, and Parveen Saini. "Carbon nanotube-based polymer composites: synthesis, properties and applications." Carbon nanotubes-current progress of their polymer composites (2016).

Index

C

D

G

H

I

N

T

For Product Safety Concerns and Information please contact our EU
representative GPSR@taylorandfrancis.com
Taylor & Francis Verlag GmbH, Kaufingerstraße 24, 80331 München, Germany

www.ingramcontent.com/pod-product-compliance
Lightning Source LLC
Chambersburg PA
CBHW071350220926
51613CB00008B/37
* 9 7 8 1 7 7 4 9 1 3 3 5 2 *